Pharmaceutical Science: Clinical Research

Pharmaceutical Science: Clinical Research

Edited by **Sean Boyd**

Callisto Reference
New York

Published by Callisto Reference,
106 Park Avenue, Suite 200,
New York, NY 10016, USA
www.callistoreference.com

Pharmaceutical Science: Clinical Research
Edited by Sean Boyd

International Standard Book Number: 978-1-63239-675-4 (Hardback)

Printed in China.

Contents

Preface

This book was inspired by the evolution of our times; to answer the curiosity of inquisitive minds. Many developments have occurred across the globe in the recent past which has transformed the progress in the field.

This book elucidates new techniques and applications of pharmaceutical science in a multidisciplinary approach. It discusses the fundamentals as well as modern approaches of this field. Pharmaceutical science is an interdisciplinary field that has elements of chemometrics, mathematics, epidemiology, statistics, physics, chemical engineering, chemistry and biology. It mainly deals with the composition, manufacturing, delivery, and disposal of drugs. Clinical pharmacy, compounding pharmacy, pharmaceutics, medicinal chemistry, pharmacotherapy, pharmacokinetics, clinical pharmacology, pharmacogenetics, pharmacogenomics, toxicology are some of the topics discussed in this extensive book. Such selected concepts that redefine the field of pharmaceutical science have been presented herein. In this book, using case studies and examples, constant effort has been made to make the understanding of the difficult concepts as easy and informative as possible, for the readers.

This book was developed from a mere concept to drafts to chapters and finally compiled together as a complete text to benefit the readers across all nations. To ensure the quality of the content we instilled two significant steps in our procedure. The first was to appoint an editorial team that would verify the data and statistics provided in the book and also select the most appropriate and valuable contributions from the plentiful contributions we received from authors worldwide. The next step was to appoint an expert of the topic as the Editor-in-Chief, who would head the project and finally make the necessary amendments and modifications to make the text reader-friendly. I was then commissioned to examine all the material to present the topics in the most comprehensible and productive format.

I would like to take this opportunity to thank all the contributing authors who were supportive enough to contribute their time and knowledge to this project. I also wish to convey my regards to my family who have been extremely supportive during the entire project.

Editor

1

Biochemical Effects of Methanolic Extracts of *Vernonia amygdalina* and *Gongronema latifolia* on Alloxan-induced Diabetic Rats

Patrick Emeka Aba[1*] and Chidiebere Peace Okenwa-Ani[1]

[1]*Department of Veterinary Physiology and Pharmacology, University of Nigeria, Nsukka, Enugu State, Nigeria.*

Authors' contributions

This work was carried out in collaboration between both authors. Author PEA designed the study, wrote the protocol and analyzed the data while author CPO carried out the experimental processes and managed the literature searches. Both authors read and approved the final manuscript.

Article Information

Editor(s):
(1) Salvatore Chirumbolo, Clinical Biochemist, Department of Medicine, University of Verona, Italy.
Reviewers:
(1) Dhastagir Sheriff, Benghazi University, Libya.
(2) Sema Kalkan Uçar, Ege University, Turkey.
(3) Shahedur Rahman, Jessore Science & Technology University, Bangladesh.

ABSTRACT

Aim: The study investigated effects of combined methanol extracts of *Gongronema latifolium* and *Vernonia amygdalina* on fasting blood glucose (FBG) levels, oxidative stress markers and some haematological indices of alloxan-induced diabetic rats.

Methodology: Twenty five (25) albino wistar rats were assigned into 5 groups of 5 rats per group. Diabetes was induced in groups 2-5 by a single intraperitoneal injection of alloxan monohydrate (160 mg/kg) while group 1 rats served as normal control. Upon establishment of diabetes, group 2 rats were treated with 200 mg/kg of *G. latifolium* extract; group 3 rats with a combination of 100 mg/kg of *G. latifolium* and 100 mg/kg of *V. amygdalina*; group 4 rats with 200 mg/kg of *V. amygdalina* while group 5 rats were treated with 2 mg/kg glibenclamide. All treatments were daily through the oral route for 21 days. The FBG levels of the rats were assessed at 2 h, 6 h and on days 7, 14 and 21 days post-treatment while blood for clinical chemistry [Catalase, Superoxide dismutase (SOD) and Malondialdehyde (MDA)] and haematological [Red blood cell (RBC) count,

*Corresponding author: E-mail: patrick.aba@unn.edu.ng, patrickaba@yahoo.com

packed cell volume (PCV) and Haemoglobin (Hb) concentration)] analyses were collected on day 21 post-treatment.
Results: Results showed that the FBG level of the rats treated with combined extract decreased significantly ($P < 0.05$) from 203.66±1.85 on day zero to 48.00±3.57 on day 21. The mean catalase activity and MDA levels of the rats that received the combined treatment (group 3 rats) were statistically comparable to that of glibenclamide-treated rats. The SOD activity, RBC count, PCV levels and Hb concentration of the rats in group 3 were significantly ($P < 0.05$) higher than those of the negative control group.
Conclusion: Treatment of diabetic rats with 100 mg/kg each of methanol extracts of *G. latifolium* and *V. amygdalina* exhibited hypoglycaemic, anti-oxidant and anti-anaemic potentials.

Keywords: Gongronema latifolium; Vernonia amygdalina; biochemical; haematology diabetic rats.

1. INTRODUCTION

Diabetes mellitus is derived from the Greek word 'diabetes' meaning siphon (to pass through) and the Latin word 'mellitus' meaning honeyed or sweet. It was known in the 17th century as the 'pissing evil' [1]. Diabetes mellitus commonly referred to as diabetes is a group of metabolic diseases in which a person or animal has high blood sugar, either because the pancreas does not produce enough insulin, or because the body's cells do not respond to the insulin that is being produced [2]. This high blood sugar (hyperglycaemia) produces the classical symptoms of polyuria (frequent urination), polydipsia (increased thirst) and polyphagia (increased appetite or hunger).

Diabetes was the cause of 4.9 million deaths in 2014 (as against 1.5 million in 2012), implying that every seven seconds, a person died from diabetes. It was also estimated that 1 in 12 people were living with diabetes including diagnosed and undiagnosed cases [3]. In animals, diabetes is most commonly encountered in dogs and cats. Middle-aged animals are most commonly affected. Female dogs are twice as likely to be affected as males while according to some sources, male cats are also more prone than females. In both species, all breeds may be affected but some small dog breeds are particularly likely to develop diabetes such as Miniature Poodles, Dachshunds, Cairn Terriers and Beagles, but any breed can be affected [4].

In developing countries, few people have access to the conventional diabetes management drugs, thus, many people use plant for treatment of diabetes. Also, the inadequacies associated with the conventional medicines have led to a determined search for alternative natural therapeutic agents.

Vernonia amygdalina commonly called bitter leaf is a perennial shrub that belongs to the family Asteraceae and grows throughout tropical Africa [5]. Extracts from *V. amygdalina* have been shown to posses anti-diabetic, hepato-protective, serum lipid modulation, and other properties [6]. According to [7] in a study conducted on the effect of *V. amygdalina* extract on blood glucose levels of diabetic rats, there was a remarkable decrease in blood glucose level from mean value 4.44±0.2 to 1.66±0.2 mMol/L. Other researchers [8,9] have also confirmed hypoglycemic effects of this shrub. *Gongronema latifolium* is a herbaceous, non-woody plant from the family Asclepiadaceae. It produces milky clear latex and is widespread in the tropical and subtropical regions especially in Africa and South America, with a moderate representation in Northern and South Eastern Asia [10]. Pharmacological studies have also shown that *G. latifolium* has hypoglycemic properties [11,12]. In Nigeria, these two plants are used culinarily and there is a dearth of information on some biochemical effects of their combined usage.

The available synthetic drugs have complicated mode of intake and they are expensive with serious side effects. There is therefore the need to search for an alternative source of therapy thus this study. This study therefore was to investigate possible haemato-biochemical changes that may be associated with the combined usage of these two shrubs on alloxan-induced diabetic rats.

2. MATERIALS AND METHODS

2.1 Materials

2.1.1 Plant materials

The leaves of *Gongronema latifolium* (GL) and *Vernonia amygdalina* (VA) were purchased from

Ogige market in Nsukka Local Government Area both in Enugu State, Nigeria and were identified by a Botanist in the Botany Department, University of Nigeria, Nsukka.

2.1.2 Chemical, reagents and drugs

Methanol, alloxan monohydrate (SIGMA ALDRICH, U.K.), Red blood cell (RBC) and white blood cell (WBC) diluting fluids and Drabkin's reagent, Malondialdehyde (MDA), superoxide oxide dismutase (SOD) and Catalase reagents Glibenclamide (Hovid®, Hong Kong) were used.

2.1.3 Animals

Male albino Wistar rats weighing between 150-200 g were obtained from the Department of Veterinary Physiology and Pharmacology, University of Nigeria, Nsukka laboratory animal house. The rats were acclimatized for two weeks. The environmental temperature where the animals were housed varied between 28 - 32℃. The animals were kept in stainless wire mesh cages and provided with good clean water *ad libitum*. They were fed with Vital feed® (grower).

2.2 Methods

2.2.1 Preparation of the plant extract

Cold maceration method of extraction was employed. The leaves of *G. latifolium* and *V. amygdalina* were air dried at a very low intensity of sunlight to avoid denaturation of the active ingredient. They were pulverized and stored in an air tight container pending its usage. About 2 kg of each of the pulverized leaves were soaked separately in 10 liters of 80% methanol with intermittent shaking every 2 h for 48 h. The mixtures were filtered using Whatmann No 1 filter paper. The filtrates were concentrated using rotary evaporator and the extract stored at 4℃.

2.2.2 Experimental design

Twenty five (25) adult male albino wistar rats weighing between 150 -200 g were assigned into 5 groups of 5 rats per group. Diabetes was induced in rats of groups 2-5 while group 1 rats served as normal control. Upon establishment of diabetes, (rats with fasting blood glucose values above 7 mmol/L (126 mg/dl) were considered diabetic.), the rats were treated as shown below:

Groups	Treatment
1	Normal control + 10 ml/kg distilled water
2	Diabetic + 200 mg/kg GL
3	Diabetic + 100 mg/kg GL and 100 mg/kg VA
4	Diabetic + 200 mg/kg VA
5	Diabetic + 2 mg/kg Glibenclamide

The treatment was through the oral route daily for 21 days. The FBG levels were assessed 2 h, 6 h, 7 days, 14 days and 21 days post treatment. On the 21st day, blood samples were collected into EDTA bottles for haematological (red blood cell, white blood cell, packed cell volume, and haemoglobin concentration) analyses while plasma was used for biochemical (superoxide dismutase, catalase and malondialdehyde) determinations.

2.2.3 Induction of experimental diabetes mellitus

Diabetes was induced in rats using the method described by [13]. The rats were fasted for 16 h prior to induction of diabetes. Diabetes was induced by single intraperitoneal injection of alloxan monohydrate at the dose of 160 mg/kg. Diabetes was established on day two post induction on confirmation of fasting blood glucose levels above 7 mmol/l or 126 mg/dl.

2.2.4 Estimation of superoxide dismutase

Superoxide dismutase activity was assayed by the method of [14]. 0.5 ml of plasma was diluted to 1.0 ml with ice cold water, followed by 2.5 ml ethanol and 1.5 ml chloroform (chilled reagent). The mixture was shaken for 60 seconds at 4℃ and then centrifuged. The enzyme activity in the supernatant was determined as follows. The assay mixture contained 1.2 ml of sodium pyrophosphate buffer, 0.1 ml of PMS and 0.3 ml of NBT and approximately diluted enzyme preparation in a total volume of 3 ml. The reaction was started by the addition of 0.2 ml NADH. After incubation at 30℃ for 90 seconds, the reaction was stopped by the addition of 1 ml glacial acetic acid. The reaction mixture was stirred vigorously and shaken with 4 ml n-butanol. The mixture was allowed to stand for 10 minutes, centrifuged and butanol layer was separated. The colour intensity of the chromogen in the butanol layer was measured in a spectrophotometer at 520 nm. A system devoid of enzyme served as control. One unit of enzyme activity is defined as the enzyme concentration, which gives 50% inhibition of NBT reduction in one minute under assay conditions. SOD activity was expressed as U/ml of plasma.

2.2.5 Estimation of catalase

The activity of catalase was assayed by the method of [15]. To 0.9 ml of phosphate, 0.1 ml of plasma and 0.4 ml of H_2O_2 were added. The reaction was stopped after 15, 30, 45 and 60 seconds by adding 2 ml of dichromate acetic acid mixture. The tubes were kept in a boiling water bath for 10 minutes, cooled and the colour that developed was read at 530 nm. Standards in the concentration range of 20-100 µmoles was processed for the test. The activity of catalase was expressed as U/ml for plasma (U- µmoles of H_2O_2 Utilised / second).

2.2.6 Estimation of lipid peroxidation (malondialdehyde)

Lipid peroxidation was estimated by measuring spectrophotometrically, the level of the lipid peroxidation product, malondialdehyde (MDA) as described by [16]. A volume, 0.1 ml of the plasma was mixed with 0.9ml of H_2O in a test tube. A volume, 0.5 ml of 25% TCA (trichloroacetic acid) and 0.5 ml of 1% TBA (thiobarbituric acid) in 0.3% NaOH were also added to the mixture. The mixture was boiled for 40 minutes in water-bath and then cooled in cold water. Then 0.1 ml of 20% sodium dodecyl sulfate (SDS) was added to the cooled solution and mixed properly. The absorbance was taken at wavelength 532 nm and 600 nm against a blank.

$$\% \text{ TBARS} = \frac{A_{532} - A_{600} \times 100}{0.5271 \times 0.1} \text{ (mg/dl)}$$

2.2.7 Blood collection for haematological analyses

Blood samples were collected from the rats using orbital technique, that is, from the retrobulbar plexus of the median canthus of the eye. Plasma for *in vivo* antioxidant assay was obtained by centrifuging the EDTA-treated blood sample and decanting the supernatant into another clean sample bottle.

2.2.8 Determination of packed cell volume

The packed cell volume (PCV) was determined by the microhaematocrit method [17]. Micro-capillary tubes were almost filled with the anti-coagulated blood samples and one end sealed with plasticine. The filled tubes were centrifuged at 10,000 revolutions per minute for 5 minutes using a microhaematocrit centrifuge (Hawksley, England). The PCV was read as a percentage on the microhaematocrit reader.

2.2.9 Determination of haemoglobin concentration

The haemoglobin concentration (Hb) was determined by the cyanomethaemoglobin method [18]. The blood sample (0.02 ml) was added to 5 ml of Drabkins reagent in a clean test tube. This was mixed gently and kept at room temperature for 20 minutes to react. The absorbances of both sample and standard were read, against a working reagent blank at a wavelength of 540 nm using a spectrophotometer (Lab-tech, India). The haemoglobin concentration of the blood sample was obtained by multiplying the absorbance of the sample with the factor derived from the absorbance and concentration of the standard.

2.2.10 Erythrocyte count

The erythrocyte count was determined by the haemocytometer method [17]. Blood sample (0.02 ml) was added to 4 ml of red blood cell diluting fluid (sodium citrate, formaldehyde solution and distilled water) in a clean test tube, to make a 1:200 dilution. A drop of the diluted blood was charged onto the Neubaeur counting chamber and allowed to settle for 2-3 minutes. The objective (x 40) lens of the light microscope was used in carrying out the erythrocyte count, in the five groups of 16 small squares. The number of erythrocytes enumerated for each sample was multiplied by 10,000 to obtain the erythrocyte count per microlitre of blood.

2.2.11 Total leukocyte count

The total leukocyte count was determined by the haemocytometer method [17]. Blood sample (0.02 ml) of blood was added to 0.38 ml of white blood cell diluting fluid (glacial acetic acid tinged with gential violet) in a clean test tube, to make a 1:20 dilution. A drop of the diluted blood was charged onto the Neubaeur chamber and allowed to settle for 2 minutes. The x10 objective lens of the light microscope was used in making a total count of white blood cells on the four corner squares. The number of cells counted for each blood sample was multiplied by 50 to obtain the total leukocyte count per microlitre of blood.

2.3 Statistical Analysis

Data obtained from the study were analyzed using One-way Analysis of Variance (ANOVA). Duncans Multiple Range post hoc test was used to separate variant means. P (probability) values less than 0.05 were considered significant. The results were presented as mean ± Standard Error of the Mean (SEM).

3. RESULTS

3.1 Effect of the Methanol Extract of *V. amydalina and G. latifolium* on the Fasting Blood Glucose (FBG) Levels of Alloxan-induced Diabetic Rats

The pre-induction fasting blood glucose (FBG) levels of the rats in groups 1-5 were statistically comparable ($P > 0.05$). However, the post-induction FBG of the rats in groups 2-5 increased significantly ($P < 0.05$) compared to the FBG of group 1 rats (normal control).

Two hours (2 h) post-treatment, the FBG of groups 3-5 rats were statistically comparable ($P > 0.05$) but were significantly ($P < 0.05$) lower than that of the group 2 rats. The FBG of the group 1 rats were equally comparable ($P > 0.05$) to that of the group 5 rats.

On the 6th h post treatment, the FBG levels of the rats in groups 3-5 were statistically comparable ($P > 0.05$) but were still significantly ($P< 0.05$) higher than those of the group 1 rats (normal control) and significantly ($P < 0.05$) lower than those of the group 2 rats.

The FBG levels of the rats in groups 2-5 were statistically comparable ($P > 0.05$) but were significantly ($P < 0.05$) higher than those of the group 1 rats on the 7th day post-treatment.

On day 14 post-treatment however, the FBG levels of the rats in groups 1 & 3 were statistically comparable ($P > 0.05$) but were significantly ($P < 0.05$) higher than that of the group 5 rats. Rats in groups 2 and 4 had FBG levels that were comparable ($P > 0.05$) to each other but were statistically higher than that of the other groups.

On the 21st day post-treatment, the rats in group 3 had a significantly ($P < 0.05$) lower FBG level compared to other groups, the FBG levels of the rats in groups 1 & 5 were statistically comparable ($P > 0.05$), while the FBG levels of the rats in group 2 were significantly ($P < 0.05$) higher than those of the rats in the other groups.

3.2 Effect of the Methanol Extract of *Vernonia amygdalina* and *Gongronema latifolium* on Oxidative Stress Markers of Alloxan-induced Diabetic Rats

Table 2 indicates that the catalase activities of the rats in groups 2-5 were statistically comparable ($P > 0.05$) but were significantly ($P < 0.05$) lower than that of the group 1 rats.

The SOD activities of group 4 rats compared favorably with those of the other groups. However, the SOD activities of the rats in groups 1, 2 and 5 were significantly ($P < 0.05$) lower than those of the other groups while the SOD activities of the rats in group 3 were significantly ($P < 0.05$) higher than those of the other groups.

The MDA levels of the rats in group 5 were significantly ($P < 0.05$) lower than those of the other groups while those of the rats in group 2 were significantly ($P < 0.05$) higher than those of the other groups. However, the MDA levels of the rats in groups 1, 3 and 4 compared favorably with those of groups 2 and 5.

3.3 Effect of the Methanol Extract of *Vernonia amygdalina* and *Gongronema latifolium* on Some Haematological Indices of Alloxanized Rats

The Red Blood Cell (RBC) count of the rats in groups 1, 3 and 5 were statistically comparable ($P > 0.05$) while those of the rats in group 2 were significantly ($P < 0.05$) lower than those of the other groups. The RBC count of the rats in group 4 were significantly ($P < 0.05$) higher than those of the rats in group 2 but were lower than those of groups 1 and 3.

The Packed Cell Volume (PCV) levels of the rats in group 3 compared favorably with those of the rats in the other groups. The PCV levels of the rats in group 1 was significantly ($P < 0.05$) higher than those of the other groups but was statistically comparable to ($P > 0.05$) those of group 3.

The haemoglobin (Hb) levels of the rats in groups 2-5 were statistically comparable ($P > 0.05$). The Hb levels of group 1 rats compared very well with those of group 5 rats but was significantly ($P < 0.05$) higher than those of the rats in groups 2-4.

Table 1. Effect of the methanol extract of *V. amydalina and G. latifolium* on the Fasting Blood Glucose (FBG) levels of alloxan-induced diabetic rats

Group	Pre-induction FBG (mg/dl)	Post-induction FBG (mg/dl)	2 h post-treatment FBG (mg/dl)	6 h post-treatment FBG (mg/dl)	7 days post-treatment FBG (mg/dl)	14 days post-treatment FBG (mg/dl)	21 days post-treatment FBG (mg/dl)
1	78.66 ± 0.33^a	75.00 ± 1.15^a	77.66 ± 0.88^a	69.00 ± 0.57^a	75.33 ± 0.88^a	77.33 ± 4.48^b	70.66 ± 1.76^b
2	78.00 ± 2.08^a	209.33 ± 0.88^c	185.33 ± 7.53^c	157.66 ± 21.78^c	105.00 ± 2.88^b	104.33 ± 2.84^c	101.00 ± 2.08^d
3	78.33 ± 0.88^a	203.66 ± 1.85^b	135.00 ± 18.17^b	102.00 ± 1.15^b	93.66 ± 4.84^b	68.00 ± 6.80^b	48.00 ± 3.57^a
4	77.66 ± 4.91^a	204.33 ± 1.76^b	116.00 ± 7.02^b	120.66 ± 5.36^b	106.33 ± 8.76^b	93.66 ± 2.40^c	91.66 ± 2.72^c
5	78.66 ± 1.52^a	210.00 ± 0.58^c	105.55 ± 3.46^{ab}	102.33 ± 1.20^b	102.33 ± 0.88^b	53.00 ± 1.00^a	71.60 ± 6.00^b

a, b, c and d indicate significant difference at P<0.05 down the groups (down the column)

Table 2. Effect of the methanol extract of *Vernonia amygdalina* and *Gongronema latifolium* on oxidative stress markers of alloxan-Induced diabetic rats

Group	Catalase (U/ml)	SOD (U/ml)	MDA (g/dl)
1	5.00 ± 0.10^b	0.57 ± 0.03^a	4.39 ± 0.04^{ab}
2	2.73 ± 0.25^a	0.58 ± 0.05^a	5.88 ± 0.86^b
3	2.98 ± 0.26^a	0.74 ± 0.02^b	4.55 ± 0.25^{ab}
4	2.42 ± 0.62^a	0.64 ± 0.04^{ab}	5.45 ± 0.33^{ab}
5	3.18 ± 0.16^a	0.51 ± 0.04^a	4.18 ± 0.455^a

a and b indicate significant difference at P < 0.05 down the columns (across the groups); SOD- Superoxide Dismutase; MDA- Malondialdehyde

Table 3. Effect of the methanol extract of *Vernonia amygdalina* and *Gongronema latifolium* on some haematological indices of alloxanized rats

Group	RBC count($x10^6$) (millions/µl)	PCV (%)	Hb Conc. (g/dl)	WBC count($x10^3$) (thousands/µl)
1	6.92 ± 0.20^c	40.33 ± 0.33^b	13.66 ± 0.33^b	6.89 ± 0.01^a
2	4.85 ± 0.47^a	37.00 ± 0.577^a	12.66 ± 0.16^a	6.66 ± 0.33^a
3	6.44 ± 0.32^c	38.66 ± 0.33^{ab}	12.83 ± 0.16^a	6.87 ± 0.03^a
4	5.64 ± 0.16^b	37.66 ± 0.33^a	12.66 ± 0.33^a	6.64 ± 0.22^a
5	6.18 ± 0.18^{bc}	38.40 ± 0.36^a	13.16 ± 0.16^{ab}	6.61 ± 0.31^a

a, b and c indicate significant difference at P ≤ 0.05 down the columns; RBC count- Red blood cell count; PCV- Packed cell volume; Hb- Haemoglobin

The white blood cell counts of the rats in all the groups (groups 1-5) were statistically comparable ($P > 0.05$) to each other.

4. DISCUSSION

Upon the administration of alloxan monohydrate to the rats in the treatment groups (groups 2-5), there was a significant ($P < 0.05$) increase in FBG levels of the rats to levels positive for diabetes mellitus (DM) as against the normal controls. This was attributed to the effect of alloxan monohydrate. Alloxan monohydrate is a toxic glucose analogue which selectively destroys the insulin-producing β cells in the pancreas when administered to rodents and many other animal species [19]. There was a significant ($P < 0.05$) reduction in the FBG of rats treated with *Gongronema latifolium* (GL) extract from the 1st to the 21st day of treatment by 51.7%. Francis et al. [12] had earlier reported hypoglycaemic potentials of *G. latifolium*. The effect was thought to be mediated through the activation of hexokinase, phoshofructokinase, glucose-6-phosphatase dehydrogenase and the inhibition of glucose kinase in the liver [11].

Similarly, there was a significant ($P < 0.05$) reduction in the FBG of rats treated with *Vernonia amygdalina* (VA) extract. The percentage reduction from the initial hyperglycaemic level was 55%. The anti-hyperglycaemic effect of VA has been reported by other researchers [8,9]. The work of [20] suggests that VA may exert anti-diabetic or glucose-lowering action by a simultaneous suppression of gluconeogenesis and potentiation of glucose oxidation via the pentose phosphate pathway almost exclusively in the liver.

The decrease in FBG resulting from the treatment with glibenclamide (77.3%) was comparable to the decrease brought about by the treatment with the combination of VA and GL extracts (76.7%). This striking hypoglycaemic activitiy achieved by combining VA and GL could be because the phytochemical components of the different plants worked synergistically to bring about a significant ($P < 0.05$) decrease superior to either of the plants used alone.

Superoxide dismutase (SOD) is an enzyme that catalyzes the dismutation (or partitioning) of superoxide (O^{-}_2) radical into either ordinary molecular oxygen or hydrogen peroxide. Superoxide is produced as a byproduct of oxygen metabolism and if not regulated, causes many types of cell damage. Hydrogen peroxide is also damaging but less so and is degraded by other enzymes such as catalase. Thus, SOD is an important antioxidant defense in nearly all living cells exposed to oxygen [21]. The study showed that rats in the group treated with a combination of GL and VA had a significantly ($P < 0.05$) higher SOD activity compared to the other groups. A synergy in the phytochemical components of both extracts is probably responsible for this.

Catalase is a common enzyme found in nearly all living organisms exposed to oxygen (such as bacteria, plants and animals). It catalyzes the decomposition of hydrogen peroxide to water and oxygen [22]. It is a very important enzyme in protecting the cell from oxidative damage by reactive oxygen species (ROS). Catalase is frequently used by cells to rapidly catalyze the decomposition of hydrogen peroxide to less-reactive gaseous oxygen and water molecules [23]. It has been reported that a catalase deficiency may increase the likelihood of developing type 2 diabetes mellitus [24]. Studies have also shown that patients with diabetes mellitus usually have a reduced catalase activity [25]. Rats that received the combined treatment of GL and VA produced a higher catalase activity than the other treatment groups.

The Malondialdehyde levels of the rats treated with a combination of the extracts was however lower than those of the rats treated with either of the extracts signifying a less lipid peroxidative activity in this group of rats. Malondialdehyde (MDA) is the organic compound that results from the lipid peroxidation of poly unsaturated fatty acids [26] and it is therefore a marker of oxidative stress [27]. This compound is a reactive aldehyde and is one of the many reactive electrophile species that cause toxic stress in cells and form covalent protein adducts [28].

Anaemia is a common finding in patients with diabetes mellitus particularly in those with overt nephropathy [29]. Similarly, another study showed that the mean values of red blood cell (RBC) count, haemoglobin (Hb) concentration, packed cell volume (PCV) and mean corpuscular haemoglobin concentration (MCHC) for the diabetic patients were lower than the values of the control group indicating the presence of anaemia in the former group [30]. Previous report indicates that the occurrence of anaemia in DM is due to increased non-enzymatic glycosylation of RBC membrane proteins which correlates with hyperglycaemia [31]. On the other hand, research has shown that WBC counts are significantly higher among diabetics compared to non-diabetics and that there is a positive correlation between raised WBC levels and poor glycaemic control defined as hyperglycaemia [32].

The result of this study as seen in Table 3 shows that rats treated with a combination of GL and VA leaf extracts had RBC counts ($6.44\pm0.32 \times 10^6$ millions/μl) statistically comparable to those of the normal control ($6.92\pm0.2 \times 10^6$ millions/μl). The RBC counts of the rats that received the combined treatment was significantly ($P < 0.05$) higher than those of the rats that received either of the extracts alone signifying a better glycaemic control as explained by Thomas and Rampersad, [31].

The PCV of the rats in the treatment groups were statistically comparable but were significantly lower than those of the normal control. The rats that received the combined treatment however had PCV levels (38.66±0.33%) similar to those of the normal control (40.33±0.33%). This also indicates a better glycaemic control exerted by the combination of the extracts.

The study also shows that the WBC count of all the rats in the different groups were statistically comparable although those of the rats that received the combined treatment ($6.87\pm0.03 \times 10^3$ thousand/μl) was closest to those of the normal controls ($6.89\pm0.01 \times 10^3$ thousand/μl).

5. CONCLUSION

The results of the present study show that the combination of the methanol extracts of GL and VA exhibited hypoglycaemic, *in vivo* anti-oxidant effects in addition to a positive effect on haematological indices superior to either of the extracts used alone.

CONSENT

It is not applicable.

ETHICAL APPROVAL

All authors hereby declare that "principles of laboratory animal care" (NIH publication No 85-23, revised 1985) were followed, as well as specific national laws. All experimemts have been examined and approved by the appropriate ethics committee.

COMPETING INTERESTS

Authors have declared that no competing interests exist.

REFERENCES

1. Ahmed AM. History of diabetes mellitus. Saudi Med J. 2002;23(4):373-8.
2. Twari AK, Rao JM. Diabetes mellitus and multiple therapeutic approaches of phytochemicals: Present status and future prospects. Current Science. 2002;83: 30-37.
3. International diabetes federation diabetes atlas, diabetes facts and figures 6th edn update; 2014.
4. Kahn C. The merck veterinary manual. Merck and co. Inc. Whitehouse station, NJ, USA; 2005.
5. Erasto P, Grierson DS, Afolayan AJ. Bioactive sesquiterpene lactones from the leaves of *Vernonia amygdalina*. Nutr Food Sci. 2006;38:99-109.
6. Ijeh II, Ejike CECC. Current perspectives on the medicinal potential of *Vernonia amygdalina* del. J. Med. Plant Res. 2011; 5(7):1051-1061.
7. Nwaoguikpe RN. The effect of extract of bitter leaf (*Vernonia amygdalina*) on blood glucose levels of diabetic rats. International Journal of Biological and Chemical Sciences. 2010;4:3. ISSN 1991-8631.
8. Osinubi AAA. Effects of *Vernonia amygdalina* and chlorpropamide on blood glucose. Med. J. Islam. World Acad. Sci. 2007;16:115-11.
9. Fasola TR, Okeocha PC, Odetola A. Screening for the hypoglycaemic potentials of the extract of *Vernonia amygdalina*. Ethnobotanical Leaflets. 2010;14:759-765.
10. Agbo CU, Baiyeri KP, Obi IU. Indigenous knowledge and utilization of *Gongronema latifolium* benth: A case study of women in University of Nigeria Nsukka. Bio-Research Journal. 2005;3(2):66-69.
11. Ugochukwu NH, Babady NE. Antihyperglycaemic effect of aqueous and ethanolic extracts of *Gongronema latifolium* leaves on glucose and glycogen metabolism in livers of normal and streptozotocin-induced diabetic rats. Life Sciences. 2003;73(5):1925-1938.

12. Francis V Udoh, Grace A Eshiet, Joneas O Akpan (Late), Frank E Edu (Late). Hypoglycaemic effect of *Gongronema latifolium* extracts in rats. Journal of Natural Sciences Research. 2013;3:5. ISSN 2224-3186 (Paper) ISSN 225-0921 (Online).
13. Venogopal PM, Prince PSM, Pari L. Hypoglycemic activities of *Syzigium cumini* seeds effect on lipid peroxidation in alloxan diabetic rats. Journal of Ethnopharmacology. 1998;61:1-7.
14. Kakkar SB, Viswanaathan P. A modified spectrophtometric assay of superoxide dismutase. Indian J. Biochem. Biophysics. 1989;21:130-132.
15. Sinha AK. Colorimetric assay of catalase. Anal. Biochem. 1972;47(2):389-92.
16. Wallin B, Rosengren B, Shertzer HG, Camejo G. Lipoprotein oxidation and measurement of TBARS formation in a single microliter plate; its use for evaluation of antioxidants. Anal. Biochem. 1993;208: 10-15.
17. Thrall MA, Weiser MG. Haematology. in: Hendrix CM (Ed.). Laboratory procedures for veterinary technicians 4th Edn, Mosby Incorporated, Missouri, USA. 2002;29-74.
18. Higgins T, Beutler E, Doumas BT. Measurement of haemoglobin in blood in Burtis CA, Ashwood ER, Bruns DE (Eds.). Tietz fundamentals of clinical chemistry, 6th edition. Saunders Elsevier, Missouri. 2008;514-515.
19. Lenzen S. The Mechanisms of alloxan and streptozotocin-induced diabetes. Diabetologia. 2008;51(2):216-226.
DOI: 10.1007/s00125-0070886-7
PMID: 18087688
20. Atangwho Item Justin, Khoo Boon Yin, Muhammad Ihtisham Umar, Mariam Ahmad, Mohd Zaini Asmawi. *Vernonia amygdalina* simultaneously suppresses glucose oxidation via the pentose phosphate pathway in streptozotocin-induced diabetic rats. BMC Complementary Altern Med. 2014;14:426.
21. Borgstahl GE, Parge HE, Hickey MJ, Johnson MJ, Boissinot M, Hallewell RA, Leprock JR, Cabelli De, Tainer JA. Human mitochondrial manganese superoxide dismutase polymorphic variant ile58thr reduces activity by destabilizing the tetrameric Interfere. Biochemistry. 1996;35(14):4287-97.
DOI: 10.1021/bi951892w
PMID: 8605177
22. Chelikani P, Fita L, Loewen PC. Diversity of structures and properties among catalases. Cell Mol. Life Sci. 2004;61(2): 192-208.
DOI: 10.1007/s00018-003-3206-5
PMID: 14745498
23. Gaetani GF, Ferraris AM, Rolfo M, Managerini R, Arena S, Kirkman HN. Predominant role of catalase in the disposal of hydrogen peroxide within human erythrocytes. Blood. 1996;87(4): 1595-9.
PMID: 8608252
24. Goth L. Catalase deficiency and type 2 diabetes. Diabetes Care. 2008;24(10): e93-e93.
DOI: 10.2337/dc08-1607
PMID: 19033415
25. Cojocaru IM, Cojocaru M, Musuroi C, Botezat M, Lazar L, Druta A. Lipid peroxidation and catalase in diabetes mellitus with and without ischemic stroke. Rom J Intern Med. 2004;42(2):423-9.
PMID: 15529632.
26. Davey MWI, Stals E, Panis B, Keulemans J, Swennen RL. High-throughput determination of malondialdehyde in plant tissues. Analytical Biochemistry. 2005; 347(2):201-207.
DOI: 10.1016/j.ab.2005.09.041
PMID: 16289006
27. Del Rio D, Stewart AJ, Pellegrini N. A Review of recent studies on malondialdehyde as toxic molecule and biological marker of oxidative stress. Nutr Metab Cardiovasc Dis. 2005;15(4):316-28.
DOI: 10.1016/j.numed.2005.05.003
PMID: 16054557
28. Farmer EE, Davoine C. Reactive electrophile species. Curr. Opin. Plant Biol. 2007;10(4):380-6.
DOI: 10.1016/j.pbi.2007.04.019
PMID: 17646124
29. Oyedemi SO, Yakubu MT, Afolayan AJ. Antidiabetic activities of aqueous leaves extract of *Leonotis leonurus* in streptozotocin induced diabetic rats. J Med Plant Res. 2011;5:119-125.
30. Ruchi Kothari, Pradeep Bokariya. A comparative study of haematological parameters in type 1 diabetes mellitus patients and healthy young adolescents. Int J Biol Med Res. 2012;3:2429-2432.

31. Thomas S, Rampersad M. Anaemia in diabetes. Acta Diabetol. 2004;41(Suppl1): 13-17.
32. Uko EK, Erhabor O, Isaac IZ, Abdulrahaman Y, Adias TC, et al. Some haematological parameters in patients with type 1 diabetes in Sokoto, North Western Nigeria. J. Blood Lymph. 2013;3(1):110. DOI: 10.4172/2165-7831.1000110 ISSN: 2165-7831

2

In vitro Efficacies of Some Nigerian Medicinal Plant Extracts against Toxigenic *Aspergillus flavus*, *A. parasiticus* and *A. ochraceus*

Yemisi Adefunke Jeff-Agboola[1*] and Anthony Kayode Onifade[2]

[1]Department of Biological Sciences, Ondo State University of Science and Technology, P.M.B 353 Okitipupa, Nigeria.
[2]Department of Microbiology, Federal University of Technology, P.M.B 704, Akure, Nigeria.

Authors' contributions

This work was carried out in collaboration between both authors. Author YAJA designed the study, wrote the protocol, analyze the study and wrote the first draft of the manuscript. Author AKO managed the literature searches, managed the experimental process and identified the species of plant. Both authors read and approved the final manuscript.

Article Information

Editor(s):
(1) Dongdong Wang, Department of Pharmacogonosy, West China College of Pharmacy, Sichuan University, China.
Reviewers:
(1) Norbert De Kimpe, Ghent University, Belgium.
(2) Antonello Santini, University of Napoli Federico II, Italy.
(3) Atef Mahmoud Mahmoud Attia, National Research Centre, Egypt.
(4) Daniela Hanganu, Hatieganu University of Medicine and Pharmacy Cluj-Napoca, Romania.

ABSTRACT

The aim of this work was to find an alternative to chemical fungicides currently used in the control and prevention of activities of toxigenic *Aspergillus flavus, A. parasiticus and A. ochraceus* in food and feed. The antifungal activity of extracts of five medicinal plants used in native medicine in Nigeria is reported. All plant extracts were screened for their minimum inhibitory concentration (MIC) against toxigenic *Aspergillus flavus, A. parasiticus and A. ochraceus*. Antifungi efficacies of the medicinal Plant extracts showed that maximum antifungal activity was demonstrated by ethanolic, hot and cold water extracts of *Borreria verticillata, Lactuca capenisi, Colocasia esculenta, Jatropha gossy and Ageratum conyzoide*. Leaves part of the five medicinal plants were investigated for antifungal activities against toxigenic *Aspergillus flavus* using radial growth technique. The plant extracts of *Borreria verticillata* inhibited the growth of the test organisms. *Borreria verticillata*

**Corresponding author: Email: yjeffagboola@yahoo.com*

appears to be more effective as an antifungal agent than other plant extracts. The ethanolic extracts were more effective than the cold and hot water extracts against the tested organism.

Keywords: Antifungi; toxigenic Aspergillus spps; medicinal plant.

1. INTRODUCTION

Fungal deterioration of stored seeds and grains is a chronic problem in the Nigeria storage system because of the tropical hot and humid climate. Harvested grains are colonized by various species of Aspergillus, under such conditions leading to deterioration and mycotoxin production. Aspergilli are the most common fungal species that can produce mycotoxin in food and feedstuffs. Aflatoxins are primarily produced by the fungi *Aspergillus flavus* and *Aspergillus parasiticus*, which contaminate a wide variety of food and feed commodities including maize, oilseeds, spices, groundnuts, tree nuts, milk and dried fruits [1]. Presence of aflatoxins in food chain is associated with decrease in quality and quantity of food and feed materials. In addition, consumption of aflatoxin-contaminated products can pose a risk of development of various diseases in human and animals. Aspergillus can attack crops at different times, in the field, during harvest, transport and storage. Today, there are strict regulations on chemical pesticide use, and there is political pressure to remove the most hazardous chemicals from the market [2].

The known success of traditional medicine has guided the search for new chemotherapeutic alternatives to eliminate the infections caused by drug-resistant microbes and to reduce the harm caused by antibiotic [3,4].

Medicinal Plants are rich in a wide variety of secondary metabolites, such as tannins, terpenoids, alkaloids, flavonoids, phenols and quinones [5-7]. Which have been used worldwide in traditional medicine to treat several diseases and infection [8-10]. Many studies all over the world have shown that these plants and their extract have multi-antimicrobial properties [11-13].

Many of the plant materials used in traditional medicine are readily available in rural areas and this has made traditional medicine relatively cheaper than modern medicine [14].

Over Sixty percent of Nigeria's rural population depends on traditional medicine for their healthcare need [15]. Medicinal plants contain pharmacologically active principles which over the years have been exploited in traditional medical practice for the treatment of various ailments [14]. Medicinal plants play a paramount role in the management of various ailments in rural communities considering the vast potentiality of medicinal plant as sources for antimicrobial agents.

Although restrictions are being imposed to protect food quality and the environment, chemicals are still our only recourse at present to prevent diseases of food crops. In recent years, the need to develop disease control measures as alternative to chemicals has become a priority of scientists worldwide. Therefore, it is important to find a practical, cost effective and non-toxic method to prevent fungal deterioration of field crop. Use of natural plant extracts and biocontrol agents provides an opportunity to avoid chemical preservatives. Therefore, the present study was designed to evaluate the in vitro antifungal activity of some plant extracts against toxigenic strains of *A. flavus, A. parasiticus* and *A. ochraceus*.

2. MATERIALS AND METHODS

2.1 Collection of Plant Material

The leaves of five medicinal plants (Plates 1-5) of *Borreria verticillata, Lactuca capenisi, Colocasia esculenta, Jatropha gossy and Ageratum conyzoide* were collected from Akure metropolis in Nigeria. The leaves were collected in sterile resealable bags. The leaves were washed under tap water, dried in hot air oven at 60℃ for 4 days and grounded to powder to pass through 20 mesh sieves and stored in sterile resealable bags.

2.2 Preparation of Aqueous Extracts from the Plant Leaves

Fifty gram (50 g) sample of each powder was weighed separately into 200 mL of hot and cold distilled water respectively and allowed to stand for 24 hrs. The extracts were then filtered through a millipore filter into different conical flasks. The extracts obtained were evaporated to dryness using a rotary evaporator. The extracts were assayed against the test organisms to determine the antifungal properties as described by [16]

2.3 Preparation of Ethanolic Extracts from the Plant Leaves

For the preparation of ethanolic extract, a modified method [17] was used. Fifty grams (50 g) sample of each powder was weighed separately into 200 mL ethanol (SDH Chemical Ltd), water and allowed to stand for 24 hrs. The extracts were then filtered through a millipore filter into different conical flasks. The extracts obtained from ethanolic extract were evaporated to dryness using a rotary evaporator. The extracts were assayed against the test organisms to determine the antifungal properties.

2.4 Collection of Toxigenic *Aspergillus flavus, A. parasiticus and A. ochraceus* Strain and Culture Conditions

Mycotoxin producing *A. flavus, A. parasiticus* and *A. ochraceus* were previously isolated from poultry feed samples.

All the test organisms were collected from the Food Microbiology Lab of Food Science and Technology Department, Federal University of Technology, Akure, Nigeria.

Spore suspension was prepared by growing the fungi on Petri dishes for 7 days with potato dextrose agar (PDA) containing 50 mg/L of streptomycin. After incubation at 25℃, spores were harvested by adding mixture of sterilized distilled (10 mL for each plate) water and 10μl of

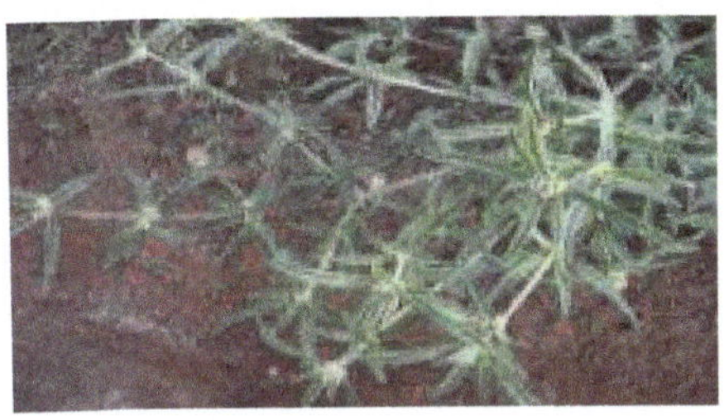

Plate 1. Photograph showing fresh leave of *Borreria verticillata* on the ground

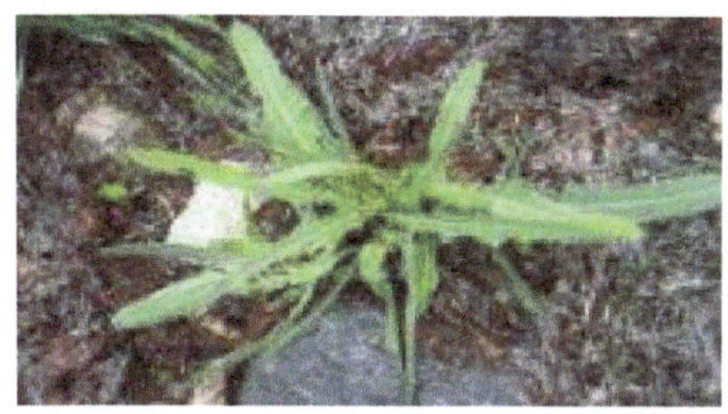

Plate 2. Photograph showing fresh leave of *Lactuca capenisi* on the ground

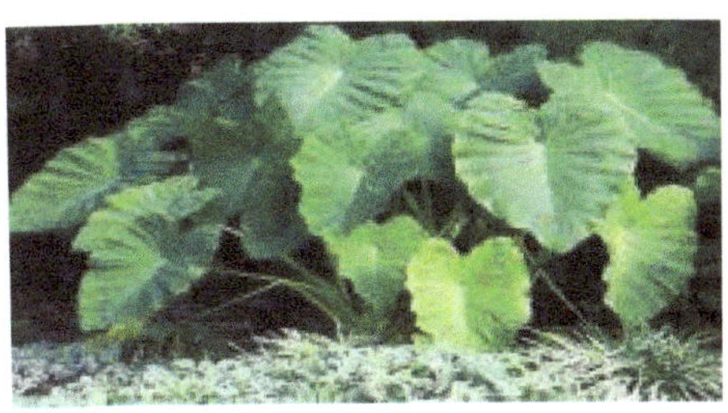

Plate 3. Photograph showing fresh leaves leaves of *Colocasia esculenta*

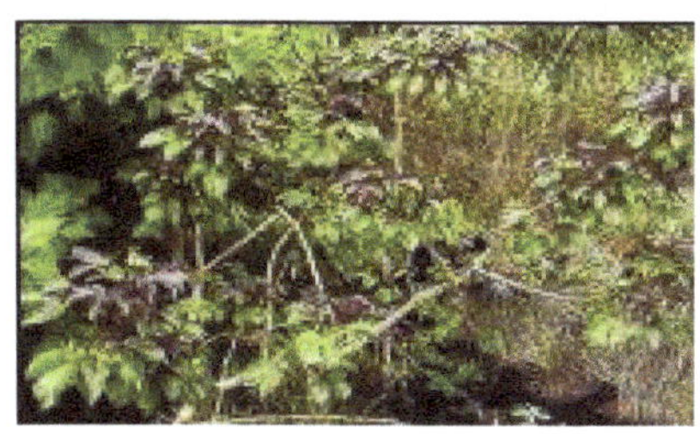

Plate 4. Photograph showing fresh of *Jatroph agossy* on the ground

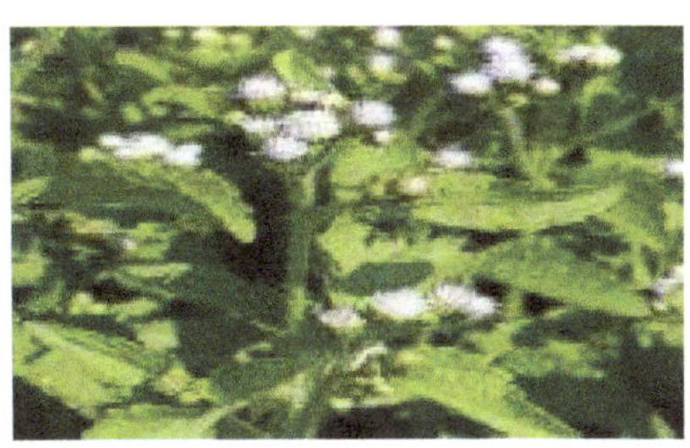

Plate 5. Photograph showing fresh leaves of *Ageratum conyzoide*

tween twenty on each plate. The spore suspension thus obtained was filtered using cheesecloth, and spores were counted using a haemocytometer and brought to a final concentration of 10^6conidia/ml.

2.5 Determination of Minimum Inhibitory Concentrations (MIC)

The MIC was determined as the concentration above which the fungal growth was totally suppressed and below which the fungus resumed growth. The MIC at which no mycelia growth of the test fungus was seen or 100 percent inhibition of the fungus growth was determined. Study was carried out by poisoned food technique using different concentrations of extracts against all the test fungi.

2.6 Procedure of MIC

A culture of the test fungi was grown on Potato Dextrose Agar (PDA) medium for certain period (generally 7 days) at the optimum temperature (25±2℃) for growth. PDA supplemented with different plant extracts at four concentrations (0.5, 1.5, 2.5 and 3.5%) was poured in the Petri plates under aseptic conditions. After solidification, small dish (0.5 cm dia.) of the fungus culture was cut with a sterile cork borer and transferred aseptically upside down at the center of petri dish. Suitable checks were maintained, where the culture discs were grown under same conditions on PDA without extract. Solvent checks were maintained to check out the inhibitory effect of solvent on fungi in which PDA was mixed with solvent (a solvent, which is used for dissolving extracts). Petri plates were incubated at 25±2℃. The radial five fungi were selected for bioassay viz. *Borreria verticillata, Lactuca capenisi, Colocasia esculenta, Jatropha gossy and Ageratum conyzoide leaves.* Growth of fungus colony was measured after every 24h till the fungus in the control plates completely occupied it. Three replications were maintained for each treatment. The antifungal activity was evaluated by measuring the relative growth of fungus in treatment vis-à-vis control. To maintain aseptic condition (the word aseptic means without microorganisms) throughout the experiment is very important. The percent growth inhibition over control was worked out using the formula. I = C-T/C x 100 Where, I is inhibition percent, C is colony diameter in control (cm) and T is colony diameter in treatment (cm) [17,18].

2.7 Data Analysis

The experiment was conducted using a completely randomized design. Standard errors of means of three replicates were computed using computer software Microsoft Excel.

3. RESULTS AND DISCUSSION

The results of antifungal screening of extracts of *Borreria verticillata, Lactuca capenisi, Colocasia esculenta, Jatropha gossy and Ageratum conyzoide* are given in Tables 1-5.

The results in Table 1 show that ethanolic, hot and cold water extract were effective against *A. ochraceus* but have no effect on *A. flavus and A. parasiticus* with maximum mean value concentration from hot water extract (49.23%) compared with ethanolic extract (42.84%) and cold water extract (30.22%). The result in Table 2 shows that ethanolic extract of *Jatropha gossy* has the highest mean concentration (40.85%) than hot water extract (30.12%) and cold water extract (23.61%) against *A. flavus* but have no inhibitory concentration against the other fungi used.

Ethanolic extract of *Colocasia esculenta* was more effective against *A. flavus and A. paraciticus* (Table 3). The highest mean concentration of the extract that inhibited the growth of *A. flavus* was observed with ethanolic extract (45.37%) compared with the hot water extract (24.27%) and cold water extract (26.36). Also the ethanolic extract was able to inhibit the growth of *A. parasiticus* at mean concentration of 29.77% while the hot and cold water extract had no inhibitory effect on *A. parasiticus.* It was also observed that the three extract had no inhibitory effect on *A. ochraceus.*

The result of the effect of different concentrations of ethanolic, hot and cold water extracts of *Lactuca capenisi* on the radial growth of fungi (Table 4) shows that the maximum inhibitory effect was observed from ethanolic extract against *A. flavus* (56.20%) and *A. parasiticus* (62.76%) compare to hot water extract (44.83, 57.13)% and cold water extract (41.30, 42.4)% respectively. All the extracts of *Lactuca capenisi* had no inhibitory effect on *A. ochraceus.*

Table 1. Effect of different concentrations of ethanolic, hot and cold water extracts of *Ageratum conyzoide* on the radial growth of fungi

Fungus species	Concentration/Growth inhibition (%) ethanolic extract						Concentration/Growth inhibition (%) hot water extract						Concentration/Growth inhibition (%) cold extract					
	Control	0.5	1.5	2.5	3.5	Mean	Control	0.5	1.5	2.5	3.5	Mean	Control	0.5	1.5	2.5	3.5	Mean
Aspergillus flavus	0.00	0.00	0.00	0.00	0.00	0.00	0.00	0.00	0.00	0.00	0.00	0.00	0.00	0.00	0.00	0.00	0.00	0.00
A. parasiticus	0.00	0.00	0.00	0.00	0.00	0.00	0.00	0.00	0.00	0.00	0.00	0.00	0.00	0.00	0.00	0.00	0.00	0.00
A. ocheracus	0.00	22.35	35.25	45.00	68.75	42.84	0.00	25.50	39.25	55.00	77.15	49.23	0.00	10.15	28.26	35.23	47.25	30.22

Table 2. Effect of different concentrations of ethanolic, hot and cold water extracts of *Jatropha gossy*on the radial growth of fungi

Fungus species	Concentration/Growth inhibition (%) ethanolic extract						Concentration/Growth inhibition (%) hot water extract						Concentration/Growth inhibition (%) cold extract					
	Control	0.5	1.5	2.5	3.5	Mean	Control	0.5	1.5	2.5	3.5	Mean	Control	0.5	1.5	2.5	3.5	Mean
Aspergillus flavus	0.00	23.65	37.00	44.50	58.25	40.85	0.00	15.00	24.65	35.66	45.15	30.12	0.00	10.00	18.55	28.15	37.75	23.61
A. parasiticus	0.00	0.00	0.00	0.00	0.00	0.00	0.00	0.00	0.00	0.00	0.00	0.00	0.00	0.00	0.00	0.00	0.00	0.00
A. ocheracus	0.00	0.00	0.00	0.00	0.00	0.00	0.00	0.00	0.00	0.00	0.00	0.00	0.00	0.00	0.00	0.00	0.00	0.00

Table 3. Effect of different concentrations of ethanolic, hot and cold water extracts of *Colocasia esculenta* on the radial growth of fungi

Fungus species	Concentration/Growth inhibition (%) ethanolic extract						Concentration/Growth inhibition (%) hot water extract						Concentration/Growth inhibition (%) cold extract					
	Control	0.5	1.5	2.5	3.5	Mean	Control	0.5	1.5	2.5	3.5	Mean	Control	0.5	1.5	2.5	3.5	Mean
Aspergillus flavus	0.00	20.15	35.66	55.50	75.15	45.37	0.00	13.25	20.00	28.68	35.15	24.27	0.00	14.65	22.15	30.00	38.62	26.36
A. parasiticus	0.00	10.00	20.15	33.25	55.67	29.77	0.00	0.00	0.00	0.00	0.00	0.00	0.00	0.00	0.00	0.00	0.00	0.00
A. ocheracus	0.00	0.00	0.00	0.00	0.00	0.00	0.00	0.00	0.00	0.00	0.00	0.00	0.00	0.00	0.00	0.00	0.00	0.00

Table 4. Effect of different concentrations of ethanolic, hot and cold water extracts of *Lactuca capenisi* on the radial growth of fungi

Fungus species	Concentration/Growth inhibition (%) ethanolic extract						Concentration/Growth inhibition (%) hot water extract						Concentration/Growth inhibition (%) cold extract					
	Control	0.5	1.5	2.5	3.5	Mean	Control	0.5	1.5	2.5	3.5	Mean	Control	0.5	1.5	2.5	3.5	Mean
Aspergillus flavus	0.00	33.25	45.00	58.22	88.36	56.20	0.00	28.65	38.00	47.65	65.00	44.83	0.00	25.00	35.65	45.77	58.76	41.30
A. parasiticus	0.00	35.00	50.15	69.17	96.70	62.76	0.00	30.10	48.15	65.00	85.25	57.13	0.00	22.35	37.35	49.25	60.65	42.4
A. ocheracus	0.00	0.00	0.00	0.00	0.00	0.00	0.00	0.00	0.00	0.00	0.00	0.00	0.00	0.00	0.00	0.00	0.00	0.00

Table 5. Effect of different concentrations of ethanolic, hot and cold water extracts of *Borreria verticillata* on the radial growth of fungi

Fungus species	Concentration/Growth inhibition (%) ethanolic extract						Concentration/Growth inhibition (%) hot water extract						Concentration/Growth inhibition (%) cold extract					
	Control	0.5	1.5	2.5	3.5	Mean	Control	0.5	1.5	2.5	3.5	Mean	Control	0.5	1.5	2.5	3.5	Mean
Aspergillus flavus	0.00	45.15	68.55	88.35	105.25	76.83	0.00	40.00	65.15	79.78	97.35	70.57	0.00	32.45	55.36	70.15	88.95	61.73
A. parasiticus	0.00	0.00	0.00	0.00	0.00	0.00	0.00	0.00	0.00	0.00	0.00	0.00	0.00	0.00	0.00	0.00	0.00	0.00
A. ocheracus	0.00	0.00	0.00	0.00	0.00	0.00	0.00	0.00	0.00	0.00	0.00	0.00	0.00	0.00	0.00	0.00	0.00	0.00

It was revealed in this study, that increase in the antifungal activity of the extracts was enhanced by increase in the concentration of the extracts. This finding agrees with the report of [19,20] that higher concentration of antimicrobial substance showed appreciation in growth inhibition. All the plant extracts tested exhibited different degrees of antifungal activity against toxigenic *A. flavus, A. parasiticus and A. ochraceus.* The maximum antimycotic activity was shown by ethanolic extract of *Borreria verticillata* against toxigenic *A. flavus* followed by hot water and cold water extract of *Borreria verticillata* against toxigenic *A. flavus.* The extract of *Borreria verticillata* was effective against fungal pathogens causing diseases in plants, human beings and animals [21] The fact that the results of this study showed that extract of the plants were effective against the test organisms may be due to the presence of active principles in the plant materials. Plants generally produce many secondary metabolites which constitute an important source of microbicides, pesticides and many pharmaceutical drugs [22] Plant products still remain the principal source of pharmaceutical agents used in orthodox medicine [22]. The MIC values of the plant extracts against the test organism showed that fungi vary widely in the degree of their susceptibility to antifungal agents. This observation therefore suggests that the antifungal substances contained in the extracts were fungistatic at lower concentrations while becoming fungicidal at higher concentrations of the extracts. Similar observations have been reported by [22]. When comparing data obtained in different studies, most publications provide generalizations about whether or not plant possesses activity against fungi. However, not all provide details about the extent or spectrum of this activity. Some publications also show the relative activity of plant and extracts by comparing results on different extracts tested against the same organism(s) [23]. It has been found that essential oils with anti-mould effectiveness is able to consistently cause morphological changes in Aspergillus species including lack of sporulation, loss of pigmentation, aberrant development of conidiophores (flattened and squashed) and distortion of hyphaes (budding, lack of cytoplasm, swelling anomalous apex bifurcation) [24]. These findings suggested that the mode of antifungal activity of plants could include an attack on the cell wall and retraction of the cytoplasm in the hyphae ultimately resulting in death of the mycelium and spore germination. The results found in this study showed fungicidal activities of *Borreria verticillata, Lactuca capenisi, Colocasia esculenta, Jatropha gossy and Ageratum conyzoide* ethanolic, hot and cold water extracts providing interesting information about rapidity and stability of its anti-Aspergillus property. It also showed that the growth and survival of food and feed -related Aspergillus species could be controlled by the use of the extracts, particularly, *Borreria verticillata* Several reports stated that the extracts of medicinal plants play an important role in controlling many phytopathogenic fungi [25-30]. The inhibitory effect of tested extracts might be due to natural bioactive materials present in these extracts [24]. This may be because the bioactive compounds of these plants may differ in quantity and quality compared to other tested plants.

It was observed that the effect of different concentrations of ethanolic, hot and cold water extracts of *Borreria verticillata* on the radial growth of fungi shows that the three extracts were able to inhibit the growth of *A. flavus* with the highest mean concentration observed from ethanolic extract (76.83%) followed by hot water extract (70.57%) and cold water extract (61.73%). The plant extract has no inhibitory effect on *A. parasiticus* and *A. ochraceus.*

Several workers have made similar observations by using essential oils or complex mixture from higher plants [31]. For example some water-soluble compounds may have a higher diffusion power and lower antimicrobial activity [32-35].

The inhibitory effect of some ethanolic plants extracts under in vitro condition might be due to the presence of phenolic compounds (polyphenols, phenolic acids, coumarins) in the extracts. Earlier work of [33] supports the finding where the polyphenols, phenolic acids, coumarins of plants were found to inhibit the growth and enzyme production (ligninolytic and pectinolytic enzymes) of *Botryosphaeria* spp. The Inhibitory activity of some other plants by the flower extracts of Daturainnoxia under in vitro condition was reported [33]. This also supports the presence of phenolic compounds (polyphenols, phenolic acids, coumarins) in the plant extract which cause the inhibition of enzymes activity.

The plant extracts of *Borreria verticillata* inhibited the growth of the test organisms except *Aspergillus parasiticus and A. ochraceus, Borreria verticillata* appears to be more effective as an antifungal agent than other plant extracts.

Ethanolic extracts were more effective than the cold and hot water extracts against all the test fungi.

4. CONCLUSION

The results obtained from this study show that the extracts of *Borreria verticillata*, *Lactuca capenisi, Colocasia esculenta* and *Jatropha gossy* used exhibit antifungal activity against *A. flavus and A. parasiticus*. While extracts of *Ageratum conyzoide* alone had inhibitory effect on *A. ochraceus,* Extracts of the plant used in this study could be useful in the treatment of fungal infections caused by *A. flavus, A. parasiticus* and *A. ochraceus*.

CONSENT

It is not applicable.

ETHICAL APPROVAL

It is not applicable.

COMPETING INTERESTS

Authors have declared that no competing interests exist.

REFERENCES

1. Strosnider H, Azziz-Baumgartner E, Banziger M., Bhat RV, Breiman R, Brune M. Workgroup report: Public health strategies for reducing aflatoxin exposure in developing countries. Environ. Health Perspect. 2006;114:1989-1903.
2. Pal KK, Gardener BM. Biological control of plant pathogens. The Plant Health Instructor; 2006.
3. Bull CT, Shetty KG, Subbarao KV. Interactions between Mycobacteria, plant pathogenic fungi, and biocontrol agents. Plant Dis. 2002;86:889-896.
4. Giamarellou H. Treatment options for multidrug-resistant bacteria. Expert Review of Anti-infective Therapy. 2006;4(4):601-618.
5. Al-Zubaydi SR, Al-Hmdany MA, Raesan SJ. Antibactrial effect of some medicinal plant extracts against some pathogenic bacteria strains. Journal of Duhok University. 2009;12(1):244-249.
6. Leon J, Rojo E, Sanchezerrano J. Wound signling in plants. Journal of Experimental Botany. 2001;52:1-9.
7. Cowan MM. Plant products as antimicrobial agents. Clinical Microbiology Reviews. 1999;12(4):564-582.
8. Saad B, Azaizeh H, Said O. Tradition and perspectives of Arab herbal medicine: A review. Evidence-Based Complementary and Alternative Medicine. 2005;2(4):475-479.
9. Kalemba D, Kunicka A. Antibacterial and antifungal properties of essential oils. Journal of Current Medicinal Chemistry. 2003;10(10):813-829
10. Jain SC, Sharmo R, Jain R, Sharmo RA. Antimicrobial activity of *Calotropis procera*. Fitoterapia. 1996;67(3):275-277.
11. Al-Juraifani AA. Antimicrobial activity of some medicinal plants used in Saudi Arabia. Canadian Journal of Pure & Applied Sciences. 2011;5(2):1509-1512.
12. Bocanegra-Garcia VM, Camacho-Corona M, Ramirez-Cabrera G, Garza-Gonzatez R. The bioactivity of plant extracts against representative bacterial pathogens of the lower respiratory tract. BMC Research Notes. 2011;2:95.
13. Bakht J, Tayyab M, Ali H, Islam A, Shafi M. Effect of different solvent extracted sample of *Allium sativum* (Linn) on bacteria and fungi. African Journal of Biotechnology 2011;10(31):5910-5915.
14. Shittu IAJ, Bankole MA, Ahmed T, Bankole MN, Shittu RK, Saalu CL, Soliman KM, Badeaa RI. Effect of oil extracted from some medicinal plants on different mycotoxigenic fungi. Food Chemistry and Toxicology. 2002;40:1669-1675.
15. Benkeblia N. Antimicrobial activity of essential oil extracts of various onions (*Allium cepa*) and garlic (*Allium sativum*). Lebensmittel-Wissenschaft und – Technologie. 2004;37:263–268.
16. Reichling J, Schnitzler P, Suschke U, Saller R. Essential oils of aromatic plants with antibacterial, antifungal, antiviral, and cytotoxic properties. An overview. Forsch Komplementmed. 2009;16:79-90.
17. Boklari FM. Antifungal activity of some medicinal plants used in Jeddah, Saudi Arabia. Mycopathologia. 2009;7(1):51-57
18. Janssen AM, Scheffer JJC. Antimicrobial activity of essential oil: 1976-86 literature review aspect of test methods. Planta Med. 1986;53:395-398.

19. Barrata TM, Dorman HJD. Antimicrobial and antioxidant properties of some commercial essential oils. Flavour Fragr. J. 1998;13:335-244.
20. Freiburghaus F, Kaminsky R, Nkunya MH H, Brun R. Evaluation of African medicinal plants for their in vitro trypanocidal activity. Journal of Ethnopharmacology. 1996;55: 1-11.
21. Elagayyar M, Draughon FA, Golden DA. Antimicrobial activity of essential oil from plants against selected pathogenic and saprophytic microorganisms. Journal of Food Protection. 2001;4:1019-1024.
22. De Billerberk VG, Roques CG, Bessiere JM, Fonvieille JL, Dargent R. Effects of *Cymbopogon nardus* (L.) W. Watson essential oil on the growth and morphogenesis of *Aspergillus niger*. Canadian Journal of Microbiology. 2001; 47:9-17.
23. McKey DL, Blumberg JB. A review of the bioactivity and potential health benefits of chamomile tea (*Matrcaria recutita* L.). Phytotherapy Research. 2006;20:519-530.
24. Rasooli I, Abyaneh MR. Inhibitory effect of Thyme oils on growth and afltoxin production by *Aspergillus parasiticus*. Food Contaminant. 2004;15:479-483.
25. Lin CH, Zon WX, Lin H, Tan RX. Antifungal activity of Artemisia annua endophytic cultures against phytopathogenic fungi. Journal of Biotechnology. 2001;88:277–282.
26. Okemo PO, Bais HP, Vivanco JM. In vitro activities of *Maesa lanceolata* extracts against fungal plant pathogens. Fitoterapia. 2003;74:312–316.
27. Choi GJ, Jang KS, Kim JS, Lee SW, Cho JY, Cho KY, Kim JC. In vivo antifungal activities of 57 plant extracts against six plant pathogenic fungi. Plant Pathology Journal. 2004;20:184–191.
28. Reichling J, Schnitzler P, Suschke U, Saller R. Essential oils of aromatic plants with antibacterial, antifungal, antiviral, and cytotoxic properties. An overview Forsch komplementmed. 2009;16:79-90.
29. Atanda OO, Akpan I, Oluwafemi F. The potential of some spice essential oils in the control of *A. parasiticus* CFR 223 and aflatoxin production. Food Control. 2007; 18:601–607.
30. Perez-Sanchez R, Infante F, Galvez C, Ubera JL. Fungitoxic activity against phytopathogenic fungi and the chemical composition of Thymus zygis essential oil. Food Science Technology International. 2007;13:341–347.
31. Rios JL, Recio MC, Villar A. Screening methods for natural products with antimicrobial activity: A review of the literature. J. Ethnopharmacol. 1988;23: 127–149.
32. Gundidza M. Antimicrobial activities of *Helinus integrifolius*. Fitoterapia. 1987;58: 180–183.
33. Janssen M, Scheffer JJC, Svedsen AB. Antimicrobial activity of essential oils: a 1976–1986 literature review. Aspects of the test methods. Planta Med. 1987;63: 395–398.
34. Nils G, Louis M, Luc V, Mai V, Duong A, Norbert D. *In vitro* and *in vivo* anti-leishmanial activity of triterpenoid saponins isolated from *Maesa balansae* and some chemical derivatives. J. Med. Chem. 2005;48:32-37.
35. Ina V, Patrick V, Luc V, Susana A, Norbert D. A comparison of traditional healers' medicinal plant knowledge in the Bolivian Andes and Amazon. Social Science & Medicine. 2004;59:837-849.

3

Cytotoxic Effect of Lingzhi Extracts on Gefitinib-resitant Lung Cancer Cells

Nguyen Hai Dang[1*], Pham Thanh Binh[1], Nguyen Thi Tham[1], Bui Thi Mai Anh[1], Nguyen Phuong Dai Nguyen[2] and Nguyen Tien Dat[1*]

[1]Insitute of Marine Biochemistry, Vietnam Academy of Science and Technology, 18-Hoang Quoc Viet, Cau Giay, Hanoi, Vietnam.
[2]Department of Biology, Faculty of Natural Science and Technology, Tay Nguyen University, 567 Le Duan, Dac Lac City 630000, Vietnam.

Authors' contributions

This work was carried out in collaboration between all authors. Authors NHD and NTD designed the study and prepared the manuscript. Authors PTB, NTT and BTMA performed the sample extraction and biological assay. Author NPDN collected and identified mushroom samples. All authors read and approved the final manuscript.

Article Information

Editor(s):
(1) Dongdong Wang, Department of Pharmacogonosy, West China College of Pharmacy, Sichuan University, China.
Reviewers:
(1) Eduardo Bernardi, Universidade Federal de Pelotas, Brazil.
(2) G. Krishna, Kakatiya University, India.

ABSTRACT

Aims: The present study was carried out to investigate the cytotoxicity of extracts from *Ganoderma* and *Amauroderma* lingzhi species collected in Tay Nguyen, Vietnam.
Methods: Mushroom samples were extracted by methanol and the cytotoxicity was performed by 3-(4,5-dimethyl-2-thiazolyl)-2,5-diphenyltetrazolium bromide (MTT) method.
Results: Among twelve extracts prepared from *Ganoderma* and *Amauroderma* species, six samples significantly inhibited the proliferation of gefitinib-resistant NSCLC cell lines NCI-H1975 and A549. *Amauroderma rugosum* exhibited cytotoxic effects against both cell lines in comparison with etoposide.
Conclusion: The obtained results suggested that the Tay Nguyen lingzhi could be regarded as a promising candidate for natural sources of epidermal growth factor receptor-tyrosine kinase inhibitors (EGFR-TKIs).

**Corresponding author: E-mail: nguyenhd@imbc.vast.vn, ngtiend@imbc.vast.vn*

Keywords: Non-small Cell Lung Cancer (NSCLC); EGFR-TKI; ganoderma; Amauroderma; ganodermataceae.

1. INTRODUCTION

Lung cancer continues to be the leading cause of cancer death worldwide with the rate of 1.6 million deaths yearly [1]. Lung cancer is the second deathliest cancers after liver cancer in Vietnam according to the same report of WHO. Also, it is reported about 110000 new cases of lung cancer every year. Approximately 98% of lung cancers are carcinoma, or tumors derived from transformed cells of epithelial lineage [2]. Currently, nearly four dozen different histopathological variants of lung carcinoma are recognized [3]. For clinical and treatment purposes, lung cancer can be classified into two major groups, namely small cell cancer (SCLC, about 15%) and non-small cell lung cancer (NSCLC, up to 85%). Squamous cell carcinoma, adenocarcinoma, and large cell carcinoma are subtypes of non-small cell lung cancer [4]. In the past few years, the discovery of the pivotal role in tumorigenesis of the epidermal growth factor receptor (EGFR) provided a new class of targeted therapeutic agents: The EGFR-tyrosine kinase inhibitors (EGFR-TKIs) [5]. Tyrosine kinase inhibitors (TKIs) are an emerging class of anticancer therapies that have shown promising clinical activity. Gefitinib (Iressa) and erlotinib (Tarceva) inhibit the epidermal growth factor receptor (EGFR) kinase and have been used to treat non–small cell lung cancers (NSCLCs) that have activating mutations in the EGFR gene [6-7]. Although most EGFR-mutant NSCLCs initially respond to EGFR inhibitors, the vast majority of these tumors ultimately become resistant to the drug treatment. In about 50% of these cases, resistance is due to the occurrence of a secondary mutation in EGFR (T790M) [8]. Other secondary EGFR gene mutations such as D761Y [9], L747S [10], and T854A [11] mutations have been reported. The frequency of such mutations appears to be low in comparison with the T790M mutation. Currently, EGFR-TKIs are known to contribute considerably to the extension of progression-free survival in prognosis for NSCLC.

Mushrooms belonging to the genera *Ganoderma* and *Amauroderma* (Ganodermataceae) have been used in traditional Vietnamese medicine for longevity and health promotion since ancient times. Various biological activities of these mushrooms have been reported. They are mostly useful for inhibiting tumor growth, modulating immune response and increasing hematopoietic activity [12]. The anticancer effects of the mushrooms of these genera, especially, *G. lucidum*, commonly referred to as Lingzhi (Linh Chi in Vietnamese), have been widely reported in both *in vitro* and *in vivo* studies [13]. Triterpenes and polysaccharides are the major bioactive substances that have been reported for the anticancer properties of the mushroom. The biological pathways which exert their anticancer activity have recently been reported [13]. However, the *Amauroderma* species have not been well investigated for their biological activities as well as their chemical compositions. In this paper, we investigated the cytotoxic effects of mushroom extracts of *Ganoderma* and *Amauroderma* species on the NSCLC cell lines with special focus on the EGFR resistant lung cancers.

2. MATERIALS AND METHODS

2.1 Materials

A total of 12 mushroom samples belonging to the genera *Ganoderma* and *Amauroderma* were collected from different regions in the Northern part of Tay Nguyen, Vietnam. The samples were identified conventionally according to their macroscopic and microscopic features by one of the author (NPDN). Voucher of specimens was deposited at the Department of Natural Sciences and Technology, Tay Nguyen University.

2.2 Preparation of Extracts

After drying by an oven (50℃ for 24 h), the samples (approximately 10 g of each sample) were extracted with methanol (50 mL x 30 min x 3 times) at room temperature by sonication-assisted solvent extraction. The combined extracts were concentrated under reduced pressure to obtain crude extracts.

2.3 Cell Lines and Cell Culture

A549 (Human lung carcinoma), NCI-H1975 (Human lung adenocarcinoma), NCI-H1650 (Human lung adenocarcinoma), NCI-H1299 (Human lung large cell carcinoma), NCI-H358 (Human bronchiolalveolar carcinoma) were kindly provided by Prof. Jeong-Hyung Lee, Department of Biochemistry, College of Natural Sciences, Kangwon National University, Korea.

The cells were cultured at 37℃ in RMPI1640 medium supplemented with 10% fetal bovine serum (FBS), 100 U/ml penicillin, and 100 μg/ml streptomycin in a 5% CO_2 incubator. Cells between 5 and 20 passages were used for the assays.

2.4 Cell Proliferation Assay

An MTT [3-(4,5-dimethyl-2-thiazolyl)-2,5-diphenyltetrazolium bromide] assay was used to measure the viability of cells after extract treatment. Cells were seeded in 96-well plates at a density of 2.0×10^5 cells/ml. Cells were treated with various concentrations of lingzhi extracts (1, 3, 10, 30 and 100 μg/ml) and then incubated at 37℃ for 24 h in fresh RMPI1640. Cells were subsequently incubated at 37℃ with MTT (0.5 mg/ml) for 4 h. After removal of supernatant, formazan crystals were dissolved in isopropanol and the optical density was measured at 570 nm. Etoposide was used as a positive control.

2.5 Statistics

Results are given as the mean standard error for the mean (SEM). Statistical analyses were performed with GraphPad Prism Software.

3. RESULTS AND DISCUSSION

In order to investigate the anticancer activities of lingzhi, 12 different mushrooms belonging to the genera *Ganoderma* and *Amauroderma* were collected in different regions of the northern part of Tay Nguyen. The results of sample collection and identification were presented in Table 1. All samples were extracted with MeOH by using sonication.

A panel of five NSCLC cell lines was divided into three groups: group #1, no mutation of EGFR (A549 and NCI-H1299), group #2, EGFR mutation and TKI-resistance inducing mutation (NCI-H1975 and NCI-H1650), group #3, EGFR mutation, sensitive to TKI inhibitors (NCI-H358).The cellular proliferation of this panel of 5 NSCLC cell lines was examined by MTT over 24 h in the presence of increasing concentrations of a variety of mushroom extracts. Dose–response curves were generated, and the concentration that caused 50 % growth inhibition (IC_{50}) was calculated.

The primary screening results indicated that at concentration 100 μg/ml, the methanol extracts of *Ganoderma* and *Amauroderma* have almost no effects on the gefitinib-sensitive NCI-H358. The same results were obtained for the effects of *Ganoderma* and *Amauroderma* extracts on NCI-H1299, a wild type of EGFR and NCI-H1650, an EGFR mutant. Interestingly, at the tested concentration, the extracts LC7 and LC11 showed positive inhibitory activity against the growth of A549, a human lung carcinoma cell line. The extracts LC2, LC3, LC4, LC11 and LC12 showed notable anti-proliferation effect on the human lung adenocarcinoma NCI-H1975 cell line (Table 2).

Table 1. List of Lingzhi samples

No.	Species	Sample code
1	*Ganoderma flexipes*	LC1
2	*Ganoderma tropicum*	LC2
3	*Ganoderma capense*	LC3
4	*Ganoderma multiplicatum*	LC4
5	*Ganoderma lobatum*	LC5
6	*Ganoderma applanatum*	LC6
7	*Ganoderma* sp.	LC7
8	*Ganoderma australe*	LC8
9	*Amauroderma* sp.	LC9
10	*Amauroderma rude*	LC10
11	*Amauroderma rugosum*	LC11
12	*Amauroderma subresinosum*	LC12

Lingzhi has long been known as a potential medicament for several major human cancers. Their mechanisms of action on different cancer cell lines have been demonstrated elsewhere [14]. However, the potential anti-proliferation effect of these mushrooms combined with EGFR-TKIs on NSCLC has not been investigated. In this study, we showed that five extracts of *Ganoderma* and two extracts of *Amauroderma* selectively inhibited the growth of A549 (EGFR wild type, TKI resistant) and H1975 (EGFR mutant, TKI-resistant) cell lines (Table 2). Tyrosine kinase domain of the EGFR was discovered from the patient with NSCLC. This domain has a remarkable clinical response to the treatment with tyrosine kinase inhibitors (TKI) like gefitinib or erlotinib [7]. Recently, there has been increasing case reports on the resistance of gefitinib treatment, especially on the patients with wild-type EGFR and acquired mutation in EGFR T790M. Our findings suggest the potential application of the *Ganoderma* and *Amauroderma* mushrooms in EGFR-TKIs therapy in NSCLC patients with different EGFR status.

Table 2. The inhibition of proliferation of NSCLC cells by mushroom extracts (100 μg/ml)

Sample code	Wild type of EGFR and TKI-resistance		Mutation of EGFR and TKI-resistance		Mutation of EGFR, sensitive to TKI inhibitors
	A549	H1299	H1650	H1975	H358
LC1	-	-	-	-	-
LC2	-	-	-	+	-
LC3	-	-	-	+	-
LC4	-	-	-	+	-
LC5	-	-	-	-	-
LC6	-	-	-	-	-
LC7	+	-	-	-	-
LC8	-	-	-	-	-
LC9	-	-	-	-	-
LC10	-	-	-	-	-
LC11	+	-	-	+	-
LC12	-	-	-	+	-

The IC_{50} values of the extracts against the growth of A549 and NCI-H1975 cell lines were determined by using Graphpad Prism software (Table 3). Accordingly, NCI-H1975 seems to be more sensitive to the mushroom extracts than does the A549 cell line. There have been a number of reports on the bioactive constituents of the mushroom with anticancer properties, in which polysaccharides and triterpenes are among the most active components. A phytochemical study should, therefore, be conducted on the active extracts to find potential substances with potent anticancer activity.

Table 3. Inhibition concentrations 50% (IC_{50}) values for mushroom extracts towards A549 and NCI-H1975 cells

Sample code	A549 (μg/ml)	H1975 (μg/ml)
LC2	>100	42.9±3.25
LC3	>100	51.2±0.86
LC4	>100	42.1±1.76
LC7	68.0±2.12	>100
LC11	62.0±0.52	47.6±1.60
LC12	>100	45.7±1.89
Etoposide (μM)	57.8±0.71	64.5±1.35

4. CONCLUSION

Our findings suggest that the crude extracts of *Ganoderma* and *Amauroderma* species, mushrooms generally well-tolerated with few side effects, may be promising materials for treatment of gefitinib resistant NSCLCs. This is the first report on the anti-proliferative effects of these mushrooms on different EGFR TKI resistant and sensitive lung cancer cell lines. Further phytochemical studies on the active extracts to determine the bioactive components will be carried out in future works.

CONSENT

It is not applicable.

ETHICAL APPROVAL

It is not applicable.

ACKNOWLEDGEMENTS

The authors acknowledge the financial support from the Vietnam Academy of Science and Technology (project code VAST.UDCN.02/14-15).

COMPETING INTERESTS

Authors have declared that no competing interests exist.

REFERENCES

1. Bernard W. Stewart and Christopher P. Wild (Eds.). World Cancer Report 2014. International Agency for Research on Cancer; 2014.
2. Gadepalli VS, Deb SP, Deb S, Rao RR. Lung cancer stem cells, p53 mutations and MDM2. Subcellular Biochemistry. 2014;85: 359-370.
3. Travis WD, Travis LB, Devesa SS. Lung cancer. Cancer. 1995;75:191-202.
4. Travis WD, Brambilla E, Muller H, Konrad H. pathology and genetics of tumours of the lung, pleura, thymus and heart. World

Health Organization Classification of Tumours, IARC Press, Lyon; 2004.
5. Milovancev A, Stojsic V, Zaric B, Kovacevic T, Sarcev T, Perin B, Zarogoulidis K, Tsirgogianni K, Freitag L, Darwiche K, Tsavlis D, Zissimopoulos A, Stratakos G, Zarogoulidis P. EGFR-TKIs in adjuvant treatment of lung cancer: To give or not to give. Onco Targets Ther. 2015;8:2915-21.
6. Raz DJ, He B, Rosell R, Jablons DM. Bronchioloalveolar carcinoma: A review. Clinical Lung Cancer. 2006;7:313-322.
7. Bencardino K, Manzoni M, Delfanti S. Epidermal growth factor receptor tyrosine kinase inhibitors for the treatment of non-small-cell lung cancer: Results and open issues. Intern Emerg Med. 2011;2:3-12.
8. Kosaka T, Yamaki E, Mogi A, Kuwano H. Mechanisms of resistance to EGFR TKIs and development of a new generation of drugs in non-small-cell lung cancer. J Biomed Biotech. 2011;2011:165214.
9. Balak MN, Gong Y, Riely GJ. Novel D761Y and common secondary T790M mutations in epidermal growth factor receptor-mutant lung adenocarcinomas with acquired resistance to kinase inhibitors. Clinic Cancer Res. 2006;12:6494-6501.
10. Costa DB, Halmos B, Kumar A - BIM mediates EGFR tyrosine kinase inhibitor-Induced apoptosis in lung cancers with oncogenic EGFR mutations. PLoS Medicine. 2007;4:1669-1680.
11. Bean J, Riely GJ, Balak M. Acquired resistance to epidermal growth factor receptor kinase inhibitors associated with a novel T854A mutation in a patient with EGFR-mutant lung adenocarcinoma. Clinic Cancer Res. 2008;14:7519-7525.
12. Xie JT, Wang CZ, Wicks S, Yin JJ, Kong J, Li J, Li YC, Yuan CS. *Ganoderma lucidum* extract inhibits proliferation of SW 480 human colorectal cancer cells. Exp Oncol. 2006;28:25-29.
13. Sliva D. *Ganoderma lucidum* (Reishi) in cancer treatment. Integr Cancer Ther. 2003;2:358-364.
14. Kao CHJ, Jesuthasan AC, Bishop KS, Glucina MP, Ferguson LR. Anti-cancer activities of *Ganoderma lucidum*: Active ingredients and pathways. Func Foods Health Disease. 2013;3:48-65.

4

Development, Characterization and *Ex vivo* Evaluation of Various Liposome-encapsulated Aceclofenac Formulations

Fathy Ibrahim Abd-Allah[1*]

[1]*Department of Pharmaceutics and Industrial Pharmacy, Faculty of Pharmacy, Al-Azhar University, Nasr City, Cairo, Egypt.*

Author's contribution

The sole author designed, analyzed and interpreted and prepared the manuscript.

Article Information

Editor(s):
(1) Abdelwahab Omri, Department of Chemistry and Biochemistry and Departments of Biomolecular Sciences, Laurentian University, Canada.
Reviewers:
(1) Hazem Mohammed Shaheen, Damanhour University, Egypt.
(2) Nkpaa K.W, University of Port Harcourt, Nigeria.
(3) Syed Umer Jan, University of Balochistan, Quetta, Pakistan.

ABSTRACT

Aim: Formulation of aceclofenac (ACE) into liposomal gel, improving its skin permeation and potentiate its local anti-inflammatory effect.

Methodology: ACE liposomes were fabricated by lipid film hydration technique. The prepared formulations were traditional liposomes containing cholesterol (F1), ultra-deformable liposomes containing Tween 60 (F2) and modified liposomes containing both cholesterol and Tween 60 (F3). All formulations were incorporated in 1% carbopol 974 as gelling agent. The developed liposomal formulations were evaluated for its particle size, zeta potential, drug entrapment efficiency percent and stability for 90 days at 4℃. While the developed liposomal gel formulations were characterized for its *in vitro* ACE release and *ex vivo* permeation through rat skin. Anti-inflammatory effect of ACE gel formulations were evaluated in rats using carrageenan induced paw edema.

Results: The prepared liposomes had a mean vesicle size of 577 nm, 218 nm and 332 nm for F1, F2 and F3 respectively and entrapment efficiency percent of 76.8%, 58.3% and 66.2% for F1, F2 and F3 respectively. The stability study revealed that F1 vesicles have the highest physical stability followed by F3, while F2 showed the lowest stability in terms of vesicles size and entrapment

**Corresponding author: Email: fabdalla73@yahoo.com*

efficiency percent. The *in vitro* and *ex vivo* results showed higher drug release and permeability from F2 and F3 than that of F1. In addition, ACE liposomal formulations have significant higher anti-inflammatory effect than that of marketed product Bristaflam cream®.

Conclusion: All liposomal gel formulations have the ability to enhance ACE anti-inflammatory effect in rats paw edema in comparison with marketed product Bristaflam cream®.

Keywords: Aceclofenac; ultra-deformable liposomes; modified liposomes; In vitro and Ex vivo evaluation.

1. INTRODUCTION

Non-steroidal anti-inflammatory drugs (NSAIDs) possess analgesic and anti-inflammatory effect against pain of mild to moderate intensity. They provide effective analgesia in patients after minor and major surgery [1]. While oral NSAIDs are useful in the treatment of variety of acute and chronic inflammatory diseases, their oral administration may associate with severe systemic adverse effects predominantly gastrointestinal disorders [2].

ACE is an analgesic, antipyretic, and anti-inflammatory drug and is indicated in rheumatoid arthritis, osteoarthritis, and ankylosing spondylitis. It acts on COX-2 to reduce the production of inflammation mediators [3,4]. ACE has also showed glycosaminoglycan synthesis stimulation in human osteoarthritic cartilage. It shows side effects relating to GIT, liver, and kidney functions as well as disturbance of platelets function [5,6]. It is practically water insoluble, having a molecular weight of 354.19, pKa value 4.7. It is BCS class II compound for whom oral bioavailability is decided by dissolution rate in GIT. These factors make it appropriate to formulate it in transdermal formulation [5,7].

Transdermal delivery of NSAIDs proved to be a convenient route of administration for variety of clinical indications [8]. Unfortunately, the majority of drugs do not penetrate the skin at a rate sufficiently enough for therapeutic efficacy because of the barrier function of the stratum corneum. Transdermal absorption of a medicinal substance depends on its physicochemical properties, its behavior when placed in a pharmaceutical vehicle and skin condition [9]. Therefore, pre-formulation studies are generally necessary in order to optimize drug release from the vehicle and skin permeation. There were many attempts to increase drugs flux through stratum corneum by using suitable formulation and penetration enhancers. Most of NSAIDs are lipophilic molecules which impose a big challenge in drug development and formulation to provide effective transdermal delivery systems [10].

For many years, liposomes have been used as an approach to formulate lipophilic molecules [11]. Liposomes have been shown to be a promising transdermal drug delivery system for variety of drugs especially lipophilic ones. They may act as drug penetration enhancer by increasing drug concentration in the epidermis and dermis layers [12].

Edge activators such as surfactants provide elasticity to liposomal vesicles membrane. Ultra-deformable liposomes have high deformability and could transport active agents more effectively through the stratum corneum into the deeper layers of the skin than traditional liposomes [13]. Ultra-deformable liposomes are prepared by replacing cholesterol (CH) in traditional liposomes with surface active agent.

So the aims of this work were to formulate ACE liposomal formulations in order to enhance their skin penetration, investigate the effect of Tween 60 as edge activator on liposomes (ultra-deformable liposomes) and in combination with CH (modified liposomes) on the physicochemical properties, stability, *in vitro* release rate and *ex vivo* permeability through rats' skin after incorporating ACE liposomal formulations in 1% carbopol 974 in comparison with ACE commercial cream. As well as to evaluate the anti-inflammatory effect of ACE gel formulations employing carrageenan induced paw edema model in rats.

2. MATERIALS AND METHODS

2.1 Materials

Aceclofenac was kindly provided by Copad Pharm Company, (Cairo, Egypt). Soybean L-α - Phosphatidylcholine (PC), Carrageenan, Triethanolamine and Cholesterol (CH) were obtained from Sigma-Aldrich, St. Louis, MO, (USA). Chloroform, Carbopol 974 and Tween 60 was purchased from BDL laboratory Ltd., Poole, England, (UK). All solvents used in chromatographic assay were HPLC-grade and other used chemicals and solvents were commercially available products of reagent grade and used as received. Marketed formulation was Bristaflam cream® (containing ACE 1.5% w/w) manufactured by Smithkline Beecham, El Haram, Giza, Eygpt.

2.2 Methods

2.2.1 HPLC assay method for determination of ACE concentrations

HPLC method using reverse phase adsorption chromatography was used for determination of drug concentration. The instrument consisted of a Shimadzu LC-10ATVP pump, a SIL-10AF autoinjector, an SPD-10AVUV-VIS detector, and an SCL-10A VP system controller (Shimadzu, Japan). The column was Shim-pack VP-ODS, having 4.6 mm I.D. and 150 mm bed length with adsorbent particle size 5 μm (Shimadzu, Japan). The sample was prepared in methanol and 20 μL was injected into the column. The column was eluted isocratically with Acetonitrile, methanol, and pH 7.4 phosphate buffer (20:40: 40, v/v/v) at 1 ml/min. The detection wavelength was set at 275 nm [14].

2.2.2 Preparation of ACE liposomal formulations

Lipid film hydration method was used to formulate the nanovesicles as per Table 1. The drug and lipids were accurately weighed and dissolved in a mixture of methanol and chloroform (1:2, V/V), in around bottom flask. The organic solvent system was slowly removed under reduced pressure, using a rotary evaporator (Bibby Sterilin Ltd., Stone Staffordshire, UK) at 40℃ and 150 rpm, such that a thin film of dry lipids was formed on the inner surface of the flask. The dry lipid film was slowly hydrated with 10 ml of phosphate buffered saline (PBS) pH 7.4 for 1 h. The resulting liposomal suspension was mechanically shaken for 1 h using a thermostatically controlled mechanical shaker (Kottermann, Hanigsen, Germany) at 60 rpm and 40℃ leading to the formation of liposomes. The liposomal suspension was left to mature overnight at 4℃, to ensure hydration of the lipid [15-17].

Table 1. Composition of liposomal formulations of ACE

Formulation No.	Contents (mg)		PC
	CH	Tween 60	
F1 (traditional)	20	-	80
F2 (ultra-deformable)	-	10	90
F3 (modified)	7.5	2.5	90

2.2.3 Characterization of ACE liposomal dispersion

2.2.3.1 Vesicle size and zeta potential

The mean vesicular size, size distributions expressed as the resultant polydispersity indices (PDIs) and zeta potential were determined by Zetasizer Nano series (Malvern Instruments Ltd., UK). Liposomal dispersions were diluted 10 times with phosphate buffer saline before analysis. Analysis was performed at ambient temperature. Each reported value was the average of three measurements.

2.2.3.2 Entrapment Efficiency percent (EE%)

Ultracentrifugation method was employed for determining the entrapment efficiency. An aliquot of formulation was centrifuged at 12000 rpm using ultracentrifuge (Centrifuge model no. D-7200 from Hitachi Company New Zealand) and content of drug was estimated separately in the sediment and the supernatant [18]. The entrapment efficiency was estimated as follows:

$$(T - C / T) \times 100$$

Where T is the total drug content and C is the drug content in supernatant.

2.2.4 Physical stability of ACE liposomal dispersion

Physical stability of ACE liposomal vesicles was determined by monitoring the variations in particle size and EE% during storage at 4±0.2℃, for 3 months [15,19]. The results of stability study are shown in Figs. 1 and 2.

2.2.5 Preparation of ACE liposomal gel formulations

ACE nanovesicles were formulated into gel for ease in application. Carbopol 974 was dispersed in distilled water and dispersion (1%) was prepared. The dispersion was mechanically stirred for 10 min at 150 rpm using an overhead stirrer (overhead stirrer Stuart, bioCote, UK) and then neutralized by drop wise addition of triethanolamine solution (0.5%) until pH 5.5. The neutralized dispersion was kept overnight to remove any air bubble. Then nanovesicles were incorporated into the gel base and stirred for 1 h and stored at 4°C for further investigations [20]. A control formulation of marketed product Bristaflam cream® was used for comparison (F0).

2.2.6 Evaluation of the prepared ACE liposomal gel

2.2.6.1 Physical investigations

The prepared gels were tested for their color, odor, texture, phase separation or bleeding as well as the feel upon application (stiffness, grittiness, greasiness) once the preparation is applied on the skin and also after 2 min of

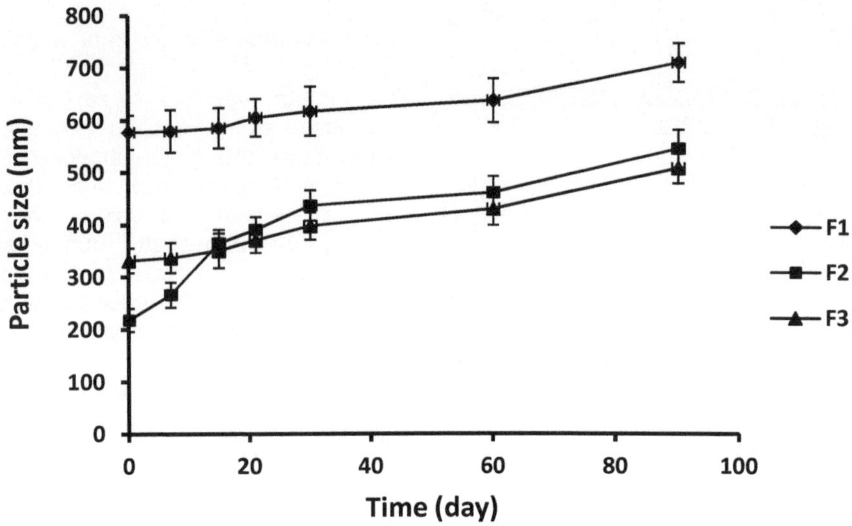

Fig. 1. Change in liposomes particle size upon storage at 4°C for 90 days

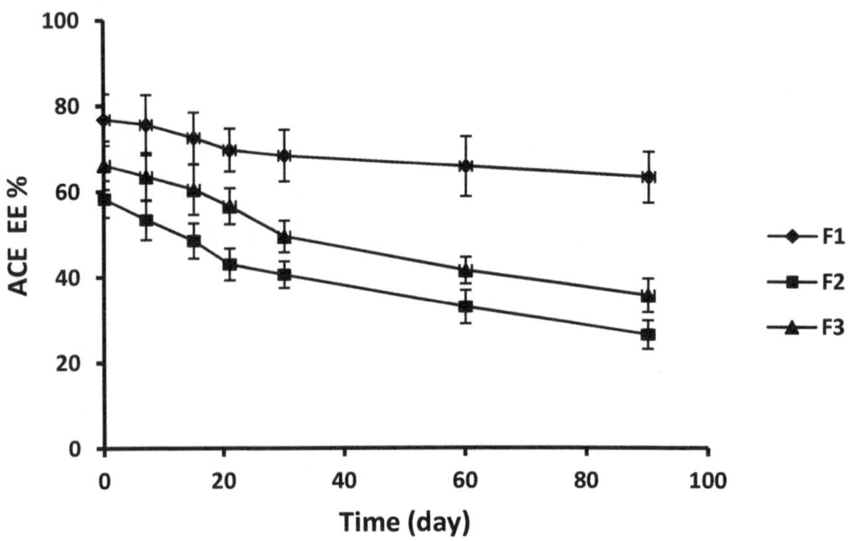

Fig. 2. Variation in ACE EE% upon storage at 4°C fo r 90 days

application. Briefly, the homogeneity of the prepared gel can be evaluated by pressing 100 mg of gel between the thumb and the index finger to notice its consistency and freedom from any coarse particles attached or detached on finger. Also, the washability can be assessed by rubbing 100 mg of gel on the skin of the back of the hand, then washed with water and observed whether it is washable or not [21]. In addition, the pH of the prepared gels (1 g of each gel formula diluted with 9 g of calibrated distilled water and mixed well) was measured by using pH meter (Jenway 3510, UK). Measurement of pH was performed in triplicates [22].

2.2.7 *In vitro* release of ACE from liposomal gel

Cellulose acetate dialysis membrane (Spectra Por® Dialysis membrane, Spectrom Medical Industries, Inc., USA) was utilized for the *in vitro* study. The membrane was soaked in phosphate buffer saline of pH 7.4 for 12 h before use. Dialysis membrane was mounted between the donor and the receptor compartments of Franz diffusion cells (Logan instruments corporation NJ, USA).The receptor compartment was filled with phosphate buffer of pH 7.4 maintained at 32±0.5℃ and constantly stirred by small magnetic bar in order to ensure its homogeneity. The Franz diffusion cell had an effective permeation surface area of 1.76 cm^2.

A Known weight from each formula equivalent to 1% of ACE was added to the donor compartment. One ml of the receptor solution was withdrawn periodically over 12 h and replaced with an equivalent volume of fresh and preheated phosphate buffer saline of pH 7.4. The samples were analyzed for ACE content by the previously mentioned HPLC method against blank liposomal gels that processed similarly [14]. Experiments were carried out in triplicate and the mean of results were reported and represented in Fig. 3.

2.2.8 ACE *Ex vivo* permeability through rat skin

Regarding permeation study, abdominal skin of adult Albino rat weighing 192±17 g was used. Appropriate skin parts were mounted between the donor and the receptor compartments of the Franz diffusion cells with the stratum corneum facing upward into the donor compartment and the dermal side of the skin allowed to contact with constantly stirred phosphate buffer saline of pH 7.4 maintained at 32±0.5℃. A specific amount of each gel formulation equivalent to 1% of ACE was added to the donor compartment. One ml of the receptor solution were withdrawn periodically over 24 hr and replaced with an equivalent volume of phosphate buffer saline of pH 7.4, [17,23]. The samples were analyzed for ACE content. Data are shown in Fig. 4.

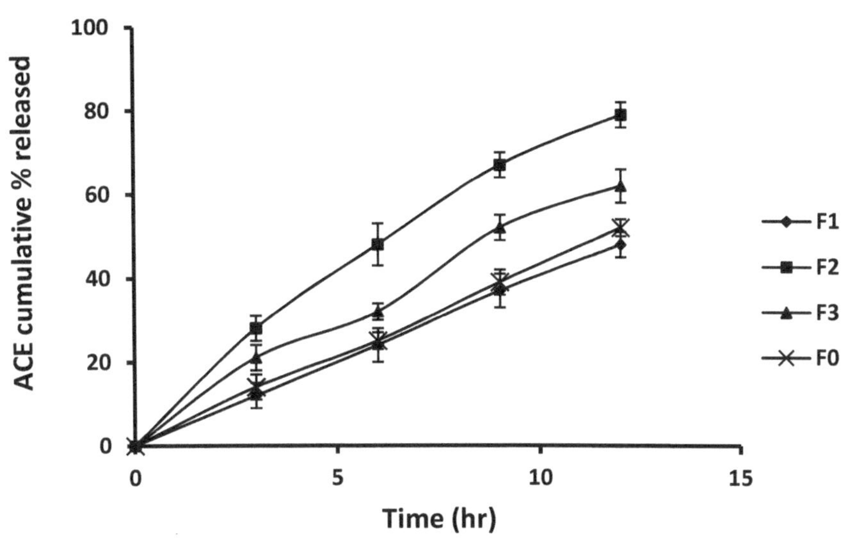

Fig. 3. Dissolution profile of ACE from different gel formulations

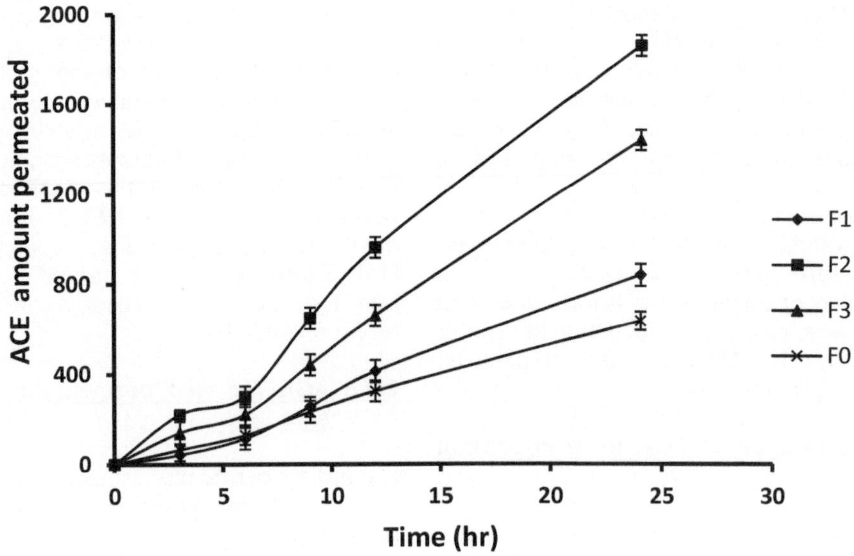

Fig. 4. ***Ex vivo*** **permeation of ACE from gel formulations through rats' skin**

2.2.9 Pharmacodynamics' evaluation of ACE gel formulations

2.2.9.1 Animals and design

Adult male Albino rats (192±17 g) were used for this experiment. The animals were maintained under standard laboratory conditions (light period of 12 h/day and temperature maintained at 25±2°C), with free access to food and water. Thirty animals were divided into five groups, six animals each. The first group (control) was received no treatment. The second group was treated with F0. The third group was treated with F1. The fourth group was treated with F2, and the last group was treated with F3. All studies were approved by the Ethical Committee of the Faculty of Pharmacy, Al-Azhar University, Cairo, Egypt, and followed the Legislation for the protection of animals used for scientific purposes [24] and Guiding Principlein Care and Use of Animals [25].

2.2.10 Anti-inflammatory activity of ACE formulations

Carrageenan-induced hind paw edema model was used for determination of anti- inflammatory activity of ACE gel formulations [25,26]. Half an hour after dermal application of ACE formulations (1 g) on rats in each treated group (F0, F1, F2 and F3), the rats were injected with 0.1 ml of 1% W/V carrageenan solution in normal saline into the subplantar tissue of the left hind paw to produce acute inflammation. The paw volume was recorded before carrageenan injection (zero time) and at intervals of 0.5, 1, 2, 3, 4 and 6 hr after injection of carrageenan solution. The right hind paw was served as the control and received an injection of saline (0.9% w/v, NaCl, 0.1 ml).The paw volume was measured by water displacement method using Plethysmometer having 0.01 ml resolution (Ugo Basile, Italy). The increase in paw edema of the treated groups was compared with that of the control one (Fig. 5). The relative effect of ACE formulations was calculated based upon the percentage inhibition of the inflammation.

The percent inhibition of inflammatory edema induced by carrageenan was calculated for each group using the following equation:

% of edema inhibition (anti-inflammatory activity) = $(1 - E_t/E_c) \times 100$

Where, E_t is the edema volume of treated group and E_c is the edema volume of control group at the same time point [27]. Fig. 6 shows the percent inhibition of paw edema after application of ACE gel formulations.

2.3 Statistical Analysis

All values were expressed as the mean ± standard deviation (SD) and the results were analyzed statistically by one way analysis of variance (ANOVA) followed by Tukey

Comparison Test. $P = .05$ was considered to be statistically significant.

3. RESULTS AND DISCUSSION

3.1 Preparation of ACE Liposomal Formulations

Tween 60 and CH were used in preparing liposomes for their interesting properties such as biodegradability, biocompatibility and low toxicity and derivation form easily available materials. They have been tested in various pharmaceutical drug delivery systems. All studied liposomal formulations were able to form vesicles. Liposomes appeared as translucent white dispersions that showed no sedimentation.

3.2 Vesicle Size and Zeta Potential

As shown in Table 2, the employed method in preparing ACE liposomes obtained nanovesicles of different particle size. Incorporation of Tween 60 resulted in decreasing the particles size of the liposomes as shown in F2 (218±28 nm) while presence of CH increases liposomes particle size as in case of F1 and F3. All liposomal vesicles showed a narrow size distribution as indicated by the low values of PDIs [28,29].

Regarding the zeta potential, the surface charge of the vesicles affects the stability of liposomes [30]. Increasing the electrostatic repulsion forces between the vesicles prevents its coalescence. Zeta potential was determined after dilution of liposomes with phosphate buffer saline and the values were shown in Table 2. As was expected, presence of CH increases the rigidity of the membrane bilayer structure hence CH improves the physical stability of liposomal systems. It was reported that presence of CH in liposomes improves the stability [31,32]. In the other hand, F2 showed the lowest zeta potential value (29.7±2.1 mV) due to the absence of CH in this formulation.

3.3 Entrapment Efficiency

ACE liposomes were prepared by lipid film hydration technique. This method was proven to obtain high drug encapsulation efficiency [15,17]. The results in Table 2 indicated that, incorporation of CH in liposomal formulations improves the EE% of the formulations. The absence of CH in F2 showed the lowest EE% of value 58.3±4.3. It was also reported that addition of surfactant provides deformability to the vesicles membrane and reduces drug EE% in liposomal formulations [13].

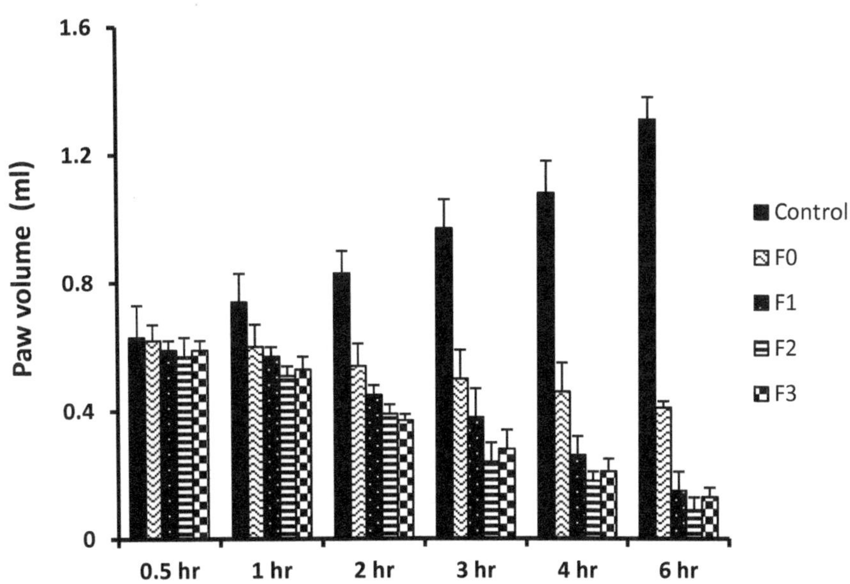

Fig. 5. Paw edema volume (ml) after application of ACE gels in different rats' groups compared with control one

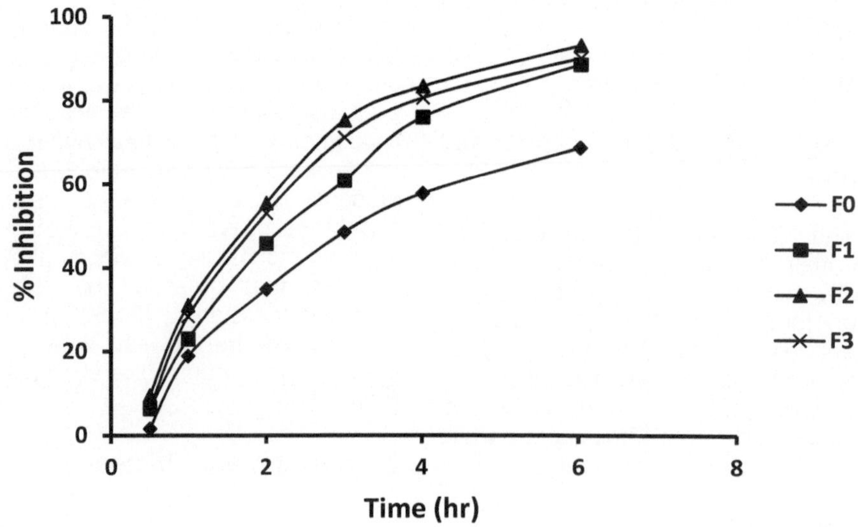

Fig. 6. Percent inhibition of paw edema after application of ACE gel formulations

Table 2. Physical evaluation of ACE liposomal gel formulations

Parameter	F1	F2	F3	F0
Particles size (nm)	577±39	218±28	332±33	-
EE%	76.8±5.9	58.3±4.3	66.2±5.1	-
PDI	0.219±0.18	0.284±0.31	0.273±0.37	
Zeta potential(mV)	38.4±1.4	29.7±2.1	34.2±2.6	-
Lag time (h)	2.28±0.2	0.38±0.1	2.50±0.2	0.77±0.1
Permeability coefficient (cm/h)	$5.54X10^{-3}$	$11.24X10^{-3}$	$9.56X10^{-3}$	$3.92X10^{-3}$

3.4 Physical Stability of ACE Liposomal Dispersion

At the end of storage period, all liposomal formulations showed significant changes in particle size from initial states (Fig. 1). The vesicles sizes of F1 were relatively constant at 4°C for 90 days. By the end of the storage period F1 vesicles gain 23% in size. Stability of F3 liposomes at the test conditions revealed 53% increase in vesicles size compared to the initial state. While F2 showed up to 150% increase in vesicles size which suggesting high tendency to aggregate in comparison with F1 and F3. The stability study revealed that F1 vesicles showed the highest physical stability followed by F3, while F2 showed the lowest stability among the tested liposomes. The presence of CH in F1 and F3 could be the reason of the higher physical stability of these formulations.

The encapsulated ACE tended to leak out from the bilayer structure during storage. A direct relationship between the percentage leaking of the drug out of all the vesicles and aging was observed compared to initial drug EE% (Fig. 2). The drug leakage from F1 and F3 were lower than F2 at all-time points (*P* = .05) which indicated high stability of F1 and F3. Encapsulation loss was always associated with an increase in vesicle size, which is a thermodynamically more stable status [33]. Inclusion of CH in liposomes improved the fluidity of the bilayer membrane and reduced the permeability of ACE through the membrane [31,32]. This effect lessened the leakage of the entrapped drug from the liposomes and resulted in a higher stability of the formulation.

3.5 Evaluation of the Prepared ACE Liposomal Gels

3.5.1 Physical investigations

It is obvious that all formulations have a white viscous creamy smooth texture with homogeneous appearance and ease of spreading without any separation or bleeding. All gel formulations have pH values in the range of 6.02–7.19 which is suitable for topical application without skin irritation.

3.6 *In vitro* Release of ACE from Liposomal Gels

Generally, *in vitro* release profile revealed important information on the structure and behavior of the formulation, possible interactions between the drug and carrier composition, and their influence on the rate and mechanism of drug release [34,35].The dialysis release method was a well-established and useful technique to study *in vitro* release from micro- and nano-particulate delivery systems. This technique has been used to study a variety of formulations, including liposomes and Nanoparticles [36].

ACE release profile demonstrated gradual and sustained release rate from the prepared liposomal formulations. The highest ACE percent released was from F2 (83% over 12 h) followed by F3 (66% over 12 h). While the lowest drug percent released was from F1 and F0.

From the results it seems that formulation ingredients play a major role in determining drug release. As it mentioned before, presence of CH results in obtaining rigid bilayer membrane which hinder drug release rate. As CH content decrease, as shown in F3, or even diminished as in case of F2 drug release rate improved (Fig. 3).

3.7 ACE *Ex vivo* Permeability through Rat Skin

For *ex vivo* ACE permeation study, abdominal rat skin model was used because it is comparable to human skin in stratum corneum thickness and water permeability [37,38]. ACE permeation from liposomal gel formulations through rat skin not only affected by each formulation composition but also affected with vesicles size as well. Fig. 4 and Table 2 show the results of ACE ex *vivo* permeability through rat skin. Two mechanisms have been proven to enhance drug permeation from ultra-deformable liposomes. The first one is the ability to deform its shape and hence the vesicles capable of penetrating via narrow spaces delivering the drug to subcutaneous tissues [39]. The second mechanism is what so called trans-epidermal osmotic gradient. In which ultra-deformable liposomes dry over the skin due to water evaporation so the vesicles withdrawn to subcutaneous tissue rich with water content [40]. These and the smaller vesicles size explain why F2 and F3 had the higher ACE permeability through rat skin which came in agreement with other research works [40-42]. There was significant difference in permeation between F2 and F3 (P = .05), probably due to presence of Tween 60 in F2 which provide elasticity to the vesicles and hence high drug permeation. On the other hand, the relatively higher vesicles size (577±36 nm) as well as the higher CH content (20 mg) in F1 hindered and delayed ACE permeability from this formulation.

3.8 Assessment of Anti-inflammatory Activity of ACE Gel

Inflammation is a pathophysiological response of living tissue to injuries that leads to local accumulation of plasmatic fluid and blood cells [43]. Edema induced by phlogistic agents is widely accepted model for evaluation of anti-inflammatory effect of drugs. Carrageenan induced rat paw edema assay is believed to be one of the most reliable and also the most widely used test for evaluating the anti-inflammatory activity of active ingredients. Development of edema induced by carrageenan is commonly correlated with the early exudative stage of inflammation, one of the important processes of inflammatory pathology. At the beginning of carrageenan injection (phase one), there is sudden elevation of paw volume as a consequence of histamine and/or serotonin liberation from the cells [44]. After 1 h the inflammation increases gradually and is elevated after 3–6 hr. This second phase is mediated by prostaglandins, cyclooxygenase products [45].

All ACE gel formulations showed no effect on phase 1 (0.5-1 h after carrageenan injection) which was expected since ACE as NSAID has no histamine and/or serotonin inhibitory effect. On the other hand, in the biphasic process of inflammation the effect of all ACE liposomal gel formulations (F1, F2 and F3) and ACE commercial cream (F0) showed significant inhibition of edema at 1-6 h of the study in comparison to control. That could be explained by the reduction of prostaglandin synthesis via inhibiting enzymes of cyclooxygenase pathway [46]. There was significant different between all ACE liposomal gel formulations and F0 (P = .05) after one hour of carrageenan injection. This study has shown that F1, F2 and F3 enhanced ACE anti-inflammatory activity in carrageenan induced paw edema method over F0.

4. CONCLUSION

All ACE liposomal formulations have nano size particles range and high EE%. Incorporation of Tween 60 in ACE liposomal formulations decrease the particles size of the obtained vesicles and improves the *in vitro* and *ex vivo* ACE permeation while decreases physical stability of ACE liposomes. On contrary, incorporation of CH either in modified formulation or in traditional liposomes increases ACE EE% and enhances physical stability of the obtained vesicles. The prepared ACE liposomal formulations significantly improved ACE skin penetration and potentiated its anti-inflammatory effect in comparison with marketed product Bristaflam cream®.

CONSENT

It is not applicable.

ACKNOWLEDGEMENTS

The author would like to extend their sincere appreciation to Dr. Ahmed M. Mansour, Associate Professor of Pharmacology and Toxicology, Faculty of Pharmacy, Al-Azhar University, for his valuable collaboration and technical support throughout the in vivo part of this work.

COMPETING INTERESTS

Author has declared that no competing interests exist.

REFERENCES

1. Hanada S, Fujioka K, Futamura Y, Manabe N, Hoshino A, Yamamoto K. Evaluation of anti-inflammatory drug-conjugated silicon quantum dots: Their cytotoxicity and biological effect. Int J Mol Sci. 2013;14: 1323-34.
2. Whitehouse MW. Anti-inflammatory glucocorticoid drugs: Reflections after 60 years. Inflammopharmacology. 2011;19:1-19.
3. Legrand E. Aceclofenac in the management of inflammatory pain. Expert OpinPharmacother. 2004;5:1347–57.
4. Shavi G, Nayak U, Averineni RK. Multiparticulate drug delivery system of Aceclofenac: Development and *in vitro* studies. Drug Dev Ind Pharm. 2009;35: 252–8.
5. Seyda AA, Figen T. A nonsteroidal anti-inflammatory drug: Aceclofenac. J Pharm Sci. 2010;35:105–18.
6. Insel PA. Analgesic-antipyretics and anti-inflammatory agents: Drugs employed in the treatment of rheumatoid arthritis and gout, in Goodman and Gilman's the pharmacological basis of therapeutics, Gilman AG, Rall T, Nies A, Taylor P. Eds., 9th edition, Pergamon, Oxford, NY, USA; 1990.
7. Alvarez-Larena A, Piniella JF, Carrasco E, Ginebreda A, Julia S, Germain G. Crystal structure and spectroscopic study of 2-[(2,6-dichlorophenyl)amino] phenylacetoxyacetic acid (Aceclofenac). Journal of Crystallographic and Spectroscopic Research. 1992;22:323–28.
8. Cevc G, Blume G. New highly efficient formulation of diclofenac for the topical transdermal administration in ultradeformable drug carriers. Transfersomes Biochim Biophys Acta. 2001;2:191-205.
9. Karadzovska D, Brooks JD, Riviere JE. Modeling the effect of experimental variables on the *in vitro* permeation of six model compounds across porcine skin. Int J Pharm. 2013;443:58-67.
10. Rupp C, Steckel H, Müller BW. Mixed micelle formation with phosphatidylcholines: The influence of surfactants with different molecule structures. Int J Pharm. 2010;387:120-8.
11. Ali MH, Moghaddam B, Kirby DJ, Mohammed AR, Perrie Y. The role of lipid geometry in designing liposomes for the solubilisation of poorly water soluble drugs. Int J Pharm. 2013;453:225-32.
12. Pierre MB, Dos Santos MCI. Liposomal systems as drug delivery vehicles for dermal and transdermal applications. Arch Dermatol Res. 2011;303:607–621.
13. Mishra D, Dubey V, Asthana A, Saraf DK, Jain NK. Elastic liposomes mediated transcutaneous immunization against hepatitis B. Vaccine. 2006;24:4847–55.
14. Lee J, Lee Y, Kim J, Yoon M, Young WC. Formulation of microemulsion systems for transdermal delivery of Aceclofenac. Arch Pharm Res. 2005;28:1097–1102.
15. Sinico C, Manconi M, Peppi M, Lai F, Valenti D, Fadda AM. Liposomes as carriers for dermal delivery of tretinoin: *In vitro* evaluation of drug permeation and vesicle skin interaction. J Control Release. 2005;103:123–136.

16. Gaur PK, Mishra S, Gupta VB, Rathod MS, Purohit S, Savla BA. Targeted drug delivery of Rifampicin to the lungs: Formulation, characterization, and stability studies of preformed aerosolized liposome and in situ formed aerosolized liposome. Drug Dev Ind Pharm. 2010;36:638–646.
17. Gaur PK, Purohit S, Kumar Y, Mishra S, Bhandari A. Preparation, characterization and permeation studies of a nanovesicular system containing diclofenac for transdermal delivery. Pharm Dev Technol. 2014;19:48–54.
18. Paradissis A, Hatziantoniou S, Georgopoulos A, Demetzos C. Lipid analysis of Greek broad bean oil: preparation of liposomes and physicochemical characterization. European Journal of Lipid Science and Technology. 2005;107:799– 804.
19. Ishida T, Takanashi Y, Doi H, Yamamoto I, Kiwada H. Encapsulation of an antivasospastic drug, fasudil, into liposomes, and *in vitro* stability of the fasudil-loaded liposomes. Int J Pharm. 2002;232:59–67.
20. Al-Suwayeh SA, Taha EI, Al-Qahtani FM. Evaluation of skin permeation and analgesic activity effects of carbopol Lornoxicam topical gels containing penetration enhancer. Sci World J. 2014; 127495.
21. Agrawal V, Gupta V, Ramteke S, Trivedi P. Preparation and evaluation of tubular micelles of pluronic lecithin organogel for transdermal delivery of sumatriptan. AAPS Pharm Sci Tech. 2010;11:1718–25.
22. El-Nabarawi MA, Bendas ER, Abd-Elrehem TR, Abary MYS. Formulation and evaluation of dispersed paroxetine liposomes in gel. J Chem Pharm Res. 2012;4:2209–22.
23. Akhter S, Jain GK, Ahmad FJ. Investigation of nanoemulsion system for transdermal delivery of domperidone: *Ex vivo* and *in vivo* studies. Current Nanoscience. 2008;4:381–90.
24. European Parliament. Directive 2010/63/EU of the European Parliament and of the Council of 22 September 2010 on the protection of animals used for scientific purposes. Off J Eur Union L 276/33 D: 33–79; 2010.
25. Council for International Ogranization of Medical Sciences NCE, T.I.C.F.L.A.S. International Guiding Principles for Biomedical Research Involving Animals; 2012. Available:http://www.the-aps.org/mm/SciencePolicy/About/Policy-Statements/Guiding-Principles.html [last accessed 17 Mar 2015]
26. Sadeghi H, Hajhashemi V, Minaiyan M, Movahedian A, Talebi A. A study on the mechanisms involving the anti-inflammatory effect of amitriptyline in carrageenan-induced paw oedema in rats. Eur J Pharmacol. 2011;667:396–401.
27. Manosroi A, Jantrawut P, Manosroi J. Anti-inflammatory activity of gel containing novel elastic niosomes entrapped with diclofenac diethylammonium. Int J Pharm. 2008;360:156–63.
28. Pouton CW, Porter CJ. Formulation of lipid-based delivery systems for oral administration: Materials, methods and strategies. Adv Drug Deliv Rev. 2008;60: 625-37.
29. Hathout RM, Nasr M. Transdermal delivery of betahistine hydrochide Aceclofenace using microemulsions: Physical characterization, biophysical assessment, confocal imaging and permeation studies. Colloids Surf B Biointerfaces. 2013;110: 254-60.
30. Gershanik T, Benita S. Self-dispersing lipid formulations for improving oral absorption of lipophilic drugs. Eur J Pharm Biopharm. 2000;50:179-88.
31. Song J, Shi F, Zhang Z, Zhu F, Xue J, Tan X. Formulation and evaluation of celastrol-loaded liposomes. Molecules. 2011;16: 7880-92.
32. Junyaprasert VB, Singhsa P, Suksiriworapong J, Chantasart D. Physicochemical properties and skin permeation of Span 60/Tween 60 niosomes of ellagic acid. Int J Pharm. 2012;423:303-11.
33. Fang JY, Lin HH, Hsu LR, Tsai YH. Characterization and stability of various liposome-encapsulated enoxacin formulations. Chem Pharm Bull. 1997;45: 1504–9.
34. D'Souza SS, DeLuca PP. Methods to assess in vitro drug release from injectable polymeric particulate systems. Pharm. Res. 2006;23:460–74.
35. Hitzman CJ, Wiedmann TS, Dai H, Elmquist WF. Measurement of drug release from microcarriers by microdialysis. J. Pharm. Sci. 2005;94: 1456–66.

36. Gupta M, Goyal AK, Paliwal SR, Paliwal R, Mishra N, Vaidya B. Development and characterization of effective topical liposomal system for localized treatment of cutaneous candidiasis. J. Liposome. Res. 2010;20:341–350.
37. Taha EI. Lipid vesicular systems: Formulation optimization and *ex vivo* comparative study. J. Mol. Liq. 2014;196: 211-216.
38. Kong M, Xi G, Chen D, Keon K, Hyun JP. Investigations on skin permeation of hyaluronic acid based nanoemulsion as transdermal carrier. Carbohydr Polym. 2011;86:837–843.
39. Jain S, Jain P, Umamaheshwari B, Jain K. Transfersomes A novel vesicular carrier for enhanced transdermal delivery: Development, characterization, and performace evaluation. Drug Dev Ind Pharm. 2003;29:1013–26.
40. Bragagni M, Mennini N, Maestrelli F, Cirri M, Mura P. Comparative study of liposomes, transfersomes and ethosomes as carriers for improving topical delivery of celecoxib, Drug Deliv. 2012;19:354-61.
41. Benson HA. Elastic liposomes for topical and transdermal drug delivery. Curr Drug Deliv. 2009;6:217-26.
42. Jain SK, Gupta Y, Jain A, Rai K. Enhanced transdermal delivery of acyclovir sodium via elastic liposomes. Drug Deliv. 2008;15: 141-7.
43. Panda BB, Gaur K, Kori ML, Tyagi LK, Nema, RK, Sharma CS. Anti-inflammatory and analgesic activity of *Jatropha gossypifoliain* experimental animal models. Glob J Pharmacol. 2009;3:1-5.
44. Georgewill OA, Georgewill UO. Evaluation of the anti-inflammatory activity of extract of *Vernonia amygdalina*. Asian Pac J Trop Med. 2010;3:150-1.
45. Kalpanadevi V, Shanmugasundaram R, Mohan VR. Antiinflammatory activity of seed extract of Entadapursaetha DC against carrageenan induced paw edema. Sci Res Reporter. 2012;2:69-71.
46. Seibert K, Zhang Y, Leahy K, Hauser S, Masferrer J, Perkins W. Pharmacological and biochemical demonstration of the role of cyclooxygenase-2 in inflammation and pain. Proc Natl Acad Sci USA. 1994;91: 12013-17.

5

Antimicrobial, Antioxidant and Anticancer Activities of *Turnera ulmifolia* (Yellow Alder) Callus

K. Kalimuthu[1*], V. Chinnadurai[1], R. Prabakaran[2], P. Subramaniam[3] and Y. Sarmila Juliet[1]

[1]Department of Botany, Plant Tissue Culture Division, Government Arts College (Autonomous), Coimbatore-641018, Tamil Nadu, India.
[2]Department of Botany, PSG College of Arts and Science (Autonomous), Coimbatore- 641014, Tamil Nadu, India.
[3]Government Boys Higher Secondary School, Chinna Thadagam, Coimbatore, India.

Authors' contributions

This study was carried out in collaboration between all authors. Author KK designed the study and corrected the manuscript. Author RP wrote the first draft of the manuscript. Author VC analysis the different activities of the callus. Author PS carried out callus induction experiment and author YSJ collected the literature and identified the species of plant. All authors read and approved the final manuscript.

Article Information

Editor(s):
(1) Dongdong Wang, Department of Pharmacogonosy, West China College of Pharmacy, Sichuan University, China.
Reviewers:
(1) Daniela Hanganu, Iuliu Hatieganu University of Medicine and Pharmacy Cluj-Napoca, Romania.
(2) Lorna T. Enerva, Polytechnic University of the Philippines, Philippines.

ABSTRACT

Aim: The current work aims to study the effect of ethanolic and methanolic extracts of *Turnera ulmifolia* callus on antimicrobial, antioxidant and anticancer activities.
Study Design: The Five grams of leaf derived 30 days old callus powder was soaked in 10 ml of ethanol and methanol overnight and then filtered through Whatman filter paper No. 41 along with 2 gms sodium sulphate to remove the sediments and traces of water in the filtrate. Before filing the filter paper along with sodium sulphate is wetted with ethanol. The filtrate was then concentrated by bubbling nitrogen gas in to solution and reduces the volume to one ml.
Place and Duration of Study: Plant Tissue Culture Division, PG and Research Department of Botany, Government Arts College (Autonomous), Coimbatore-641018, Tamil Nadu, India.

**Corresponding author: Email: k_kalimuthu@rediffmail.com*

Methodology: Ethanolic and methanolic callus extracts were evaluated for antimicrobial, antioxidant (DPPH & FRAP) and anticancer activities (MTT assay).
Results: The ethanolic and methanolic callus extracts of *Turnera ulmifolia* showed rich sources of antimicrobial, antioxidants, anticancer and can be incorporated into the drug formulations.
Conclusion: This study conformed the use of callus instead of wild plant for herbal medicine. Further studies are needed for isolation and identification of compounds.

Keywords: Antimicrobial; antioxidant; anticancer; Turnera ulmifolia; breast cancer cell.

1. INTRODUCTION

India is in a unique position to be a major global player in medicine field because of our rich heritage of flora and centuries of experience in the use of traditional system. Due to the side effect and higher cost of allopathic medicine, the plant based medicines has been over wheming in the recent times. Increasing the usage of herbal medicine, the Global market for medicinal plants is also increasing rapidly. The plant based drugs have the advantage of being simple, effective and broad spectrum of activity. Rapid increase in the demand poses a threat to their population in the natural habitats. In this regard, *in vitro* culture can provide alternative source of supply that will reduce the pressure of collecting from the wild.

Turnera ulmifolia Linn. or Damiana (Turneraceae) it is already known to be of medicinal value, being used popularly as an anti-inflammatory, as an expectorant and in the treatment of several problems [1,2]. The plant has an antioxidant, antimicrobial activity [3]. It also has phytoconstituents like toosendanin, phenylmethanone phytfluene etc [4]. Researchers have detected flavonoids, alkaloids, tannins, and phenolic compounds in preparations from this plant [5,6,4].

T. ulmifolia is used as tonic, against indigestion and bronchitis in Mexico (Martinez. 1969). It is also used as a remedy against swellings, pains, fever, respiratory and pulmonary disorders, laxative, carminative, tonic expectorant, abortive agent and fertility related applications [7-11]. *Turnera ulmifolia* is used as expectorant, antidiabetic, anticancer agent [12-14].

To the best of our knowledge the antioxidant antimicrobial and anticancer properties of leaf callus extract of this plant is not yet reported. Hence to reduce the pressure on collection of wild plant it was worth to evaluate the antioxidants, antimicrobial and anticancerous potential of callus of this plant.

2. MATERIALS AND METHODS

2.1 Source of Plant Materials

Plants of *Turnera ulmifolia* L. var. elegans (Otto) Urb. (= *Turnera subulata* Sm.) were collected from garden and being identified by Botanical Survey of India (BSI) Coimbatore (Reference No: BSI/SRC/5/23/2013-14/Tech/408) and maintained in earthen pots in shade house at Government Arts College, Coimbatore.

2.2 Extraction from *in vitro* Callus

The leaf derived 30 days old callus collected from our laboratory was air dried and powdered and stored in room temperature. Five grams of powder was soaked in 10 ml of ethanol and methanol overnight and then filtered through Whatman filter paper No. 41 along with 2 gms sodium sulphate to remove the sediments and traces of water in the filtrate. Before filing the filter paper along with sodium sulphate is wetted with ethanol. The filtrate was then concentrated by bubbling nitrogen gas into the solution and reduces the volume to one ml [15,16].

2.3 Antimicrobial Activity

2.3.1 Test microorganisms

The test organisms used were clinical isolates *viz., Streptococcus pyogenes, Staphylococcus aureus, Escherichia coli* and *Klebsiella pneumoniae.* The human fungal pathogens like *Candida albicans and Trichoderma viride,* which were obtained from Department of Microbiology, Hindusthan College of Arts and Science Coimbatore. The bacterial and the fungal cultures were maintained on nutrient agar medium and potato dextrose agar (PDA) medium respectively.

2.3.2 Growth and maintenance of test microorganism for antimicrobial studies

The bacterial cultures were maintained on nutrient broth (NB) at 37°C and fungus was maintained on Potato dextrose agar (PDA) at 28°C.

2.3.3 Preparation of inoculum

The gram positive bacteria *Streptococcus pyogenes*, *Staphylococcus aureus* and gram negative bacteria *E. coli* and *Klebsiella pneumoniae* were pre-cultured in nutrient broth overnight in a rotary shaker at 37°C, centrifuged at 10,000 rpm for 5 min, pellet was suspended in double distilled water and the cell density was standardized spectrophotometrically (A_{610}nm). The fungal inoculums *Candida albicans*, *Trichoderma viride* were prepared from 5 to 10 day old culture grown on Potato dextrose agar medium. The Petri dishes were flooded with 8 to 10 ml of distilled water and the conidia were scraped using sterile spatula. The spore density of each fungus was adjusted with spectrophotometer (A_{595}nm) to obtain a final concentration of approximately 10^5 spores/ml.

2.3.4 Antibacterial activity [17]

The *in vitro* callus extracts of *T. ulmifolia* were tested against bacteria by the well diffusion method. Different concentration of the extracts (20, 40, and 60 µg/ml) was prepared by reconstituting with ethanol and methanol. The test microorganisms were seeded into respective medium by spread plate method 10 µl (10 cells/ml) with the 24 h cultures of bacteria growth in nutrient broth. After solidification the filter paper wells (5 mm in diameter) impregnated with the extracts were placed on test organism-seeded plates. Streptomycin (10 µg) used as standard for antibacterial test. The antibacterial assay plates were incubated at 37°C for 24 hrs. The diameters of the inhibition zones were measured in mm.

2.3.5 Antifungal activity [18]

The antifungal activities of ethanol and methanol *in vitro* callus extracts were tested by well diffusion method. The potato dextrose agar plates were inoculated with each fungal culture (10 days old) by point inoculation. The filter paper wells (5 mm in diameter) impregnated with 20, 40 and 60 µg/ml concentrations of the extracts were placed on test organism-seeded plates. Streptomycin (10 µg) used as positive control. The activity was determined after 72 hrs of incubation at 28°C. The diameters of the inhibition zones were measured in mm.

2.4 Antioxidant Activity

2.4.1 DPPH radical scavenging activity [19]

Various concentrations of ethanol and methanol extracts of the sample (0.5-2.5 mg/ml) were mixed with 1.0 ml of ethanolic and methanolic solution containing DPPH radicals, resulting in the final concentration of DPPH being 0.2 mM. The mixture were shaken vigorously and left to stand for 30 min, and the absorbance was measured at 517 nm. Ascorbic acid was used as control. The percentage of inhibition in DPPH radical scavenging activity was calculated as follows;

$$\% \text{ Inhibition} = A0- A1/A0 \times 100$$

2.4.2 FRAP assay [20]

The stock solution of 10 mM 2, 4, 6-tripyridyl-s-triazine (TPTZ) in 40 mM HCl, 20 mM $FeCl_3.6H_2O$ and 0.3 M acetate buffer (pH 3.6) was prepared. The FRAP reagent contained 2.5 ml TPTZ solution, 2.5 ml ferric chloride solution and 25 ml acetate buffer. It was freshly prepared and warmed to 37°C. Then, 900 µl FRAP reagent was mixed with 90 µl water and 30 µl test sample/ ethanol/ methanol/ distilled water/ standard antioxidant solution. The reaction mixture was then incubated at 37°C for 30 minutes and the absorbance was recorded at 593 nm. An intense blue colored complex were formed when ferric tripyridyl triazine (Fe^{3+}-TPTZ) complex were reduced to ferrous (Fe^{2+}) form. The absorption at 540 nm was recorded. The calibration was plotted with absorbance at 593 nm vs concentration of ferrous sulphate in the range 0.1 mM both aqueous and ethanol solutions. The concentrations of $FeSO_4$ were in turn plotted against concentration of standard antioxidants L-ascorbic acid.

2.5 *In vitro* Cytotoxicity Assay

2.5.1 Methodology

The human breast cancer cell line (MCF 7) was obtained from National Centre for Cell Science (NCCS), Pune and grown in Eagles Minimum Essential Medium (EMEM) containing 10% fetal bovine serum (FBS). All cells were maintained at 37°C, 5% CO2, 95% air and 100% relative humidity. Maintenance cultures were passaged weekly, and the culture medium was changed twice a week.

2.5.2 Cell treatment procedure

The monolayer cells were detached with trypsin-ethylene diaminetetraacetic acid (EDTA) to make single cell suspensions and viable cells were counted by tryphan blue exclusion assay using a hemocytometer. The cell suspension was diluted with medium containing 5% FBS to give final density of $1x10^5$ cells/ml. One hundred microlitres per well of cell suspension were seeded into 96-well plates at plating density of 10,000 cells/well and incubated to allow for cell attachment at 37°C, 5% CO_2, 95% air and 100% relative humidity. After 24 h the cells were treated with serial concentrations of the test samples. They were initially dispersed in phosphate buffered saline (PBS) and diluted to twice the desired final maximum test concentration with serum free medium. Additional four, 2 fold serial dilutions were made to provide a total of five sample concentrations. Aliquots of 100 µl of these different sample dilutions were added to the appropriate wells already containing 100 µl of medium, resulted the required final sample concentrations. Following drug addiction the plates were incubated for an additional 48 h at 37°C, 5% CO_2, 95% air and 100% relative humidity. The medium containing without samples were served as control and triplicate was maintained for all concentrations.

2.5.3 MTT assay

3-[4,5-dimethylthiazol-2-yl]2, 5-diphenyltetrazolium bromide (MTT) is a yellow water soluble tetrazolium salt. A mitochondrial enzyme in living cells, succinate-dehydrogenase, cleaves the tetrazolium ring, converting the MTT to an insoluble purple formazan. Therefore,the amount of formazan produced is directly proportional to the number of viable cells. After 48 h of incubation, 15 µl of MTT (5 mg/ml) in phosphate buffered saline (PBS) was added to each well and incubated at 37°C for 4 h. The medium with MTT was then flicked off and the formed formazan crystals were solubilized in 100 µl of DMSO and then measured the absorbance at 570 nm using micro plate reader. The % cell inhibition was determined using the following formula.

% Cell Inhibition = 100- Abs (sample)/Abs (control) x100.

Nonlinear regression graph was plotted between % Cell inhibition and Log concentration and IC_{50} was determined using Graph Pad Prism software.

3. RESULTS

3.1 Antimicrobial

The antimicrobial activity of *T. ulmifolia* ethanolic and methanolic callus extracts against various microbial strains and standard Streptomycin with respect to various concentrations (20, 40 and 60 µl) were presented in Tables 1 & 2. From the Table values, it was reported that the test extracts and standard Streptomycin have significant antimicrobial action against all the microbial stains *Escherichia coli, Streptococcus pyogenes, Staphylococcus aureus, Klebsiella pneumonia* and *Trichoderma viride.*

The zone of inhibition of test concentration was compared with standard Streptomycin (10 µg/ml). Figs.-1 A, B, C, D, E and F shows the zone of inhibition of different concentrations of ethanolic extract along with Streptomycin. Among the four different bacterial strains used, higher zone of inhibition (18 mm) was observed in 60 µl concentration of ethanol in *S. aureus* against the control (8 mm) followed by 20 µl and 40 µl concentrations (16 mm and 15.5 mm respectively). In the case of *E. coli, S. pyogenes* and *K. pneumoniae,* the zone of inhibition is higher in 60 µl concentration (12 mm, 11.5 mm and 10.5 mm respectively) against control (6, 8 and 8 mm) respectively. But the effect of ethanol extracts on fungal stains was less (8 and 6 mm) when compared to standard (10 and 8 mm).

Table 1. Anti-microbial activity of ethanol extract of leaf callus of *T. ulmifolia*

S.no	Pathogens	Ethanol extract zone of inhibition (mm)			Standard (streptomycin)
		20 µl	40 µl	60 µl	
1.	*Streptococcus pyogenes*	10	11	11.5	8
2.	*Staphylococcus aureus*	16	15.5	18	8
3.	*Escherichia coli*	8	12	12	6
4.	*Klebsiella pneumoniae*	8.5	10	10.5	8
5.	*Candida albicans*	4	5.5	8	10
6.	*Trichoderma viride*	5.5	5.5	6	8

The result of Table 2 revealed that all the four bacterial strains were found to be resistant to standard Streptomycin but the methanolic extract was very effective control in the growth of the four bacterial strains. Interestingly the zone of inhibition was found to be increased by 10.5 to 22 mm in the four strains of bacteria in 60 μl concentration against standard. In the present study the zone of inhibition (22 mm) is higher in *Klebsiella pneumoniae* at 60 μl concentration followed by 40 μl concentration (20 mm) and 20 μl concentration (18 mm) against control (8 mm) (Fig- 2 B). In the case of *S. aureus* the maximum zone of inhibition (20 mm) was observed in 60 μl followed by 40 μl concentration (18 mm) and 20 μl concentration (16 mm) against the value of standard Streptomycin(8 mm) (Fig- 2 C). In *E. coli* and *S. pyogenes* also the maximum inhibition zone (12, 10.5 mm respectively) was observed in 60 μl concentration followed by 40 μl concentration (8.5, 10 mm respectively) (Figs. - 2 A and D). Here the inhibition zone observed in Streptomycin was 6 mm. In all the four strains of bacteria the concentration increases the zone of inhibition also increases. Whereas, the effect of the methanol extract of callus against two fungal strains *C. albicans* and *T. viride* were equal (8, 10 mm) to the standard Streptomycin (8, 10 mm respectively) (Figs. 2 E and F).

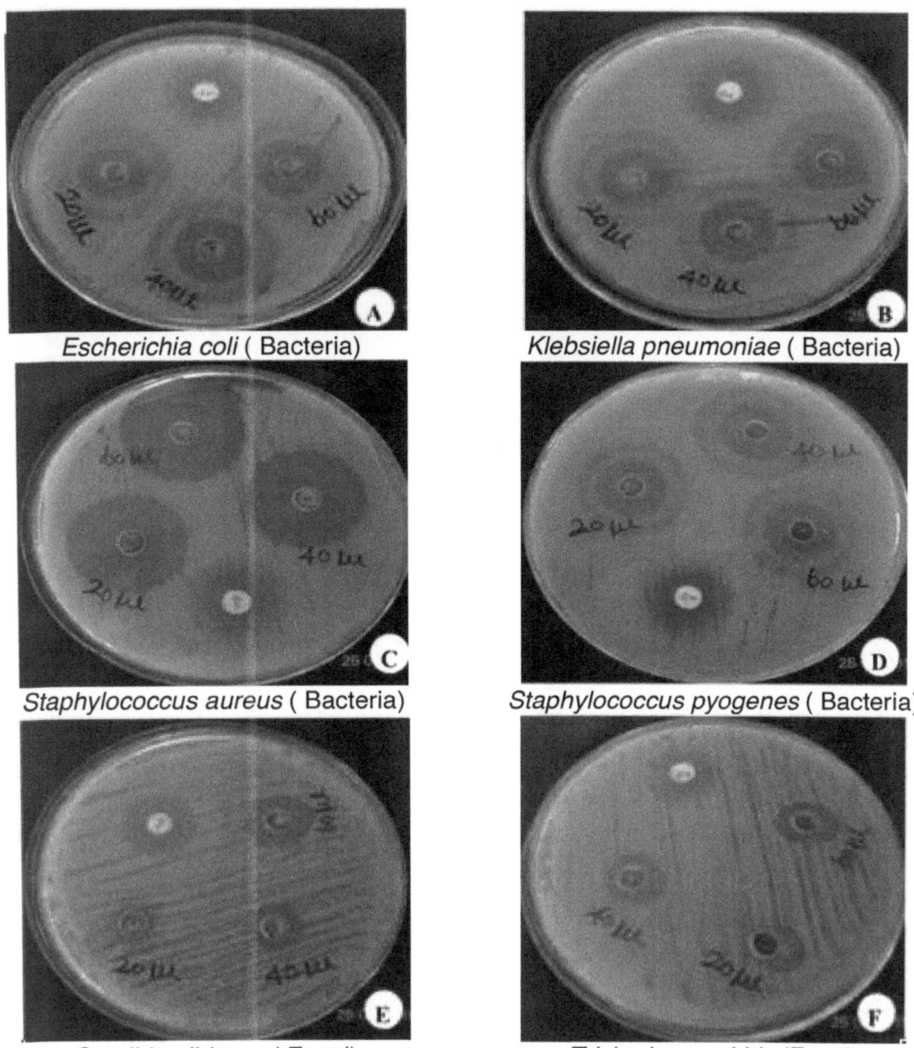

Escherichia coli (Bacteria) — *Klebsiella pneumoniae* (Bacteria)

Staphylococcus aureus (Bacteria) — *Staphylococcus pyogenes* (Bacteria)

Candida albicans (Fungi) — *Trichoderma viride* (Fungi)

Fig. 1. Antimicrobial activity of ethanolic leaf callus extract of *Turnera ulmifolia*

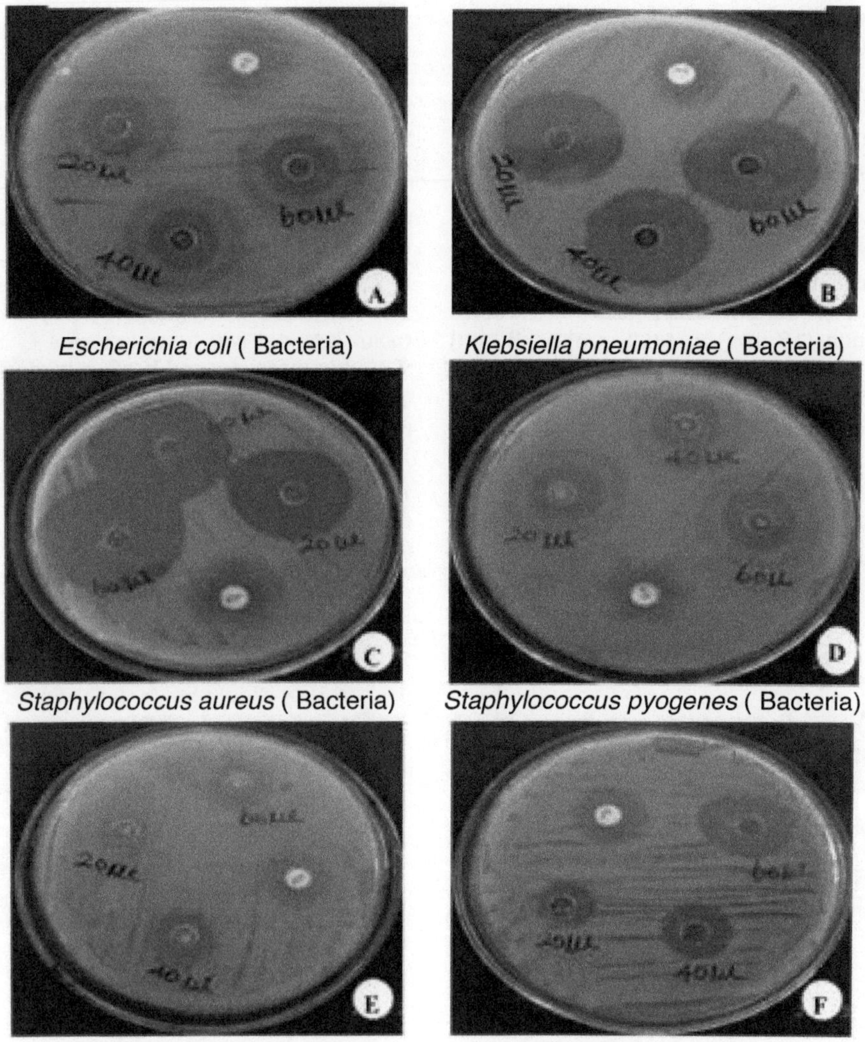

Escherichia coli (Bacteria) *Klebsiella pneumoniae* (Bacteria)

Staphylococcus aureus (Bacteria) *Staphylococcus pyogenes* (Bacteria)

Candida albicans (Fungi) *Trichoderma viride* (Fungi)

Fig. 2. Antimicrobial activity of methanolic leaf callus extract of *Turnera ulmifolia*

Table 2. Anti-microbial activity of methanol extract of leaf callus of *T. ulmifolia*

S.no	Pathogens	Methanol extract zone of inhibition (mm)			Standard (streptomycin)
		20 µl	40 µl	60 µl	
1.	*Streptococcus pyogenes*	10	10	10.5	6
2.	*Staphylococcus aureus*	16	18	20	8
3.	*Escherichia coli*	8.5	8.5	12	6
4.	*Klebsiella pneumoniae*	18	20	22	8
5.	*Candida albicans*	5.5	8	8	8
6.	*Trichoderma viride*	6	8	10	10

3.2 Antioxidant

3.2.1 DPPH scavenging activity

The antioxidant activities of *T. ulmifolia* ethanolic and methanolic callus extracts were assessed by using 2,2-diphenylpicryl-1-picrylhydrazyl (DPPH) and ferric reducing antioxidant power assay (FRAP). The DPPH activity of different concentration of solvent extracts (1 mg/ml to 5 mg/ml) along with standard ascorbic acid is presented in the Table 3. Among the five different concentration of extracts tested, the higher percentage of inhibition (56.29±0.94) was observed in 5 mg/ml of methanolic extract followed by ethanolic extract (53.27±0.99), against the standard ascorbic acid (74.25±0.56) (Fig. 3). The minimum DPPH activity 15.25±1.02 and 12.56±0.94 was noticed in 1 mg/ml concentration of ethanolic and methanolic extract respectively. The dose titration curves allowed determination of IC_{50} for the ethanolic and methanolic callus extracts towards DPPH scavenging activity. The extracts demonstrated dose dependent DPPH scavenging activity effects with IC_{50} values 4.36 mg/ml, 4.50 mg/ml and 3.10 mg/ml in methanolic, ethanolic extracts and standard ascorbic acid respectively. The result showed that the both ethanolic and methanolic extracts possess almost similar potent scavenging activity of the stable face radical DPPH.

3.2.2 FRAP activity

FRAP activity of ethanolic and methanolic extracts of *T. ulmifolia* callus were assayed by using five different concentrations (1 mg/ml to 5 mg/ml). The result of reducing power of solvent extracts is presented in Table 4 and Fig. 4. The absorbance was increased with the increasing concentrations of both methanolic and ethanolic callus extracts. In this study more absorbance (0.62±0.02 and 0.58±0.02) was observed in the concentration of 5 mg/ml of methanolic and ethanolic extracts respectively. It is followed by 4 mg/ml concentration with 0.50±0.01 and 0.45±0.01 absorbance in methanolic and ethanolic extracts respectively, where as in standard ascorbic acid the absorbance was 0.71±0.02 in 5 mg/ml concentration and 0.65±0.01 in 4 mg/ml concentration (Table 4, Fig. 4). The absorbance value of methanolic and ethanolic callus extract was almost equal.

3.3 Anticancerous Activity

To evaluate the cytotoxic activity, the extracts were tested with various doses on the human breast cancer cell line (MCF 7) and normal cells. After 48 hours, cell viability was analyzed using end point MTT assay. Some cells were beginning to detach from the plate and become rounded after 48 hours of treatment (18.75-300 μg/ml). All the samples used exhibition different levels of cytotoxicity like cell rounding, shrinkage, aggregation and cell death depending upon the concentration of the extracts (Figs. 5 and 6). At the concentration of 300 μg/ml the tested samples produced more cytotoxic effect as evidenced by the increased number of dead cells (47.00 and 33.64, methanolic and ethanolic extracts respectively). The callus extracts exhibited greater cytotoxicity on human breast cancer cells with IC_{50}> 300 mg/ml. The methanolic and ethanolic callus extracts induced cell cytotoxicity in a concentration dependent manner (Figs. 5 and 6).

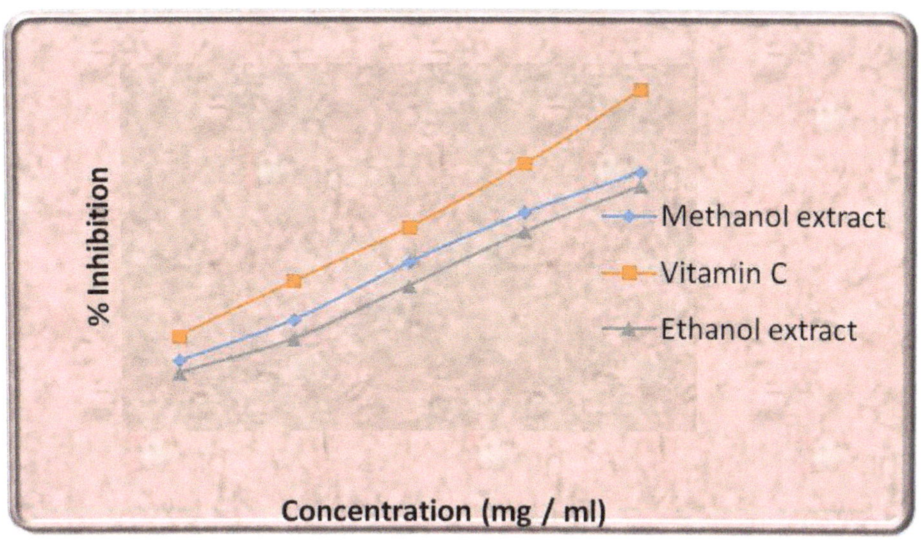

Fig. 3. Antioxidant (DPPH assay) activity of ethanolic and methanolic extracts of leaf callus of *Turnera ulmifolia*

Table 3. Antioxidant (DPPH scavenging) activity of ethanolic and methanolic leaf callus extracts of *T. ulmifolia*

S. no.		% inhibition				
		1 (mg/ml)	2 (mg/ml)	3 (mg/ml)	4 (mg/ml)	5 (mg/ml)
1	Methanol extract	15.25±1.02	24.15±0.47	36.67±0.77	47.54±0.86	56.29±0.94
2	Ethanol extract	12.56±0.94	19.88±0. 76	31.52±0.59	43.26±0.46	53.27±0.99
3	Ascorbic acid	20.66±0.49	32.58±0.80	44.25±0.76	58.16±0.83	74.25±0.96

The experiment was conducted in triplicates (n=3)

Table 4. Antioxidant (FRAP assay) activity of ethanolic and methanolic leaf callus extracts of *T. ulmifolia*

S. no		Absorbance at 593 nm				
		1 (mg/ml)	2 (mg/ml)	3 (mg/ml)	4 (mg/ml)	5 (mg/ml)
1	Methanol extract	0.19±0.01	0.29±0.02	0.38±0.009	0.50±0.01	0.62±0.02
2	Ethanol extract	0.14±0.02	0.22±0.01	0.34±0.03	0.45±0.01	0.58±0.02
3	Ascorbic acid	0.38±0.012	0.45±0.01	0.53±0.02	0.65±0.01	0.71±0.02

The experiment was conducted in triplicates (n=3)

Table 5. Anticancer activity of ethanol extracts of leaf callus of *T. ulmifolia*

Concentration	18.75 µg	37.5 µg	75 µg	150 µg	300 µg	Control
Absorbance	0.311	0.31	0.293	0.24	0.215	0.313
	0.314	0.313	0.304	0.249	0.209	0.324
	0.319	0.305	0.307	0.241	0.207	0.314
Average	0.314	0.309	0.301	0.243	0.210	0.317
Cell Inhibition %	0.73	2.41	4.94	23.23	33.64	-

IC50 value >300 µg/ml

Table 6. Anticancer activity of methanol extracts of leaf callus of *T. ulmifolia*

Concentration	18.75 µg	37.5 µg	75 µg	150 µg	300 µg	Control
Absorbance	0.319	0.304	0.268	0.200	0.175	0.313
	0.315	0.309	0.261	0.208	0.168	0.324
	0.313	0.302	0.259	0.194	0.161	0.314
Average	0.315	0.305	0.262	0.200	0.168	0.317
Cell Inhibition %	0.42	3.78	17.13	36.69	47.0	-

IC50 value >300 µg/ml

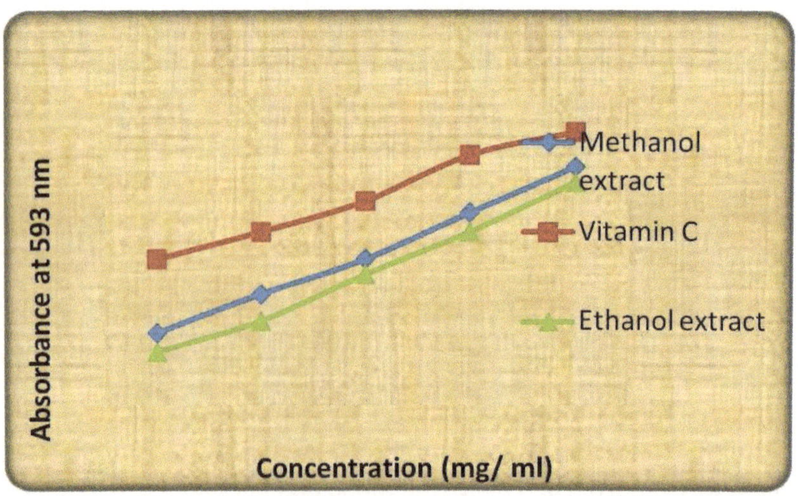

Fig. 4. Anti-oxidant (FRAP assay) activity of ethanolic and methanolic extracts of leaf callus of *Turnera ulmifolia*

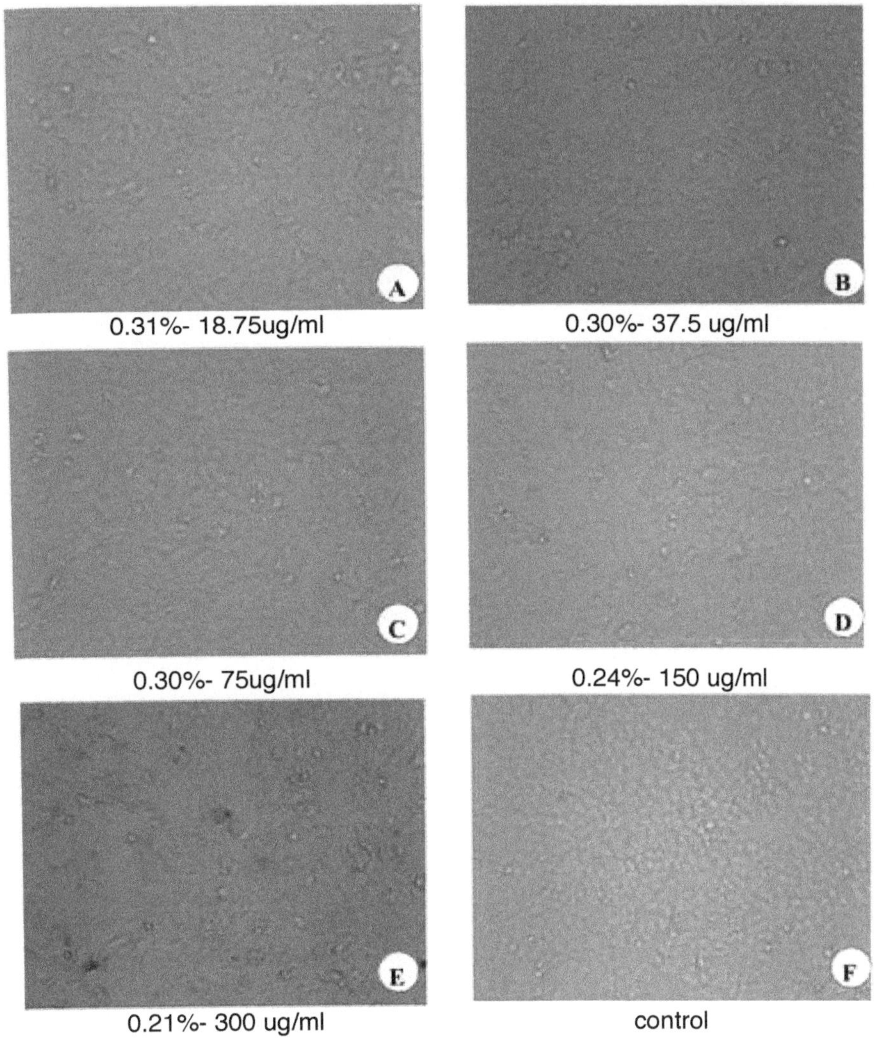

Fig. 5. MTT assay (cytotoxic activity) of the ethanolic callus extract of *Turnera ulmifolia*

4. DISCUSSION

Turnera ulmifolia leaf is considered to be a potent source of bioactive compounds. Many of the naturally occurring compounds present in plants have antimicrobial functions and could thus serve as a source of traditional drugs. Naturally occurring compounds presents in plants many have antimicrobial functions and could thus serve as a source of traditional drugs [21]. Four different bacterial stains and two fungal pathogens were used in the present work to study the effect of ethanolic and methanolic callus extracts of *T. ulmifolia*. The test extracts and standard streptomycin have significant antimicrobial action against all the microbial strains.

Among the four different bacterial strains used, higher zone of inhibition (18 mm) was observed in 60 μl concentration of ethanol in *S. aureus* against the control (8 mm) followed by 20 μl and 40 μl concentrations (16 mm and 15.5 mm respectively). In the case of *E. coli, S. pyogenes* and *K. pneumoniae,* the zone of inhibition is higher in 60 μl concentration (12 mm, 11.5 mm and 10.5 mm respectively) against control (6, 8 and 8 mm) respectively. But the effect of ethanol extracts on fungal stains was less (8 and 6 mm) when compared to standard (10 and 8 mm).

Very few articles were published focusing on pharmacological activity of the genus *Turnera* [2,22,23,4]. In *T. ulmifolia* the effect of ethanolic extracts against methicillin resistant *Streptococcus aureus* conformed the

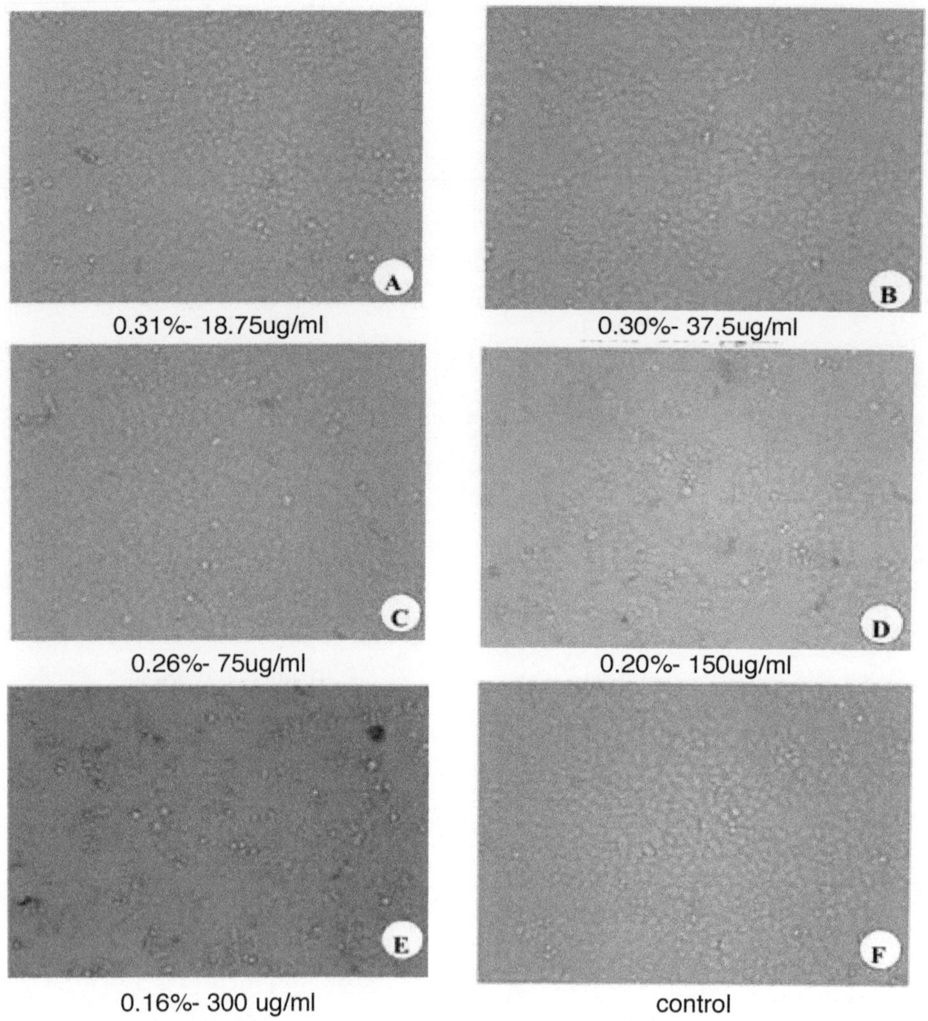

Fig. 6. MTT assay (Cytotoxic activity) of the methanolic callus extract of *Turnera ulmifolia*

antimicrobial activity [22]. Poonam Sethi [23] and Kalimuthu et al. [3] also reported the antibacterial activity of *T. ulmifolia*. As far as we know there is no report on antimicrobial activity of the callus of *T. ulmifolia*. All the reports are from *in vivo* plants extracts. In the present result confirmed the antimicrobial activity of *T. ulmifolia* callus extracts against 4 bacterial and 2 fungal strains. Among the two extracts (ethanol and methanol) tested against bacterial and fungal strains, both the extracts have almost similar effect except the strain *K. pneumoniae*. Our callus extracts results were comparable to that of earlier reports published by using *in vivo* plant extracts. From the obtained results this plant could serve as a source of plant derived natural products with antimicrobial activity to be used against microbes.

FRAP activity of ethanolic and methanolic leaf callus extracts of *T. ulmifolia,* the activity of these extracts to reduce Fe^{3+} to Fe^{2+} was determined and compared with that of standard ascorbic acid. Hence, the absorbance was increased with the increase concentrations of the extracts and decreased when compared to that of standard ascorbic acid. The present finding agrees well with the earlier report on antioxidant activity of ethanolic leaf extract of *T. ulmifolia* [3]. The present study confirmed that the *in vivo* leaf and leaf callus might have similar therapeutic properties because of the similar activities.

The value of medicinal plants lies in the potential access to extremely complex molecular structures that would be difficult to synthesize in the laboratory [26]. The limitations of the available cancer management modalities create an urgent need to screen and generate novel molecules. Despite, well-documented illustrations of phytochemicals being used for prevention and treatment of cancer, their importance in modern medicine remains underestimated. Plants are the storehouse of "pre-synthesized" molecules that act as lead structure, which can be optimized for new drug development. In practice, a large number of cancer chemotherapeutic agents that are currently available in the market can be traced back to their plant resource [27]. Leaf derived callus ethanolic and methanolic extracts of *T. ulmifolia* were tested for their antiproliferative activity. *In vitro* antiproliferative property of the extracts of *T. ulmifolia* was minimum in the present results. Morphological analysis of the cells exhibited that the extract treatment had initiated apoptotic mechanism to trigger cell death. At 300 µg/ml concentration over 17%, 25% of the cell population had been rendered apoptotic by both the extracts respectively through flow cytotoxic observation. In general both the extracts showed very less inhibition percentage. So it is confirmed that the leaf derived callus was having very less anticancerous activity.

5. CONCLUSION

In this report the antimicrobial potential of ethanolic and methanolic callus extracts of *T. ulmifolia* were evaluated against pathogenic microbes and both the extracts were found active against the strain of bacteria and fungi. Therefore these extracts could be used for antimicrobial drug development. Further these extracts showed strong antioxidant activity in both DPPH & FRAP in dose depending manner. It also had profound cytotoxic activity against human breast cancer cell line. Together, our finding showed that the callus can be used for the isolation and evaluation of bioactive compounds. This will save the wild plant from collection for herbal remedy.

CONSENT

It is not applicable.

ETHICAL APPROVAL

It is not applicable.

COMPETING INTERESTS

Authors have declared that no competing interests exist.

REFERENCES

1. Braga R, Plantas do Nordeste, Especialmente do Ceara´. ESAM (Colec¸ Mossoroense), Fortaleza, Brazil; 1976. Genus: *Turnera* L. germplasm resources information network. United States Department of Agriculture. 2010-01-27. Retrieved; 2011.
2. Hosamani KM. Fatty acids in seed oil from *Turnera ulmifolia.* Phytochemistry. 1993; 34:1363-1365.
3. Kalimuthu K, Prabakaran R, Preetha V. Antimicrobial and antioxidant activities of ethanolic crude extracts of *Turnera ulmifolia* Linn. International Journal of Pharmaceutical Sciences and Drug Research. 2014;6(4):329-333.
4. Kalimuthu K, Prabakaran R, Preetha R. Phytochemical screening and GC-MS studies on the ethanolic extract of *Turnera ulmifolia* L. Int. J. Pharm Phytopharmacol Res. 2014;4(3):179-181.
5. Antonio MA, Souza Brito AR. Oral anti-inflammatory and antiulcerogenic activities of a hydroalcoholic extract and partitioned fractions of *Turnera ulmifolia* (Turneraceae). Ethnopharmacol. 1998;6: 215-228.
6. Nascimento MA, Silva AK, Franca LC, Quignard EL, Lopez JA, Almeida MG. *Turnera ulmifolia* L. (Turneraceae): preliminary study of its antioxidant activity. Bioresour Technol. 2006;97:1387-1391.
7. Aguilar A, Camacho JR, Chino S, Jáquez P, López ME. Herbario Medicinal del Instituto Mexicano del Seguro Social. Instiuto Mexicano del Seguro Social, Mexico; 1994.
8. Coe FG, Anderson GJ. Ethnobotany of the Sumu (Ulwa) of Southeastern Nicaragua and comparisons with Miskitu plant lore. Econ. Bot. 1999;53:363-386.
9. Halberstein RA. Traditional botanical remedies on a small Caribbean Island: Middle (Grand) Caicos, West Indies. J. Altern. Complement. Med. 1997;3:227-239.
10. Kumar D, Kumar A, Prakash O. Potential antifertility agents from plants: A comprehensive review. J. Ethno-pharmacology. 2012;140:1–32.
11. Mitchell SA. The Jamaican toottonics: A botanical reference. Focus Altern. Complement. Ther. 2011;16:271–280.
12. DeAraújoBarbosa D, NuritSilva K, Fátima Agra M. Estudofarmacobotâ- nico

comparative odefolhasde *Turnerachamaedrifolia* Cambess. e *Turnera subulata* Sm. (Turneraceae). Revista Brasileirade Farmacognosia. 2007;17:396-413.

13. Almir de Araújo F, Teles Leite D, Soares Sousa LCF, de Albuquerque Fernandes A, Borges Maracajá P. Etno-botanicandetnovetin Jacusettlementin Municipality of Pompal-Paraiba-Brazil. *Revista verdede* Agroecologiae Desenvolvimento Sustentâve. 2011;16: 149-156.
14. Albuquerque UP, Medeiros PM, Almeida ALS, Monteiro JM, Neto Freitas Lins, Melo EM, Santos JP. Medicinal plants of the *Caatinga* (semi-arid) Vegetatio no FNE Brazil: aquantitati veapproach. J. Ethnopharmacol. 2007;114:325–354.
15. Jayakar B, Rajkapoor B. Efforts of *Caralluma attenuata* in normal and alloxen induced diabetic rate. J. Herb Phamacother. 2004;4:35-40.
16. Kokate CK, Purohit AP, Gokhale SB. Pharmacognosy, 29th ed. Nirali Prakashan, Pune. 2004;318-320.
17. Anonymous. Pharmacopiea of India (The Indian Pharmacopiea), 3rd Ed. New Delhi: Ministry of Health and Family Welfare; 1996.
18. Taylor RSL, Manandhar NP, Hudson JB, Towers GHN. Screening of selected medicinal plants of Nepal for antimicrobial activities. J. Ethnopharmacol. 1995;546: 153-159.
19. Shimada K, Fujikawa K, Yahara K, Nakamura T. Antioxidative properties of xanthan on the autoxidation of soybean oil in cyclodextrin emulsion. J. Agric. Food Chem. 1992;40:945-8.
20. Benzie IFF, Strain JJ. Ferric reducing ability of plasma (FRAP) as a measure of antioxidant power: The FRAP assay. Anal. Biochem.1996;239:70.
21. Kim TU, Gu BG, Jeong JY, Byun SM, Shin YC. Purification and characterization of a maltotetraose-forming alkaline µ-amylase from an alkalophilic *Bacillus* strain, GM8901. Applied and Environmental Microbiology. 1995;61(8):3105-3112.
22. Henrique DM, Coutinho José GM, Costa Edeltrudes O, Lima Vivyanne S, Falcão-Silva, José P Siqueira Júnior. BMC Complementary and Alternative Medicine. 2009;9(13):9-13.
23. Poonam Sethi. Antibacterial activity of aqueous extract of the leaves of *Turnera ulmifolia* Linn. (Turneraceae). Advance Research in Pharmaceuticals Biologicals. 2011;1(2):101-104.
24. Gülçin I. Antioxidant properties of resveratrol: A structure-activity insight. Innovative Food Sci Emer Technol. 2010; 11:210–218.
25. Kadam Balaji, Manasa G, Amarender Reddy A, Nagaraju M, Srikanth T, Saarangi Ramesh. Evaluation of *In vitro* antioxidant and cytotoxicity activity of aqueous extract of *Pergularia daemia.* Sch. Acad. J. Pharm. 2013;2(2):125-129.
26. Savita Dixit, Huma Ali. Anticancer activity of medicinal plant extract-A review. J. Chem. and Chem. Sci. 2010;1(1):79-85.
27. Heinrich M, Bremner P. Ethnobotany and Ethanopharmacy their role for anticancer drug development. Curr. Drug Target. 2006;7:239.

6

Anti-bacterial and *in vitro* Anti-diabetic Potential of Novel Isoxazole Derivatives

Lincy Joseph[1*] and Mathew George[1]

[1]*Pushpagiri College of Pharmacy, Kerala, India.*

Authors' contributions

This work was carried out in collaboration between both authors. Both authors read and approved the final manuscript.

Article Information

Editor(s):
(1) Hua Naranmandura, Department of Pharmacology, Toxicology and Biochemical Pharmaceutics,College of Pharmaceutical Sciences, Zhejiang University, China.
(2) Vasudevan Mani, Universiti Teknologi MARA (UiTM), Selangor, Malaysia.
(3) Ke-He Ruan,Director of the Center for Experimental Therapeutics and Pharmacoinformatics (CETP)Professor of Medicinal Chemistry & Pharmacology, Department of Pharmacological and Pharmaceutical Sciences, University of Houston, USA.
Reviewers:
(1) Roukia Hammoudi, Université Kasdi Merbah,Ouargla, Algeria.
(2) Volodymyr Chernyshenko, NAS of Ukraine, Ukraine.

ABSTRACT

Aim: To synthesize novel Isoxazole derivatives, characterize them and subject for screening anti-bacterial action and *in vitro* anti-diabetic activity.

Methodology: Chalcones were prepared by the reaction of aromatic aldehydes with aromatic ketones in aqueous alcoholic alkaline medium. Then these were made to react with hydroxylamine hydrochloride and sodium acetate to prepare title compounds. The prepared isoxazole compounds were subjected to *in vitro* anti-diabetic screening by yeast and enzymatic method. All compounds were screened for antibacterial action by disc diffusion method.

Results: The structure of the synthesized compounds were confirmed by IR, NMR spectral datas and screened for anti-bacterial, and anti-diabetic activities. Most effective antibacterial one possessed chlorine in the Phenyl ring attached at 5-C of isoxazole and have NH_2 substitution in phenyl ring attached at 3-C of isoxazole. Compounds with significant *in vitro* anti-diabetic action by studying the glucose uptake by yeast cell method are with Br/NO_2 substituted forR_2/R_3 in phenyl ring when R'2 is OH/NH_2.

Conclusion: Presence of halogenated aromatic ring at 5-C and amine substituted phenyl ring at 3-Cof Isoxazole exhibited moderate anti-bacterial activity. In the anti-diabetic study halogenated or nitrated phenyl ring at 5-C and hydroxyl/amine substituted phenyl ring at 3-C of isoxazole exhibited anti-diabetic action.

**Corresponding author: E-mail: mathewlincg@yahoo.com*

Keywords: Isoxazole; chalcones; aromatic aldehyde; aromatic ketones; antibacterial; in vitro anti-diabetic.

1. INTRODUCTION

Isoxazole being an azole with an oxygen atom next to the nitrogen, exhibits broad spectrum of biological activity and also forms a part of various biodynamic agents. Substituted isoxazoles are also considered to be important synthons due to their versatility towards chemical transformations to useful synthetic intermediates. A lot of modifications have been done during the last few years on isoxazole nucleus. A survey of literature revealed that substituted isoxazole possess different types of potent biological activities [1-3].

Many Isoxazole derivatives are stated to have good antimicrobial activity. Cali et al identified a series of isoxazole-3-hydroxamic acid derivatives as a new class of small, nonpeptidic inhibitors of peptide deformylase. They reported the synthesis, enzyme inhibition and preliminary investigation of the binding mode of this potential antibacterial compounds [4]. Antibacterial and antifungal studies done by Khanage et al. [5] revealed that compound containing -Cl, $-NO_2$ and $-OCH_3$ groups were found to be potent antimicrobial agents. Ravi et al. [6] synthesized novel methylene bridged benzisoxazolyl imidazo[2,1-b][1,3,4]thiadiazoles and reported antibacterial activity of synthesized compounds. Many studies indicate isoxazole derivatives improved diabetic condition. Kumar et al. [7] designed and synthesized a series of 3,5-diarylisoxazole derivatives as potential anti-hyperglycemic agents. Zhou et al. [8] synthesized fifteen new β-amino ketones containing a isoxazole moiety directly through Mannich reaction. They reported most of the compounds possess weak α-glucosidase inhibitory activity and protein tyrosine phosphatase 1B inhibitory activity in low concentration, some could activate peroxisome proliferator-activated receptors (PPAR) response element moderately [8]. In this light hereby prepared many Isoxazole derivatives which screened for anti-bacterial activity and *in vitro* antidiabetic activity.

2. METHODOLOGY

2.1 Preparation of Chalcones

0.01 mol of benzaldehyde was taken and added 0.01 mol acetophenone in 10 ml 95% ethanol in a flask. 3.5 mL 6 M NaOH solution was added to the reaction mixture stirred well for 10 minutes. Cooled in ice bath until crystal formation. 2 mL ice cold water added to it followed by 2 mL ice cold ethanol. Allow to air dry. Recrystallise from ethanol.

2.2 Cyclisation Step

The formed unstable chalcones were further cyclised with 0.015 mol of hydroxylamine hydrochloride and sodium acetate 0.015 mol in 25 mL ethanol was refluxed for 6 hrs. The mixture was concentrated and poured in to ice. The precipitate obtained was filtered washed and recrystallised from ethanol.

2.3 *In vitro* Anti-diabetic Screening

2.3.1 Glucose uptake in yeast cells [9]

Yeast cells were prepared by, commercial baker's yeast and was washed by repeated centrifugation (3,000×g; 5 min) in distilled water until the supernatant fluids were clear and a 10% (v/v) suspension was prepared in distilled water. Various concentrations of extracts (1–5 mg) were added to 1 mL of glucose solution (5, 10 and 25 mM) and incubated together for 10 min at 37°C. Reaction was started by adding 100 µl of yeast suspension, vortex and further incubated at 37°C for 60 min. After 60 min, the tubes were centrifuged (2,500 × g, 5 min) and glucose was estimated in the supernatant. The percentage increase in glucose uptake by yeast cells was calculated using the following formula-

Increase in glucose uptake (%) = Abs sample– Abs control* 100 / Abs sample

Where, Abs control is the absorbance of the control reaction (containing all reagents except the test sample), and Abs sample is the absorbance of the test sample. All the experiments were carried out in triplicates.

2.3.2 Alpha-amylase inhibitory activity [10]

The activity of α-amylase was measured using the starch-iodine method. Briefly, 20 µ l of α-amylase solution (0.030 mg/ml) was mixed with 1.3 ml of Tris-HCl buffer (0.01 M containing 0.006 M NaCl, pH 6.8) and 80 µl of the aqueous extract. After incubation at 37°C for 20 min, 100 µl of the starch solution (0.1%) was added, and the mixture re-incubated for 20 min, after which

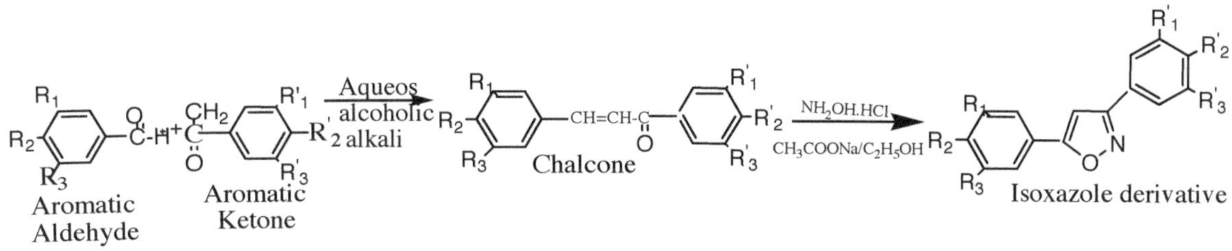

Fig. 1. Scheme of synthesis of the isoxazole derivatives

2 ml of 0.01% acidic iodine solution was added, and the absorbance measured at 565 nm. The percentage inhibition was calculated by comparing to the control which did not have the extract. Inhibition of enzyme activity was calculated as

$$\% = (A-C) \times 100 / (B-C)$$

where, A = absorbance of the sample, B = absorbance of blank (no extract), and C = absorbance of control (no starch).

2.4 Determination of Antibacterial Activity

The antibacterial activity of synthetic products was assessed against three bacteria species: *Bacillus subtilis* NCIM 2063, *Staphylococcus aureus* NCIM 2079 and *Escherichia coli* NCIM 2931. The respective cultures were prepared in nutrient broth media after incubation at 37℃ for 24 hrs. The antibacterial activity was determined by agar disc diffusion test.

2.5 Agar Disc Diffusion Test [11]

Using an aseptic technique, place a sterile swab into the broth culture of a specific organism and then gently remove the excess liquid by gently pressing or rotating the swab against the inside of the tube. Using the swab, streak the Nutrient agar plate to form a bacterial lawn. To obtain uniform growth, streak the plate with the swab in one direction, rotate the plate 90° and streak the plate again in that direction. Repeat this rotation 3 times. Allow the plate to dry for approximately 5 minutes.

Use an Antibiotic Disc Dispenser to dispense discs onto the plate and administer the respective samples onto the labelled discs. Using a flame-sterilized forceps, gently press each disc to the agar to ensure that the disc is attached to the agar. Plates should be incubated overnight at an incubation temperature of 37℃.

3. RESULTS AND DISCUSSION

None of the tested compounds are superior to Ciprofloxacin which was the standard. Most effective one possesed chlorine in the Phenyl ring attached at 5-C of isoxazole and have NH_2 substitution in phenyl ring attached at 3-C of isoxazole against Gram +ve *Bacillus subtilis, staphylococcus aureous* and Gram –ve *E. coli.* A few compounds substituted with nitro/halogen on Phenyl ring at 5-C of isoxazole and ethoxyl group on phenyl ring at 3-C of isoxazole observed to be active only against *E. coli.* Compounds with significant *in vitro* anti-diabetic action by studying the glucose uptake by yeast cell method are with Br/NO_2 substituted forR_2/R_3 in phenyl ring when R'2 is OH/NH_2.

Table 1. IR and NMR spectral details of synthesized compounds

Sample ID	IR peaks(cm^{-1})	NMR peaks (ppm)
L1	1011(N-O-stretch),1500(C-O-stretch),1243 (N-O out of pane bend)	11.663(alcoholic proton) 8-421 (2H),-CH_2-5 membered ring, 8.330, (1H)-isomer of isoxazole, 8.229, 8.2210,8.05,8.04-(4H),of Aro-H.
L2	1104(N-O- stretch),1511(C-O stretch), 1245(N-O out of pane bend)	8.404-(2H),-CH2(5-membered ring).8.357-(1H)isomer of isoxazole,8.363,8.366,8.369-(4H,Ar-H)
L3	1105(N-O stretch),1533(C-O stretch), 1350(N-O out of pane bend)	11.646-alcoholic proton., 8.424-(2H,CH2-5 membered ring),
L4	1018(N-O stretch),1500(C-O	8.337-(2H),CH2(5-membered ring)7.469-(4H) of Ar-H

Sample ID	IR peaks(cm^{-1})	NMR peaks (ppm)
	stretch),1201(N-O out of pane bend)	
L5	1018 (N-O stretch),1500(C-O stretch), 1201(N-O out of pane bend)	7.470 (4H)of Ar-H
L6	1016(N-O stretch),1530(C-O stretch), 1219(N-O out of plane bend)	11.075 – alcoholic proton peak.8.141-(2H)CH2-5-membered ring,7.959,7.955,7.875 (4H,of Ar-H)
L7	1009(N-O stretch),1550(C-O stretch), 1217(N-O out of plane bend)	11.844 alcoholic proton,8.308-(2H)CH2-5 membered ring.7.872,7.850-(4H,Ar-H)
L8	1171(N-O stretch),1517(C-O-stretch), 1245(N-O out of plane bend)	10.966-alcoholic proton,8.306-(2H,CH2-5 membered ring),8.067,7.545,7.539 (4H of Ar-H)
L9	1041(N-O stretch),1491(C-O stretch), 1295(N-O out of plane bend)	11.186-alcoholic proton peak.7.526-(2H,CH2 5-membered ring)
L10	1090(N-O stretch),1490(C-O stretch), 1219(N-O out of plane bend)	8.176-(2H,CH2-5membered ring),8.170-OH isomer of isoxazole.8.157,8.152,8.149-Ar-H
L11	1012(N-O stretch),1490(C-O stretch),1219(C-N stretch),1100(N-O out of plane)	8.175-2H (CH2-of 5-membered ring.)8.157-OH isomer of isoxazole.8.153,7.995-(4H of Ar-H)
L12	1012 (N-O stretch),1218(C-O stretch),1489(C-N stretch),1100(N-O out of plane bend)	8.175- (2H (CH2-of 5-membered ring.)8.157-OH isomer of isoxazole.8.154,7.996-(4H of Ar-H))
L13	1116(N-O stretch),1240(C-O stretch), 1550(C-O carbonyl),1100(N-O out of plane)	8.231- (2H (CH2-of 5-membered ring.)8.227-OH isomer of isoxazole.8.223,7.=8.204-(4H of Ar-H))
L14	1012(N-O stretch),1219(C-N stretch), 1490(C-N stretch)	8.177- (2H (CH2-of 5-membered ring.)8.174-OH isomer of isoxazole.8.153,7.996-(4H of Ar-H))
L15	1040(N-O stretch),1530(C-O-stretch), 1178(C-N stretch)	8.766- (2H (CH2-of 5-membered ring.)8.341-OH isomer of isoxazole.8.321,8.272,8.269-(4H of Ar-H))
L16	1008(N-O stretch),1223(C-N stretch), 1603(C-O stretch)	8.172- (2H (CH2-of 5-membered ring.)8.150-OH isomer of isoxazole.8.004,7.965-(4H of Ar-H))
L17	1016(N-O stretch),1218(C-N stretch), 1527(C-O stretch)	8.793- (2H (CH2-of 5-membered ring.)8.788-OH isomer of isoxazole.8.784,8.362-(4H of Ar-H))
L18	1047(N-O stretch),1260(C-N stretch), 1490(C-O stretch),1179(N-O out of plane)	8.173- (2H (CH2-of 5-membered ring.)8.151-OH isomer of isoxazole.7.990,7.951,7.936-(4H of Ar-H))
L19	1041(N-O stretch),1585(C-O stretch),1183(N-O out of plane)	7.746- (2H (CH2-of 5-membered ring.)7.725-OH isomer of isoxazole.7.707,7.674,7.635-(4H of Ar-H))
L20	1046(N-O stretch),1212(C-N stretch), 1507(C-O stretch),1153(N-O out of plane)	8.749- (2H (CH2-of 5-membered ring.)8.114-OH isomer of isoxazole.8.089,8.070,8.037-(4H of Ar-H))
L21	1041(N-O stretch),1264(C-N stretch), 1519(C-O stretch)	8.294- (2H (CH2-of 5-membered ring.)8.272-OH isomer of isoxazole.8.201,8.177-(4H of Ar-H))
L22	1000(N-O stretch),1507(C-O	8.052- (2H (CH2-of 5-membered ring.) 6.914--(4H of

Sample ID	IR peaks(cm^{-1})	NMR peaks (ppm)
	stretch), 1238(C-N stretch)	Ar-H))
L23	1039(N-O stretch),1129(C-Nstretch), 1492(C-O stretch)	7.503- (2H (CH2-of 5-membered ring.)7.500-OH isomer of isoxazole.7.497,7.494,7.490-(4H of Ar-H))
L24	1051(N-O stretch),1213(C-N stretch), 1507(C-O stretch)	8.320- (2H (CH2-of 5-membered ring.)7.831-OH isomer of isoxazole.7.810,7.691,7.686-(4H of Ar-H)
L25	1060-(N-O stretch),1270(C-N stretch), 1550(C-O stretch)	8.732- (2H (CH2-of 5-membered ring.)8.066-OH isomer of isoxazole.8.032,7.946,7.926-(4H of Ar-H))

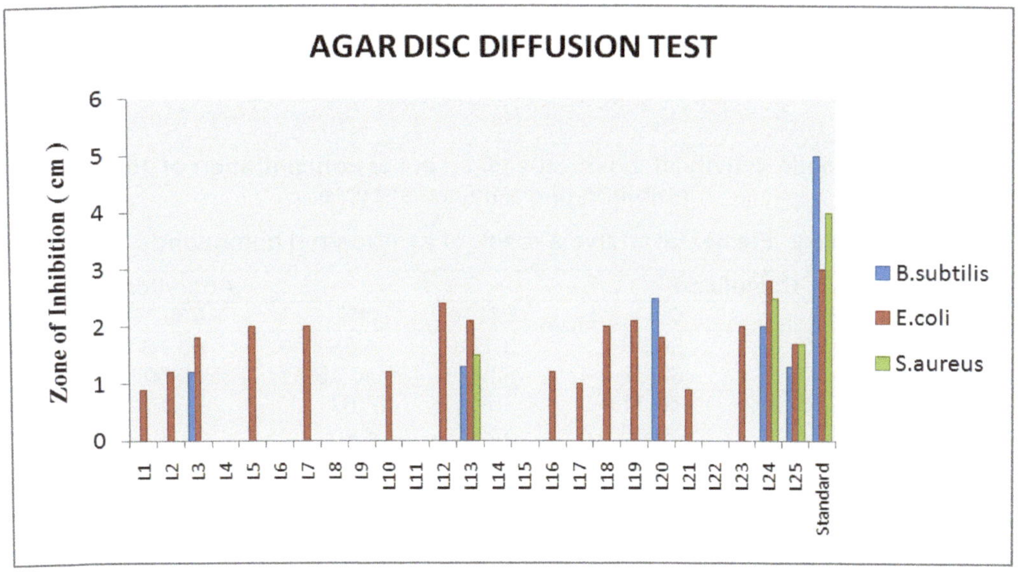

Fig. 2. Anti-bacterial activity of Isoxazole compounds (L1-25) by disc diffusion method using *Bacillus subtilis* NCIM 2063, *Staphylococcus aureus* NCIM 2079 and *Escherichia coli* NCIM 2931

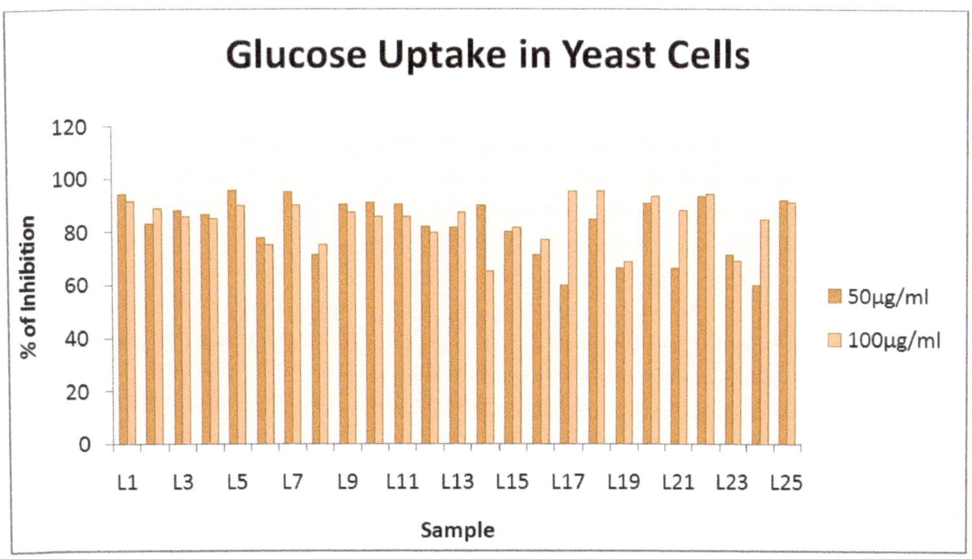

Fig. 3. Anti-diabetic activity of isoxazoles taken in the concentration of 50 µg/ml and 100 µg/ml by studying glucose uptake in living yeast cells

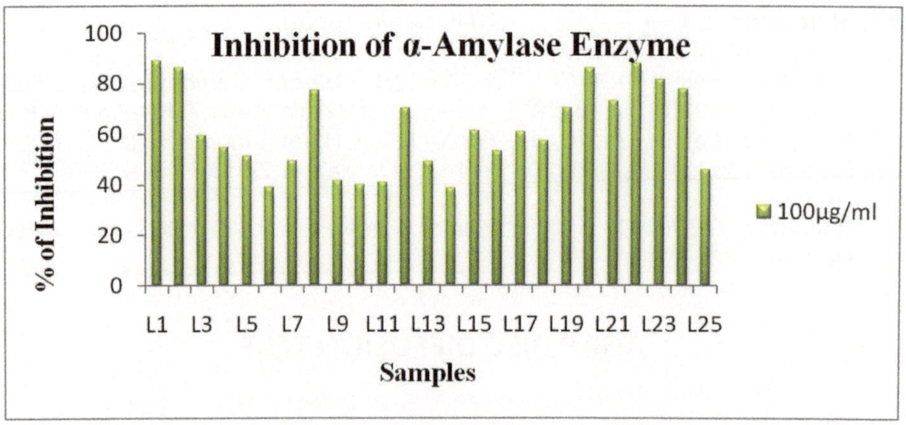

Fig. 4. Anti-diabetic activity of isoxazoles taken in the concentration of 100 µg/ml by inhibition of α amylase enzyme

Table 2. Elemental analysis result of synthesized compounds

	Calculated			Analytical		
Sample	N%	C%	H%	N%	C%	H%
L1	4.43	56.99	3.19	4.65	66.76	3.86
L2	9.92	63.83	3.57	10.59	49.60	3.81
L3	5.16	66.31	3.71	7.67	77.11	8.42
L4	5.27	76.48	5.21	8.45	51.10	3.58
L5	4.43	56.99	3.19	4.65	66.50	3.67
L6	9.92	63.83	3.57	10.64	49.87	2.79
L7	9.92	63.83	3.57	5.20	67.00	4.02
L8	4.71	68.68	5.09	4.65	66.98	4.30
L9	4.71	68.68	3.85	5.61	67.46	5.80
L10	4.58	58.85	2.96	3.80	54.30	3.60
L11	4.46	61.17	3.85	4.62	66.74	4.90
L12	9.99	68.56	4.32	10.62	49.81	3.02
L13	5.19	71.25	4.48	8.48	50,91	3.77
L14	5.62	81.90	6.06	5.19	67.85	3.75
L15	4.46	61.17	3.85	4.60	67.39	5.47
L16	9.99	68.56	4.32	10.64	68.50	6.02
L17	9.99	68.56	4.32	10.60	49.68	4.27
L18	4.07	59.32	4.10	4.10	69.71	5.16
L19	9.03	65.80	4.55	5.64	78.69	6.90
L20	4.32	61.83	4.51	3.24	59.18	4.44
L21	8.89	57.16	3.52	6.31	46.17	2.60
L22	4.89	55.71	6.08	5.96	50.98	7.98
L23	10.35	66.55	4.10	11.03	70.76	6.03
L24	10.35	66.55	4.10	10.69	68.89	6.38
L25	11.19	76.78	5.64	10.67	68.74	6.42

4. CONCLUSION

Presence of halogenated aromatic ring at 5-C and amine substituted phenyl ring at 3-Cof isoxazole exhibited moderate anti-bacterial activity. In the anti-diabetic study halogenated or nitrated phenyl ring at 5-C and hydroxyl/amine substituted phenyl ring at 3-C of isoxazole exhibited anti-diabetic action.

CONSENT

It is not applicable.

ETHICAL APPROVAL

All authors hereby declare that "Principles of laboratory animal care" (NIH publication No. 85-23, revised 1985) were followed, as well as specific national laws where applicable. All experiments have been examined and approved by the appropriate ethics committee.

All authors hereby declare that all experiments have been examined and approved by the appropriate ethics committee and have therefore been performed in accordance with the ethical standards laid down in the 1964 Declaration of Helsinki.

DISCLAIMER

Conference name: "Drug Discovery Conference" Link:"http://www.innovabalt.eu/pictures/zinas/225.pdf" (August 27-29, 2015, Riga, Latvia).

ACKNOWLEDGEMENT

The authors are acknowledge to DST-SERB – India for providing the fund and expressing thanks to STIC of Cochin University for spectral Analysis.

COMPETING INTERESTS

Authors have declared that no competing interests exist.

REFERENCES

1. Jung HK, Doddareddya MR, Cha JH, Rhim H, Cho YS, Koh HY, et al. Synthesis and biological evaluation of novel T-type Ca 2+ channel blockers. Bioorg Med Chem. 2004;12:3965–70. (PubMed)
2. Popat KH, Nirmavat KS, Kachhadia VV, Joshi HS. Synthesis and biological activity of 3-aryl-5-(3'- bromo/chlorophenyl) isoxazoles. J Indian Chem Soc. 2003;80: 707–8.
3. Norman BH, Lander PA, Gruber JM, Kroin JS. Cyclohexyl-linked tricyclic isoxazoles are potent and selective modulators of the multidrug resistance protein (MRP1) Bioorg Med Chem Lett. 2005;15:5526–30. (PubMed)
4. Calí P, Naerum L, Mukhija S, Hjelmencrantz A. Isoxazole-3-hydroxamic acid derivatives as peptide deformylase. Bioorg. Med. Chem. Letters. 2004;14(24): 5997-6000.
5. Shantaram Khanage, Popat Mohite, Ramdas Pandhare, Appala Raju, Synthesis and pharmacological evaluation of isoxazole derivatives containing 1,2,4-triazole Moiety. Marmara Phrmaceutical Journal. 2012;16:134-140.
6. Ravi SL, Nitinkumar SS, Ravindra RK, Imtiyaz MK La-mani RS, Shetty NS, Kamble, RR, Khazi IA. Synthesis and antimicrobial studies of novel methylene bridged ben- isoxazolyl imidazo[2,1-b][1,3,4]thiadiazole derivatives. EurJ Med Chem. 2009;44:2828-33.
7. Kumar A, Maurya RA, Sharma S, Ahmad P, Singh AB, Tamrakar AK, Srivastava AK. Design and synthesis of 3,5-diarylisoxazole derivatives as novel class of anti-hyperglycemic and lipid lowering agents. Bioorg Med Chem. 2009; 17:5285-92.
8. Zhou Jie-Wen, Yan Ju-Fang, Tang Xue-Mei. Synthesis and preliminary evaluation of antidiabetic activity for β-amino ketone containing isoxazole moiety. Chin. J. Org. Chem. 2010;30(04):582-589.
9. Daksha G, Chandrashekar Lobo, Yogendra R, Nilesh G. *In-vitro* antidiabetic activity of stem bark of *Bauhinia purpurea* Linn. Der Pharmacia Lettre. 2012;4(2):614-619.
10. Etoundi CB, Kuate D, Ngondi JL, Oben J, Anti- amylase, anti lipase and anti oxidant effects of aqueous extracts of some Cameroonian spices. Journal of Natural Products. 2010;3:165-171.
11. Coyle MB. Manual of antimicrobial susceptibility testing: Test methods. America Society of Microbiology. 2005;39-46.

7

Effects of Ethanol Extract of Unripe *Annona muricata* (l.) Fruits on the Haematological and Histopathological Parameters in Swiss Albino Rats Infected with *Salmonella typhi*

Olajide Sunday Faleye[1*] and Ebenezer Oluyemi Dada[1]

[1]Department of Microbiology, Federal University of Technology, Akure, Ondo State, Nigeria.

Authors' contributions

This work was carried out in collaboration between both authors. Authors OSF and EOD designed the study, wrote the protocol, and wrote the first draft of the manuscript. Author OSF managed the literature searches and various analyses performed during the study. Author OSF managed the experimental process and author EOD identified the species of plant. Both authors read and approved the final manuscript.

Article Information

Editor(s):
(1) Xiang-chun Shen, Research division of Pharmacology,Guiyang Medical University, China.
Reviewers:
(1) Humaira Zafar, Al Nafees Medical College, Islamabad, Pakistan.
(2) Muhammad Aslam, Ziauddin University, Karachi, Pakistan.

ABSTRACT

Background: In addition to the problems of resistance to commonly used antibiotics, toxicity depicts the state of adverse effects caused by the interaction of toxicants with cells. Similarly, blood components are exposed to significant concentrations of toxic compounds as they form the medium for their transport.
Aims: To study the effects of ethanol extract of unripe *Annona muricata* fruits on the haematological and histopathological parameters in Swiss albino rats infected with *Salmonella typhi.*
Place and Duration of Study: Department of Microbiology Laboratory, Federal University of Technology, Akure, Ondo State, Nigeria, between June 2014 and December 2014.
Methodology: Matured unripe fruits of *A. muricata* were collected, dried, powdered and extracted using 70% ethanol. Eighteen rats of same age between 170-220 g in weight were selected and divided into six groups containing three each. The infectivity dose (ID) was determined using the

**Corresponding author: Email: faleyeolajide@gmail.com*

clinical *Salmonella typhi* obtained from Don Bosco Catholic Hospital, Akure. The dose of the *A. muricata* fruit extract (400 mg/kg) used in this study was administered orally for 7 days. At the end of the treatment period, the rats were fasted overnight. Then blood samples were collected by cardiac puncture for haematological studies and there after sacrificed. Organs (liver, heart, kidney and spleen) were excised for relative organ weight analysis and histopathological studies.

Results: The infectious dose (ID) of *S. typhi* on experimental rats in this study was 6.8×10^6 cfu/ml while the weights of liver, heart and spleen in all groups were not significantly different from the control. However, a significant increase in the heart was observed in group given the extract and antibiotics (ciprofloxacin). The Packed Cell Volume (PCV) and Haemoglobin (Hb) of rats treated with extract and ciprofloxacin increased significantly ($p<0.05$) compared to the control while a non-significant decrease was observed in the Red Blood Cell (RBC) of rats administered only extract and ciprofloxacin after treatment. White Blood Cells (WBC) of rats given the extract significantly reduced while there was no significant difference in the lymphocyte count of rat administered the extract of *A. muricata* and ciprofloxacin. Neutrophils of rats in all groups significantly increased ($p<0.05$). However, the monocyte and eosinophil level were not significantly different from the control. Minimal disruption and reduction in nuclear clumping were observed in the liver of rats infected/treated with the extract. Similarly, there were prominent improvements in the glomerula architecture as well as the white and red pulp of the spleen after treatment with the extract of *A. muricata*.

Conclusion: The extract stimulated blood production and possessed restorative effect on various organs examined. However, excessive use might be toxic to the heart.

Keywords: Anonna muricata; Salmonella typhi; haematological; histopathological; rats.

1. INTRODUCTION

Different plants and their parts are used all over the world for various purposes. They have been reported as an efficient constituents of mostly used antioxidant, antibacterial, antifungal, antiulcer, anti-inflammatory, antiviral and anticancer agents. They have also been used for the prevention and treatment of different type of disease conditions [1]. The employment of alternative traditional medicine in the treatment of different ailments has enormously expanded in both developed and developing countries of the world due to their cheapness, efficacy and easy to come-by advantage [2]. Some plants of medicinal value are believed to also promote positive health and maintain resistance against infection by re-establishing body equilibrium and conditioning the body tissues [3].

Annona muricata (L.) also referred to as graviola, soursop or guanabana belongs to a family called *Annonaceae.* It is popularly grown across the tropical regions of the world [4]. The plant is known to produce an edible fruit that is green in colour, large, heart-shaped and 15–20 cm in diameter with a white fleshy mesocarp. The fruit is sometimes irregular, lopsided or curved due to abnormal carper formation or injury caused by insects. Soursop has a long, rich historical use in herbal medicine as well as a lengthy recorded indigenous use. Different medicinal properties and uses have been attributed to various parts of the tree. Generally, the fruit and its juice are used to combat worms and parasitic organisms, to cool fevers, increase breast milk production after birth, and as an astringent for diarrhea and dysentery. In addition, internal and external parasites, head lice, and worms are treated with crushed seeds of the plant [5].

Salmonella typhi is a non-spore forming Gram-negative bacterium. It is the causative agent of a systemic infection called typhoid fever. The clinical manifestations of the disease vary from a mild illness with low-grade fever, malaise, and slight dry cough to a severe clinical picture with abdominal discomfort and multiple complications. The infection is usually contracted by consumption of contaminated food and water [6]. Every year the disease affects at least 17million persons world-wide most of whom resides in the developing countries of South East Asia and Africa [7]. The antibacterial resistance problems associated with commonly used antibiotics as well as the re-emergence of multi-antibiotic resistant strains of this pathogen has become a possible threat to public health. Therefore, the search for effective antimicrobials is necessary [8]. Besides, toxicity is a measure of how poisonous a substance is, it shows the degree of adverse effects caused by the interaction of the toxicants with body cells. The possible effects produced depend on the chemical properties of the toxic substance and the cell membrane [9]. Similarly, blood components are exposed to significant concentrations of these toxic compounds as they form the medium for their transport. Hence, the evaluation of the toxic effects of unripe *Annona muricata* fruit extract on haematological and histopathological parameters in Swiss albino rats infected with *Salmonella typhi*.

2. MATERIALS AND METHODS

2.1 Plant Collection, Identification and Extraction of Bioactive Materials

Fresh unripe fruits of *Annona muricata* (Linn) were collected from a garden in Arimoro area of Ilesha, Osun State. The fruits were identified and authenticated by using the herbarium specimens of the Department of Crop, Soil and Pest management, Federal University of Technology, Akure (FUTA). Then the unripe *A. muricata* fruits were washed with sterile water. The peels and seeds were separated from the pulp and then cut into smaller pieces. The fruits were oven dried at 50℃ for 4 days. The dried fruits were then pulverized into fine powder by blending in a high-speed Philips Model blender. They were separately kept in an airtight container to avoid the absorption of moisture. Three hundred grams (300 g) of the powdered sample was soaked in two thousand, five hundred millilitres (2500 mL) of 70% ethanol as solvents to extract the bioactive compounds. The container was labeled appropriately and left for 72 hours (3 days). After which it was sieved using muslin cloth and then filtered using 0.45 μm micropore filter. The filtrates were vaporized to dryness using rotary evaporator and subsequently lyophilized to remove the extracting solvent. The ethanol extract was preserved in a sterile bottle at 4℃ until use [9,10].

2.2 Test Bacteria

Pure clinical isolate of *Salmonella typhi* was obtained from the stock culture of Don Bosco Catholic Hospital, Akure, Ondo State. The clinical *S. typhi* was isolated from a typhoid patient. The bacterium was further characterized in the laboratory using the methods of [11].

2.3 Experimental Animals

Forty-two Swiss albino rats (170-220 g) were obtained from Department of Animal Production and Health, Federal University of Technology, Akure, Ondo State, Nigeria. The rats were fed with standard rat pellets (Livestock Feeds, Ikeja, Lagos State) and water *ad libitum*. The animals were housed under standard laboratory conditions and were acclimatized for 7days before the treatment started. The experimental procedures involving animals were conducted in conformity with international, national and institutional guidelines as reported by [12].

2.4 Inclusion and Exclusion Criteria

Both sexes of the albino rats between 5-7 weeks old, healthy and with no previous exposure to antibiotics were used while rats that are more 7 weeks old, infected and exposed to antibiotics were excluded from this study.

2.5 Preparation of Standard Inoculum of *S. typhi* for *In vivo* Assay

The method described by [11] was employed. A 0.238 g of sodium hydrogen phosphate was dissolved in 0.019 g of potassium dihydrogen phosphate and sodium chloride respectively. The mixture was made up to 100 mL with distilled water and pH was adjusted to neutral (7). Then standard inoculum of *S. typhi* was inoculated into 1000 mL of nutrient broth and incubated for 24 hrs. After incubation, the cells were centrifuged at 2000 rpm for 10 minutes and the supernatant was discarded. Pellets were re-suspended in PBS and centrifuged again for four times. The final cell button was resuspended in PBS and serially diluted 10^1 to 10^6.

2.6 Determination of Infectious Dose (ID)

The method described by [13] was adopted. Twenty four Swiss albino rats were used to determine the ID of *S. typhi*. The rats were divided into six groups of four rats. Each group was infected with different concentrations of *S. typhi* suspension. The groups were closely monitored for seven days. The concentration of *S. typhi* suspension that produces the signs like unformed stool, weak, scattered fur, falling of hairs, stool with mucous and weight loss in animals given is taken as the infectivity dose (ID_{50}) of *S. typhi*. Also, corresponding colony-forming units per millilitres (cfu/mL) of the bacterial dilutions was determined using plate count method on *Salmonella-Shigella* agar (SSA).

2.7 *In-vivo* Bioassay

The *in-vivo* bioassay was carried out using the methods reported by [13] and [14]. A total number of eighteen rats were used and divided into six groups; Group 1 was infected with infective dose of *S. typhi* (calculated to be 6.8 X 10^6 cfu/mL) but was not treated with the extract while Group II was infected with the infective dose and then treated with the ethanolic extract of unripe *A. muricata* fruit after the infection had set in. Group III was given prophylactic dose 400 mg/mL extract of *A. muricata* for three days before being infected with *S. typhi*. Then Group IV was administered only extract of *A. muricata*; Group V was infected and treated with ciprofloxacin; while Group VI was fed with basal diet and water only. All the experimental rats in groups I, II, IV and V were observed for signs of infection before being treated.

2.7.1 Relative organ weight

After the experiment, all the animals were euthanized under chloroform anaesthesia. Organs such as heart, liver, kidney and spleen of the sacrificed animals were excised, washed with normal saline, examined for any lesions and weighed in grams to obtain the absolute organ weight [2]. The relative organ weights were calculated for each rat using;

$$Relative\ Organ\ Weight = \frac{Absolute\ organ\ weight\ (g)}{Body\ weight\ at\ Sacrifice\ (g)} \times 100$$

2.7.2 Haematological assay

Blood samples were collected before treatment through cardiac puncture while after the experiment, animals were sacrificed and incisions were quickly made in the sacrificed animal's cervical region and blood samples collected from the heart were dispensed into EDTA bottles for haematological analyses [2] and various analyses as described by [11] were carried out on the blood samples.

2.7.3 Histopathological assay

The histology of various organs was carried out using the method of [9]. The required organs were excised, weight and fixed in aqueous Bouin's solution for 48 hrs and were sequentially embedded in paraffin wax blocks according to the standard procedure, sectioned at 5 μ thickness. They were further deparaffined with xylol, and histologic observations were performed after staining with haematoxylin and eosin. The slides were examined under a light microscope and the magnified images of the tissues structure were captured.

2.8 Statistical Analysis

Mean values of replicates were reported with their standard deviations using SPSS 16.0. Analyses of Variance (ANOVA) were achieved to calculate significant differences in the treatment means, and the mean separations were achieved by Duncan's Multiple Range Test ($p \leq 0.05$).

3. RESULTS

3.1 Infectious Dose (ID) of *Salmonella typhi* on Experimental Rats

The dose of *Salmonella typhi* that produced infection signs like unformed stool, weakness, scattered fur, falling hairs, stool with mucous and weight loss in the experimental rats was 6.8 x 10^6 cfu/mL.

3.2 Effect of Treatment on Relative Organ Weights (ROW)

The effect of treatment on Relative Organ Weight (g/100 g) of the rats is shown in Table 1. The weights of liver, heart and spleen in all groups under observation were not significantly different from the control. However, a significant increase in the heart was observed in group IV and V given the extract and conventional antibiotics (ciprofloxacin).

3.3 Haematological Analysis

The results of the haematological analysis of the blood samples collected from the rats after treatment are shown in Table 2. In this study, there was no significant difference in the Erythrocyte Sedimentation Rate (ESR) level after treatment. The PCV of rats given extract (group IV) and ciprofloxacin (group V) increased significantly ($p<0.05$) compared to the control. Similarly, infected/treated group showed a significant increase in the PCV. The RBC of the rats administered with only extract and ciprofloxacin experienced an insignificant decrease. However, a significant increase ($p<0.05$) was reported for the infected/treated group. Also, the Hb significantly increased ($p<0.05$) in groups given only extract and ciprofloxacin as well as infected/treated group when compared to control after treatment.

The WBC of the group of rats given with extract (group IV) and ciprofloxacin (group V) significantly reduced ($p<0.05$) after treatment while the infected/treated group was not significantly different from the control. However, a significant increase ($p<0.05$) was observed in the group infected only with *S. typhi.*

When compared to control after treatment, the lymphocyte of rats given only extract (group IV) and infected-treated group (group V) were not significantly different while the neutrophils of rats in all groups after treatment significantly increased ($p<0.05$) when compared to the control. But the monocyte and eosinophil level were not significantly different from the control after treatment (Table 2). Basophil level significantly increased ($p<0.05$) in group administered only the extract of *A. muricata* while for other groups, the differences were not significant compared to the control.

3.4 Histological Analysis

The result of the histopathological examination carried out on the liver, kidney and spleen of the experimental rats is indicated on Plates 1A-3B. Less congested parenchyma, more distinct nuclei, improving polyhedral shape of the hepatocyte and the Kuffer's cell were observed in the infected/ treated group of rats.

Similarly, a more distinct glomerulus as well as the proximal and distal tubules filling the parenchyma, odematous space and disappearance of inflammatory cells in the glomerulus was observed in the histopathological examination of the kidney of infected/treated rats (Plate 2B).

The photomicrograph of the spleen revealed that the white and red pulp were visible. The white pulp (WP) has a centrally placed blood vessel called central arteriole while the red pulp (RP) consist of mild population of red blood cell (Plate 3A) while the white and red pulp of the infected/treated group of rats showed restoration in nuclear material and marginal zones respectively (Plate 3B).

4. DISCUSSION

Relative Organ Weight (ROW) is an important indicator of physiological and pathological status in animals. It is instrumental when diagnosing whether the organs was exposed to injury or not. In addition, heart, liver, kidney and spleen have been reported to be primary organs affected by metabolic reactions caused by toxicants [15]. The non-significant change observed in the liver, kidney and spleen weights in this study is similar to the works of [16] who reported that there was no significant change in the relative organ weights of liver, kidney and spleen of Swiss albino mice treated with hydro-methanolic extract of *Coriandrum sativum*. Similarly, [14] reported that differences in the relative weights of lungs, kidney, spleen and liver were not significant in rats administered with the extract of *Moringa oleifera* bark. Therefore, the non-significant change observed in most of these organs suggests that the extract may be virtually non-toxic. However, the slight increment observed in the relative weight of the heart in group IV and V compared to control is worthy of note. Cardiac glycosides which is the highest occurring phytochemical in the extract under study are known to improve cardiac output and reduces distention of the heart. Hence, their reported use in the treatment of congestive heart failure and cardiac arrhythmia. However, [17] reported the phytochemical to possess narrow therapeutic index and may cause intoxication at higher dose.

Table 1. Effect of treatment on relative weight of the organs

Groups	Relative organ weight (g/100 g)			
	Liver	Spleen	Heart	Kidney
Group 1	$2.93^{a}\pm0.07$	$0.84^{ab}\pm0.27$	$0.48^{ab}\pm0.05$	$1.23^{bc}\pm0.02$
Group 2	$2.79^{a}\pm0.05$	$0.64^{ab}\pm0.12$	$0.25^{a}\pm0.04$	$1.07^{b}\pm0.33$
Group 3	$2.97^{a}\pm0.08$	$0.67^{ab}\pm0.07$	$0.23^{a}\pm0.07$	$1.54^{c}\pm0.07$
Group 4	$2.79^{a}\pm0.12$	$1.02^{b}\pm0.09$	$0.58^{b}\pm0.16$	$1.15^{bc}\pm0.25$
Group 5	$3.08^{a}\pm0.08$	$0.50^{a}\pm0.17$	$0.99^{c}\pm0.02$	$0.60^{a}\pm0.09$
Group 6	$3.03^{a}\pm0.18$	$0.56^{ab}\pm0.85$	$0.28^{a}\pm0.07$	$0.99^{ab}\pm0.16$

Data are presented as Mean±S.E (n=3). Values with the same superscript letter(s) along the same column are not significantly different (P<0.05). Group 1 = Infected & untreated, Group 2 = Infected & treated with extract, Group 3= Given extract before infection, Group 4 = Given extract only, Group 5 = Infected & treated with Ciprofloxacin, Group 6 = Basal diet and water (Control)

Therefore, the increment in the relative weight of the heart reported in this study might be due to high presence of cardiac glycoside in the extract of *A. muricata*. Hence, its use should be controlled. The increased weight of the heart could also be an indication of cardiomegaly. Cardiomegaly is simply the enlargement of heart. A condition which results from stress such as high blood pressure, anaemia, cardiomyopathy and heart attack or underlying diseases suffered by the host.

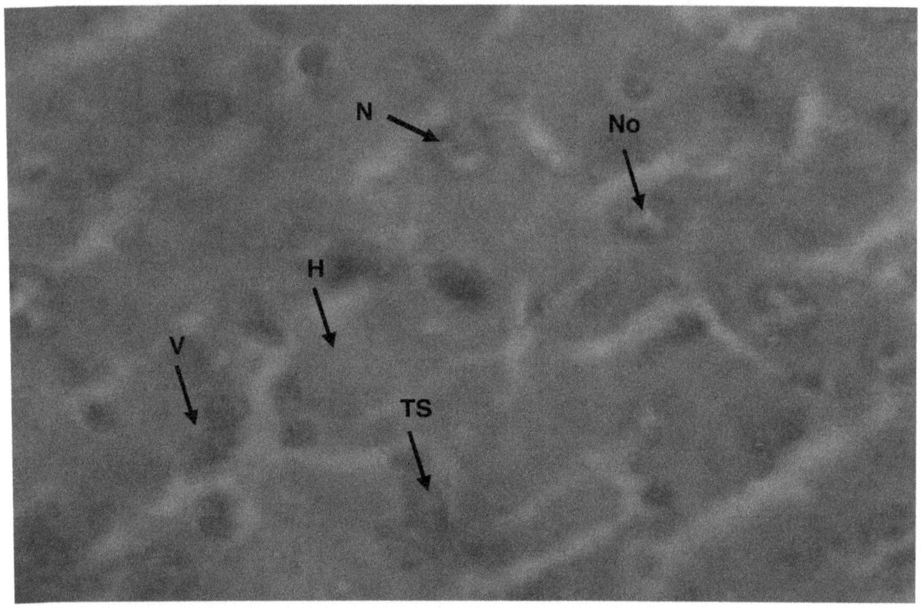

Plate 1a. Photomicrograph of a liver section of non-infected rats showing (a) polyhedral hepatocyte – h, (b) blurred trabecular structure – ts, (c) nucleus and the nucleolus -n & no, and (d) a clear intracytoplasmic lipid vacuoles in hepatocytes - v. H&e x400

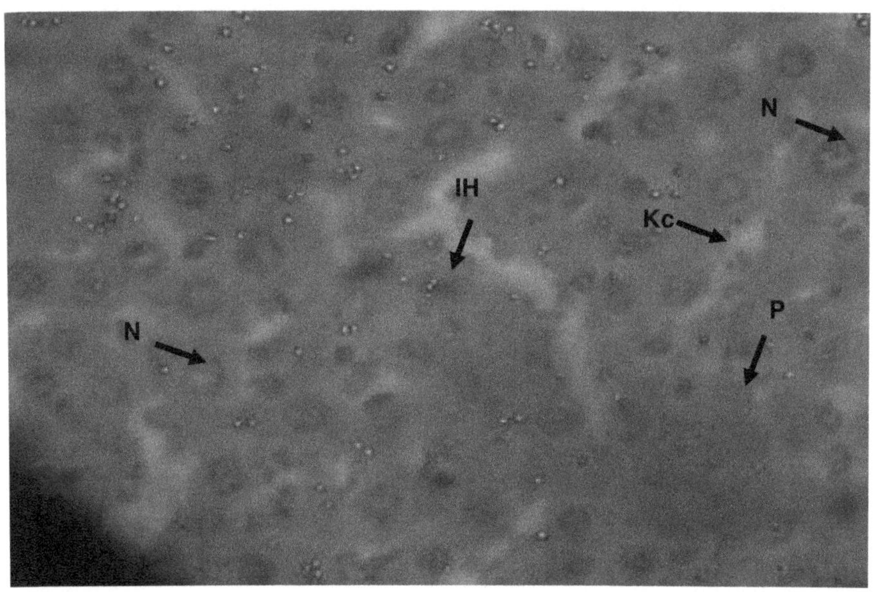

Plate 1b. Photomicrograph of a Section Liver of Rats Infected and treated with the extract of *A. muricata* showing (a) less congested parenchyma – P, (b) more distinct nucleus – N, (c) improving polyhedral shape of the hepatocyte – IH and the (d) Kuffer's cell – Kc. H&E X400

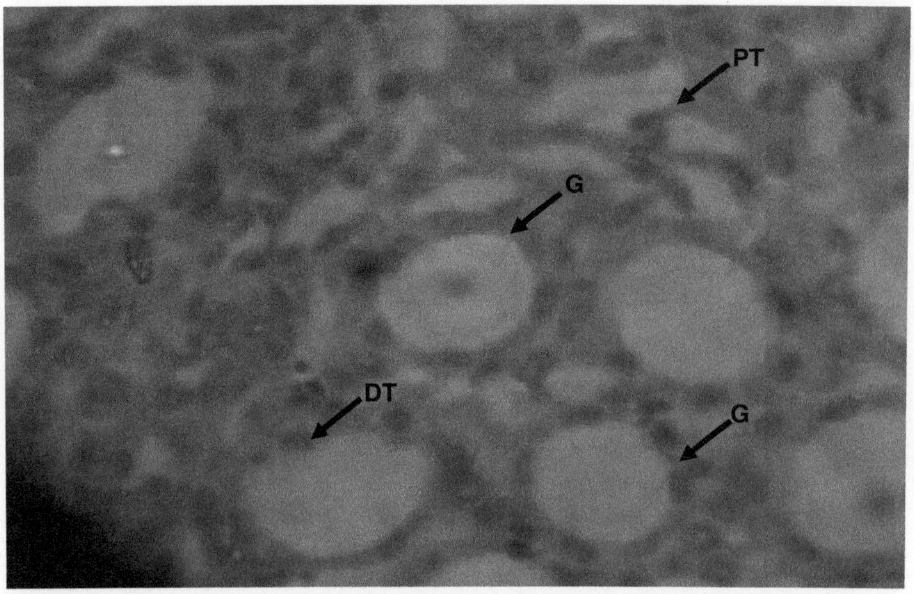

Plate 2a. Photomicrograph of a section kidney of the non-infected rats showing (a) normal glomerulus capsule - G, (b) distal tubule – DT and (c) proximal tubule. H&E x400

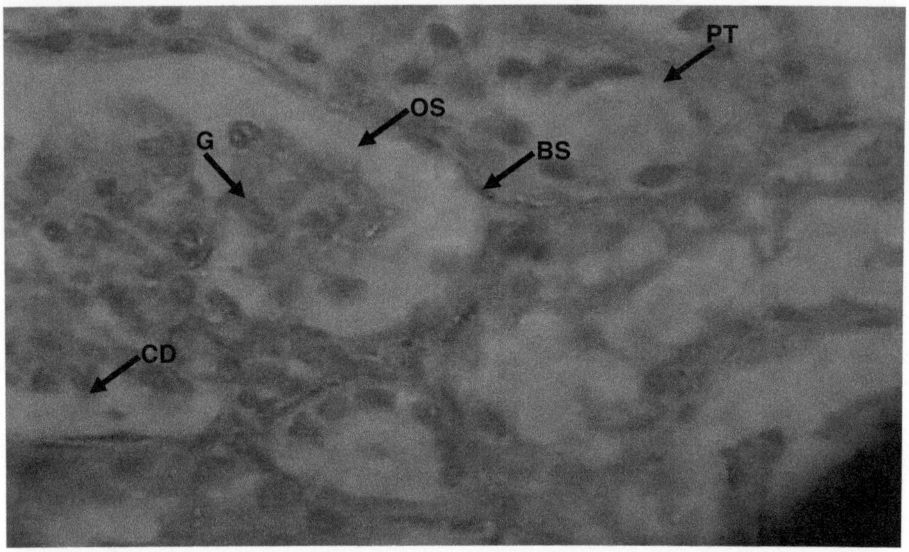

Plate 2b. Photomicrograph of a section kidney of rats infected and treated with the extract of *A. muricata* showing the (a) glomerulus – G, (b) Odematous space of the Glomerulus – OS, (c) Bowman's space – BS, (d) congested distal tubules – CD, and (e) proximal tubule – PT. H&E x 400

In this present study, the significant elevation ($p<0.05$) in the PCV and Hb of rat given only extract and the infected/treated group after the treatment corroborated the works of [18] who reported an increase in the PCV and Hb of rats treated with the leaf extract of *Voacanga africana*. However, the result differed from the findings of [19] who reported a non-significant difference in the PCV levels in the Wistar albino rats administered the ethanolic leaf extract of *Petroselinum crispum*. Odesanmi et al. [20] reported that the PCV and Hb levels of Dutch white rabbits administered the extract of *Tetrapleura tetraptera* remain unaffected. Packed Cell Volume is a measure of the volume of blood consisting of solid cells. Therefore, the increase in PCV and Hb in this study clearly indicates that the extract of *A. muricata* has a stimulatory property which ultimately results in increased blood volume. The extract possess the potential to stimulate the release of erythropoietin which is the hormonal regulator of RBC production from the kidney [21]. The stimulatory activity might be attributed to the presence of some active agents in the fruit extract of *A. muricata.* In addition, the increase in haemoglobin level observed implied an enhancement of the oxygen carrying capacity of the blood in the rats given the fruit extract of unripe *A. muricata.*

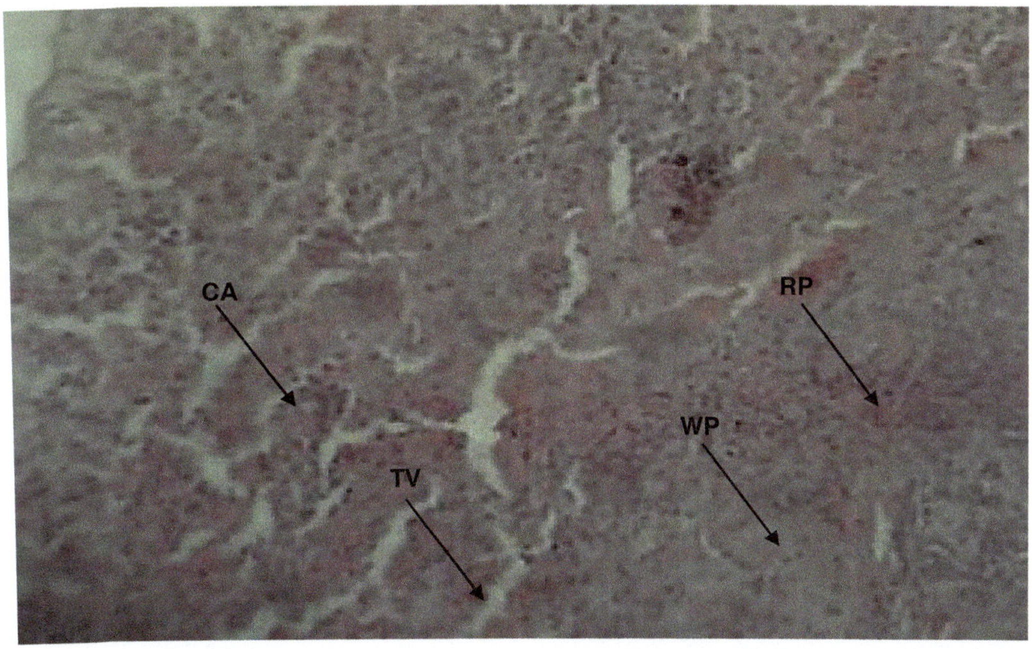

Plate 3a. Photomicrograph of a spleen section of non-infected rats showing (a) the trabecular vessel - TV, (b) white pulp - WP, (c) red pulp - RP and (d) a central arteriole - CA. H&E x400

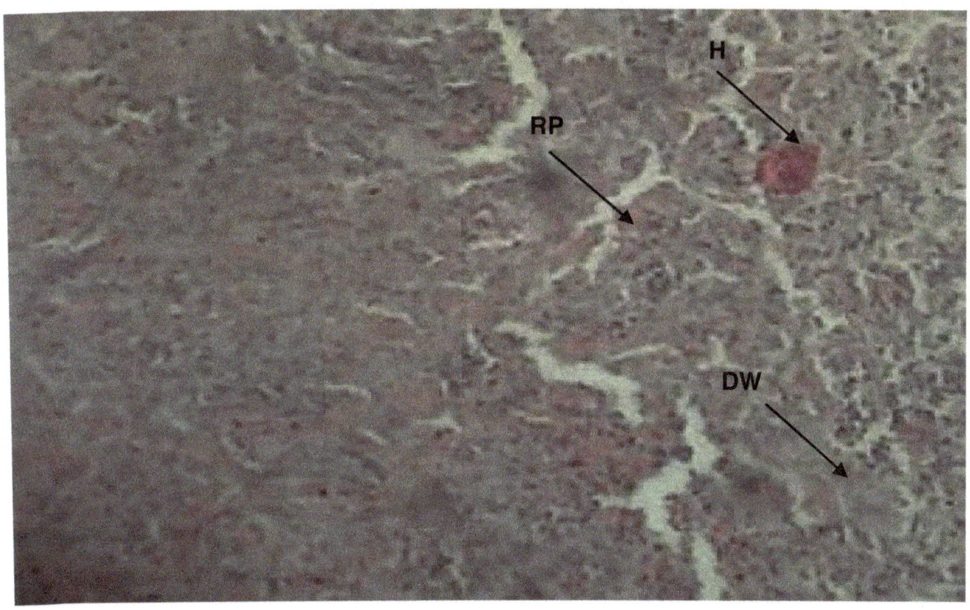

Plate 3b. Photomicrograph of a spleen section of rat infected and treated with the extract showing (a) normal structure with improvement in the red (RP) and white pulp (WP), (b) haemorrhage – H. H&E x400

Table 2. Haematological analysis after treatment

Groups	ERS (mm/hr)	PCV (%)	RBC (x10mc^3)	WBC (x10mc^3)	Hb (g/100mL)	Lymph (%)	Neutro (%)	Mono (%)	Eosin (%)	Baso (%)
Group 1	$4.00^{b}\pm0.58$	$40.00^{ab}\pm0.00$	$10.07^{c}\pm0.10$	$11.13^{e}\pm0.15$	$13.30^{ab}\pm0.17$	$66.00^{ab}\pm0.58$	$23.33^{cd}\pm0.88$	$7.33^{a}\pm0.88$	$2.33^{b}\pm0.33$	$0.35^{ab}\pm0.33$
Group 2	$1.50^{a}\pm0.28$	$42.00^{bc}\pm2.31$	$9.53^{c}\pm0.38$	$9.53^{cd}\pm0.26$	$13.88^{b}\pm0.70$	$69.00^{bcd}\pm0.58$	$21.50^{bc}\pm0.87$	$7.50^{a}\pm0.28$	$1.67^{ab}\pm0.33$	$0.67^{ab}\pm0.33$
Group 3	$2.00^{a}\pm0.00$	$40.00^{ab}\pm1.73$	$11.20^{d}\pm0.57$	$9.20^{c}\pm0.17$	$13.49^{ab}\pm0.69$	$67.00^{abc}\pm1.15$	$23.00^{bcd}\pm0.58$	$7.67^{a}\pm1.45$	$1.67^{ab}\pm0.33$	$0.67^{ab}\pm0.33$
Group 4	$2.00^{a}\pm0.00$	$43.00^{bc}\pm0.58$	$7.80^{ab}\pm0.17$	$8.10^{b}\pm0.06$	$14.86^{bc}\pm0.13$	$70.33^{cd}\pm0.33$	$19.33^{b}\pm0.33$	$8.00^{a}\pm0.58$	$1.00^{a}\pm0.00$	$1.33^{b}\pm0.33$
Group 5	$1.33^{a}\pm0.33$	$45.33^{c}\pm1.45$	$7.05^{a}\pm0.20$	$6.90^{a}\pm0.06$	$15.65^{c}\pm0.61$	$64.67^{a}\pm2.6$	$26.00^{d}\pm2.30$	$8.67^{a}\pm0.88$	$1.33^{ab}\pm0.33$	$0.33^{a}\pm0.33$
Group 6	$1.33^{a}\pm0.33$	$36.00^{a}\pm0.58$	$8.33^{b}\pm0.88$	$10.03^{d}\pm0.20$	$12.15^{a}\pm0.09$	$72.33^{d}\pm0.33$	$8.67^{a}\pm0.88$	$7.00^{a}\pm0.00$	$1.33^{ab}\pm0.33$	$0.00^{a}\pm0.00$

Data are presented as Mean±S.E (n=3). Values with the same superscript letter(s) along the same column are not significantly different ($P<0.05$).
Group 1 = Infected & untreated, Group 2 = Infected & treated with extract,
Group 3 = Given extract before infection, Group 4 = Given extract only,
Group 5 = Infected & treated with Ciprofloxacin,
Group 6 = Basal diet and water (Control)

The insignificant decrease observed in the RBCs of rats administered only the extract of *A. muricata* after treatment in this study corroborated the earlier findings of [21] who reported that the aqueous flower extract of *Hibiscus sabdariffa* had a non-significant decrease in level of RBC of rats at 400 mg/ml. However, the result is in contrast to the findings of [22] reported a significant increase in the RBC of albino rats treated with the leaf extract of *Mangifera indica*. This non-significant decrease might suggest a gradual tendency of the extract of *A. muricata* to possess an adverse effect on the bone marrow or haemoglobin metabolism in such group of rats. Similarly, saponin reported to be present in the extract [23] under study has been demonstrated to be haemolytic [24]. However, the significant increase ($p<0.05$) in RBC observed in the infected/treated group might be due to the ability of the extract to slow down the processes involved in oxidative breakdown of RBC membrane by the microorganism.

The significant increase ($p<0.05$) observed in the neutrophil level across all groups in this study is similar to the findings of [13] who reported a significant increase in all groups of rats treated with the leaf extract of *O. gratissimum*. However, this result differed from previous findings of [19] who reported a significant decrease in the level of neutrophils in Wistar albino rats when treated with leave extract of *P. crispum*. The neutrophils possess inconspicuous organelles known as primary and secondary granules which contain lytic enzymes and bactericidal substances. These granules help digest foreign materials after it is phagocytosed. They also use oxygen dependent and oxygen independent pathways that generate additional antimicrobial substances to kill ingested microorganisms [25]. Therefore, the increase observed in the neutrophil level was justified since it responds primarily to infection caused by bacteria.

Also, the insignificant change observed in the level of eosinophil and monocyte in this study agreed with the findings of [19] who reported a non-significant difference in the eosinophil levels in the Wistar albino rats administered the ethanolic leaf extract of *Petroselinum crispum*. Eosinophils are important in the defense against protozoan and helminth parasites mainly by releasing cationic peptides and reactive oxygen immediately into the extracellular fluid [25]. Hence, its non-significant change in infection involving bacteria as obtained in this study. In sub-acute oral toxicity study, non-toxic nature of extract is indicated by lack of significant changes in the blood parameters because it is one of the most sensitive targets of toxic substances [14]. Hence, this result suggests that the extract of unripe *A. muricata* did not interfere with the activities eosinophil and monocytes.

The significantly increase ($p<0.05$) in basophil level of rats administered only the extract of *A. muricata* is in agreement with the findings of [26] who reported that the basophil level of group of rats treated with aqueous fruit extract of *Solanum macrocarpum* increased significantly ($p<0.05$). Basophils are non-phagocytic cells that release specific compounds called vasoactive mediators from their cytoplasmic granules in response to different stimulations. They possess high affinity receptors for the type of antibody associated with allergic response [25]. Hence, the observed increase in basophil in this study is indicative of the likelihood of the fruit extract of *A. muricata* to possess allergic properties.

The WBC of the group of rats given the extract (group IV) and ciprofloxacin (group V) significantly reduced ($p<0.05$) after treatment. This result agreed with the works of [20] who reported a decrease in the WBC of Dutch white rabbits treated with ethanolic fruit extract of *Tetrapleura tetraptera*. However, this result differed from the findings of [18] who reported an increase in the level of WBC in rats given the extracts of *Voacanga africana*. Granulocytes regulate the proliferation, differentiation and maturation of committed stem cells responsible for the production of WBC [25]. Thus, some components of the extract might have interfered with the sensitivity of the stem cells responsible for the production of WBCs. The decrease in the WBC suggests an impairment in the ability of the extract of unripe *A. muricata* fruits to stimulate production of WBCs. However, the significant increase ($p<0.05$) in the group infected only with *S. typhi* was expected as literatures have shown that WBCs are produced rapidly in response to infection [25]. The insignificant difference observed in lymphocytes of rats given only extract (group IV) and infected/treated group (group V) could suggest the beneficial effect of the extract in improving the immunity and general well-being of the animals [2].

The result of the histopathological examination carried out on the liver, kidney and spleen of the experimental rats is indicated on Plates 1A-3B. The less congested parenchyma, more distinct nuclei, improving polyhedral shape of the hepatocyte and the Kuffer's cell observed in the group of rats infected/ treated suggests that the extract had a restorative effect on the liver architecture. This result is in agreement with the findings of [20] who reported that the extract of *Tetrapleura tetraptera* did not reveal any gross damage to tissue of the liver in experimental animals that received the dose of the extract.

The more distinct glomerulus as well as the proximal and distal tubules filling the parenchyma observed in the histopathological examination of the kidney of infected/treated rat suggests that the extract of *A. muricata* partially improved the architecture of the kidney. The improved structure of the glomerula is in agreement with a previous report that the leaf extract of *Moringa oleifera* did not produce adverse effect on the kidney of experimental animals [27]. However, odematous space observed is indicative of adverse activity. This result is comparable with the findings of [28] who reported that standardized methanolic extract of *Mitragyna speciosa* revealed some abnormal morphological characteristics in all treated rats. The partial improvement in the kidney structure after treatment may indicate that the period of treatment was not sufficient for good protection/restoration against the adverse effect of infection. It is therefore suggested that a varied period of treatment should be employed in further studies. In addition, the gradual disappearance of inflammatory cells in the glomerulus in the treated rats as against the inflammed glomerulus observed in the rats infected with *S. typhi* may be due to the anti-inflammatory activity of terpenoids detected in the extract [29].

In this study, there was not much difference in the spleen architecture of rats in the control group compared to the rats infected/treated with the extract. This suggests that the extract has a protective effect on the largest lymphoid organ of the body. This result is in agreement with works of [30] who reported that the extract of *Moringa oleifera* leaves maintained the structural integrity of the spleen tissue of murine models used. This confirmed previous reports that *A. muricata* promotes immune responses [5]. However, the haemorrhage observed on the spleen of the rats infected/treated (Plate 3B) may be due to the mechanical injury done to the tissue during excision of the organ for histopathological examination. Therefore, it is opinioned that the protective effects of detoxification carried out by the liver may explain the preserved architecture spleen in this study.

5. CONCLUSION

This present study showed that the extract of unripe *Annona muricata* fruit has stimulatory effect on the blood production and possesses restorative effect on various organs examined in this study. However, excessive use might be toxic to heart. Therefore, it is recommended that further research should be carried out using varying concentrations of the extract in order to determine its dose dependent effects.

CONSENT

It is not applicable.

ETHICAL APPROVAL

All authors hereby declare that "Principles of laboratory animal care" (NIH publication No. 85-23, revised 1985) were followed, as well as specific national laws where applicable. All experiments have been examined and approved by the appropriate ethics committee.

COMPETING INTERESTS

Authors have declared that no competing interests exist.

REFERENCES

1. Alshawsh MA, Abdulla MA, Salmah I, Zahra AA, Suhailah WQ, Hamid AH, et al. Free radical scavenging, antimicrobial and immunomodulatory activities of *Orthosiphon stamineus*. Molecules. 2012; 17:5385-5395.
2. Larbie C, Arthur FKN, Woode E, Terlabi EO. Evaluation of acute and subchronic toxicity of *A. muricata* (Linn) aqueous extract in animals. Euro. J. Exp. Bio. 2011;1(4):115-124.
3. Kumar UA, Manjunath C, Thaminzhmani T, Kran YR, Brahmaiah Y. A review on immunomodulatory activity of plants. Indian J. Novel Drug Delivery. 2012;4(2): 93-103.
4. Rajeswari DV, Gajalakshmi S, Vijayalakshmi S. Phytochemical and pharmacological properties of *Annona*

muricata: A review. Inter. J. Pharm. and Pharm. Sciences. 2012;2(4):3-6.

5. Taylor L. *Technical data report for graviola* (*A. muricata*) In: The healing power of rainforest herbs. Sage Press Inc. Austin; 2005.
6. Iroha IR, Ilang DC, Ayogu TE, Oji AE, Ugbo EC. Screening for anti-typhoid activity of some medicinal plants used in traditional medicine in Ebonyi State, Nigeria. Afri. J. Pharm. Pharmacog. 2010;4(12):860-864.
7. Khanam F, Sayeed MA, Choudhury FK, Sheikh A, Ahmed D, Goswami D, Hossain ML, Brooks A, Calderwood SB, Charles RC, Cravioto A, Ryan ET, Qadri F. Typhoid fever in young children in Bangladesh: Clinical findings, antibiotic susceptibility pattern and immune responses. PLoS. Negl. Trop. Dis. 2015;9(4):e0003619. DOI: 10.1371/journal.pntd.0003619
8. Seanego CT, Ndip RN. Identification and antibacterial evaluation of bioactive compounds from *Garcinia kola* (Heckel) Seeds. Molecules. 2012;17:6569-6584.
9. Jothy SL, Zakaria Z, Chen Y, Lau YL, Latha LY, Sasidharan S. Acute oral toxicity of methanolic seed extract of *Cassia fistula* in Mice. Molecules. 2011;16:5268-5282.
10. Nweke CN, Ibiam OFA. Pre and post harvest fungi associated with the soft rot of the fruit of *Annona muricata* and their effects on the nutrient content of the pulp. Am. J. Food & Nutri. 2012;2(4):78-85.
11. Cheesbrough M. District laboratory practice in Tropical countries. 2nd edition, Cambridge University Press, UK; 2006.
12. Adewole SO, Caxton-Martins EA. Morphological changes and hypoglycemic effects of *A. muricata* Linn. (Annonaceae) leaf aqueous extract on Pancreatic B-cells of Streptozotocin-Treated diabetic rats. Afri. J. Biomed. Res. 2006;9:173-187.
13. Dada EO, Komolafe OI.. In vivo evaluation of the inhibitory effects of *Ocimum gratissimum* on *Salmonella typhi*. Intl. J. Pharm. & Biol. Res. 2013; 4(4):185-191.
14. Reddy YRR, Lokanatha O, Ratnam KSVP, Reddy CS, Naga Raju I, Reddy CD. Acute and sub acute toxicity of *Moringa oleifera* stem bark extract in Swiss albino mice. Intl. J. Life Sci. Biotechnol. & Pharma Res. 2013;2(4):73-84.
15. Diallo A, Gbeassor M, Vovor A, Eklu-Gadegbeku K, Akilikokou K. Effect of *Tectonagrandis* on phenylhydrazine-induced anaemia in rats. Fitoterapia. 2008;79:332-336.
16. Patel D, Desai S, Devkar R, Ramachandran AV. Acute and sub-chronic toxicological evaluation of hydro-methanolic extract of *Coriandrum sativum* L. Seeds. EXCLI Journal. 2012;11:566-575.
17. Patel RP, Patel, MP. Cardiotonic activity of isolated cardiac glycoside from the fruits of *Corchorus aestuans* (Linn). Intl. Res. J. Pharm. 2012;3(7):239-242.
18. Omodamiro OD, Nwankwo CI. The effects of *Voacanga africana* leaf extract on serum lipid profile and haematological parameters on albino wistar rats. Euro. J. Exp. Biol. 2013;3(3):140-148.
19. Awe EO, Banjoko SO. Biochemical and haematological assessment of toxic effects of the leaf ethanol extract of *Petroselinum crispum* (Mill) Nyman ex A.W. Hill (Parsley) in rats. BMC Complem. & Altern. Med. 2013;13:75-80.
20. Odesanmi SO, Lawal RA, Ojokuku SA. Haematological effects of ethanolic fruit extract of *Tetrapleura tetraptera* in male Dutch witch rabbits. Res. J. Med. Plants. 2010;4(4):213-217.
21. Ejere VC, Nnamonu EI, Chukwuka CO, Ugwu GC, Ejim AO, Asogwa CN. Effect of aqueous extract of *Hibiscus sabdariffa* calyces on haematological characteristics of *Rattus novergicus*. Anim. Res. Intl. 2013;10(3):1809-1816.
22. Ogbe RJ, Adenkole AY, Anefu E. Aqueous ethanolic extract of *Mangifera indica* stem bark effect on the biochemical and haematological parameters of albino rats. Arch. Appl. Sci. Res. 2012;4(4):1618-1622.
23. Dada, EO, Faleye, OS. Studies on the phytochemical and proximate properties of the extract of unripe *Annona muricata* (L.) fruit. Intl. J. Pharm. & Biosci; 2015. (In press).
24. Okwu DE. Phytochemicals, vitamins and mineral content of two Nigerian medicinal plants. Intl. J. Mol. & Adv. Sci. 2005;1:375-381.
25. Willey JM, Sherwood LM, Woolverton CJ. Microbiology. 7th edition. McGraw Hill Publisher, New York; 2008.
26. Sodipo OA, Abdulrahman FI, UK Sandebe, Wanpana B. Comparative haematological parameters of aqueous fruit extracts of *Solanum macrocarpum*, α-solanidine and standard lipid lowering agents on triton-induced hyperlipidaemic rats. Wudpecker

J. Pharm. & Pharmacol. 2013;2(1):006-014.
27. Ezejindu DN, Udemezue OO, Akingboye AJ. Protective effects of *Moringa oleifera* leaf extract on the kidneys of adult wistar rats. Am. J. Eng. Res. 2014;3(2):157-161.
28. Harizal SN, Mansor SM, Hasnan J, Tharakan JKJ, Abdullah J. Acute toxicity study of the standardized methanolic extract of *Mitragyna speciose* Korth in Rodent. J. Ethnopharm. 2010;131:404-409.
29. Al- Harbi HA, Tarek RR, Abu Zinadah OA. Histological and histochemical studies on the effect of *Rhzya stricta* extract on the mice and the possible protective role against *Leuris quinquestriatus* scorpion Venam. Global Adv. Res. J. Environ. Sci. & Toxicol. 2012;1(9):226-234.
30. Owolabi JO, Ogunnaike PO. Histological evaluation of the effects of Moringa leaf extract treatment on vital organs of murine models. J. Med. and Medical Sci. 2014; 2(10):245-257.

8

Formulation and Evaluation of Dexibuprofen Transdermal Films in Rabbits

Boushra Mohamed El-Houssieny[1], Esmat Zein El-Dein[2] and Hussien Mohamed El-Messiry[1*]

[1]Department of Pharmaceutics, National Organization of Drug Control and Research, Giza, Egypt.
[2]Department of Pharmaceutical Technology, Faculty of Pharmacy, Tanta University, Tanta, Egypt.

Authors' contributions

This work was carried out in collaboration between all authors. Authors BMEH, EZED and HMEM designed the experiments. Author HMEM carried out the study and wrote the first draft of the manuscript. All authors read and approved the final manuscript.

Article Information

Editor(s):
(1) Syed A. A. Rizvi, Department of Pharmaceutical Sciences, College of Pharmacy, Nova Southeastern University, USA.
Reviewers:
(1) Eugenio Ragazzi, University of Padova, Italy.
(2) Syed Umer Jan, University of Balochistan, Quetta, Pakistan.

ABSTRACT

Dexibuprofen is a practically water-insoluble nonsterodial anti-inflammatory drug. Following previous experience on enhancing the solubility of the drug, a mixed hydrotropic solubilization technique was here applied in order to improve the aqueous solubility of the drug so that a soluble form of dexibuprofen was prepared and then could be used as a main active ingredient in transdermal films. Nine formulae were prepared applying 3^2 full factorial design using different amounts of hydroxypropylmethylcellulose (HPMC) and polyvinylpyrrolidone K30 (PVP K30). The prepared formulae were evaluated for their physical properties, loading efficacy and *In-vitro* dissolution studies adopting the USP XXII dissolution method type V paddle over disk apparatus method. Permeation studies were done for best three films showing higher dissolution rate using Franz cell apparatus and also bioavailability study was carried out on the best formula to compare the absorption of dexibuprofen from the prepared film (treatment A) to commercial tablets (treatment B) following administration of a single dose to rabbits. The prepared films were off-white color, opaque, smooth, moist and non-sticky. Increasing the amounts of HPMC and PVP K30 lead to increasing weight, folding endurance, tensile strength, moisture content and moisture

**Corresponding author: E-mail: hussienelmessiry@hotmail.com*

absorption. Transdermal films containing higher concentrations of PVP K30 and lower concentration of HPMC showed higher rate and amount of dexibuprofen released from dissolution medium and Franz cell. The bioavailability study showed that (T_{max}) in treatments A and B is 3 hours and 2 hours respectively. The average peak plasma concentration values (C_{max}) were 28.98±3.36 and 34.67±0.61 ug/mL, respectively and the $AUC_{0\text{-}\infty}$ values were 145.82±13.09 and 117.44±3.15 μg·h/mL, respectively. There were significant differences between treatments A and B in C_{max}, $t_{(1/2)}ab$, K_{el}, $t_{(1/2)}el$, *TCR*, $AUC_{0\text{-}8}$, $AUC_{0\text{-}\infty}$, $AUMC_{0\text{-}8}$, $AUMC_{0\text{-}\infty}$, and *MRT*. While the difference was insignificant in K_{ab}.

Keywords: Dexibuprofen; transdermal films; bioavailability; rabbits.

1. INTRODUCTION

Being the largest organ in the body, skin plays an important role by offering selective entrance of molecules and preventing access of noxious matters through it though having nano level of span. Therefore, the administration of drug particles topically has attracted researchers for developing an effective and suitable drug delivery system [1]. Transdermal drug delivery offers many important advantages, for instance, it is easy and painless, it protects the active compound from gastric enzymes, and it avoids the hepatic first-pass effect, controls absorption rate, variations in delivery rates, interference due to the presence of food, increases patient compliance, suitable for unconscious patients and enables fast termination of drug delivery, if needed. However, skin is a natural barrier, which is mainly composed of lipids & proteins and only a few drugs can penetrate the skin easily and in sufficient quantities to be effective [2]. Dexibuprofen ((S)-(+)-ibuprofen), which has better anti-inflammatory effects than ibuprofen and less gastric damage potential belongs to class II of the Biopharmaceutical Classification System (BCS) having low water solubility which is the rate limiting step in absorption of drug [3,4]. Following previous experience of our laboratory [5], the aim of the present work was to prepare and evaluate a transdermal film containing a soluble form of dexibuprofen as a main active ingredient.

2. MATERIALS AND METHODS

2.1 Materials

Dexibuprofen ((S)-(+)-ibuprofen) standard was purchased from Sigma-Aldrich (St. Louis, MO, USA). Dexibuprofen raw material was a gift from Future Pharmaceutical Industries (FPI) (Badr city, Cairo, Egypt). Distilled water was prepared in Central Nervous System (CNS) lab, National Organization of Drug Control and Research (NODCAR) (Dokki, Giza, Egypt). Acetonitrile HPLC grade, hydroxylpropylmethylcellulose (HPMC), dibutyl phethalate (DBP), methanol AR, ethanol, acetone and polyvinylpyrrolidone K30 (PVP K30) were purchased from Sigma-Aldrich (Taufkirchen, Germany). Acetic acid, sodium citrate dihydrate, ethylenediaminetetraacetic acid (EDTA) and urea were purchased from Medex (Medical Export Co Ltd, Near Naseby, Northamptonshire, UK).

2.2 Equipment

Analytical balance (Sartorius AG, Goettingen, Germany). Dissolution Test Station (Hanson Research, SR8 Plus, Chatsworth, USA). Drying Oven Digit (Raypa - R. Espinar, S.L., Barcelona, Spain). Hot plate and stirrer (Jenway, Dunmow, Essex, UK). pH meter (Jenway, Dunmow, Essex, UK). Ultrasonic water bath (Crest Ultrasonics Shanghai Ltd., Song Jiang, Shanghai, China). UV-VIS spectrophotometer (UV-2450, Shimadzu, Nakagyo-ku, Kyoto, Japan), Franz cell apparatus (Hanson Research, Variomag-Telemodul 40-S, USA), High performance liquid chromatography (HPLC) (Agilent 1200 series, USA).

2.3 Preparation of Soluble form of Dexibuprofen

Soluble form of dexibuprofen was prepared applying mixed the hydrotropic solubilization technique [5]. As hydrotropic agents, sodium citrate and urea were used to solubilize dexibuprofen in ratio (1: 3: 7.5). A minimum possible quantity of distilled water at 80-85°C contained in a 250 mL beaker was used to dissolve the urea and sodium citrate. Then, dexibuprofen was added at 30-40°C and stirred in beaker using a magnetic stirrer, maintaining the temperature at 30-40°C. Dexibuprofen was completely solubilized. Stirring was continued until a semisolid mass was obtained in the beaker. The semisolid mass obtained was spread on several watch glasses in thin layers at 40℃ for drying. When the mass became pulverizable, it was triturated with the help of mortar and pestle and again kept in oven for drying. After almost complete drying, the powder of the solid dispersion was passed through sieve #100 and was kept for 6 days in a desiccator containing silica gel and stored in air-tight containers.

2.4 Preparation of Transdermal Films

Transdermal films were prepared by solvent casting technique [6,7]. A 3^2 full factorial design (Table 1) was applied to formulate the matrix type transdermal film and to determine the effect of each polymer on release pattern of drug from transdermal drug delivery system. HPMC and dexibuprofen soluble form (230 mg equivalent to 20 mg dexibuprofen) were dissolved in 10 ml water. PVP K30 and 0.1 ml dibutyl phethalate were dissolved in 5 ml blend of acetone and ethanol (50:50). Then, both solutions were mixed and stirred on magnetic stirrer to accomplished homogeneous mixture. After vortexing the homogenous mixture was poured into a plastic mold (40 mm diameter lubricated previously using minute amount of glycerin for the easy removal of the films). The plastic mold was then kept in a clean room for solvent evaporation and after 48 hours, the films were withdrawn and stored in a desiccator until further use.

Table 1. Full factorial experimental design layout

Batch	HPMC (mg)	PVP K30 (mg)
F1	100	25
F2	100	50
F3	100	75
F4	150	25
F5	150	50
F6	150	75
F7	200	25
F8	200	50
F9	200	75

2.5 Evaluation of Transdermal Films

2.5.1 Physical properties

The physical properties test were done in triplicate, mean and standard deviation (SD) were calculated.

2.5.1.1 Physical appearance

The prepared films were evaluated for their physical appearance-opaque/ transparent, smooth/ wrinkled, moist/dry, flexible/tough, sticky/non-sticky [8].

2.5.1.2 Uniformity of weight

Weight variation was studied by individually weighing 10 randomly selected patches and calculating the average weight/cm^2 [9].

2.5.1.3 Folding endurance

Folding endurances were measured to determine the ability of patch to withstand or rupture. Folding endurance of films was determined by continually folding a small strip of film (2cm × 2 cm) at the same place until it broke. The number of times film can be folded at the same place without breaking was the folding endurance value of that prepared transdermal film [10].

2.5.1.4 Tensile strength

The tensile strength was determined by using a modified pulley system. It contains two clamps, one fixed and other movable. The strip of the patch (2×1 cm^2) was cut and hold between these two clamps. Weight was gradually increased on the pan, to increase the pulling force until the patch broke. The force required to break the film was considered as a tensile strength and it was calculated as kg/cm^2 [11].

2.5.1.5 Flatness

Three longitudinal strips were cut from each film at different portions like one from center, other one from left side and another one from right side. The length of each strip was measured, and then it was kept for 2 hours [12] and the variation in length was measured by determining percent constriction by using formula [7]: Flatness = $(L1-L2)/L1 \times 100$ where L1 is the initial length of each strip and L2 is the final length of each strip. Zero percent constriction is equivalent to 100 percent flatness.

2.5.1.6 Percent moisture content

To determine the percentage of moisture content, the films were weighed individually and kept in desiccators containing activated silica at room temperature for 24 hours. Individual films were weighed repeatedly, until they showed a constant weight. The percentage of moisture content was calculated as the difference between initial and final weight with respect to initial weight, Percentage moisture content= [(initial weight -final weight) /initial weight] X 100 [13].

2.5.1.7 Percent moisture absorption

The percent moisture absorption test was carried out to check the physical stability of the transdermal films at high humid conditions. In the present study the moisture absorption capacity of the films was determined as follows. Three 1.00 cm diameter films were cut out and weighed accurately then the films were placed in desiccator containing saturated solution of aluminum chloride keeping the humidity inside the desiccator at 79.5%; after 3 days the films were removed, weighed and percentage moisture was calculated. Average percentage moisture absorption of the three films was found. Percentage moisture absorption= [(final weight - initial weight) /initial weight] X 100 [14].

2.5.2 Determination of loading efficacy

Accurately weighted 20 mg of pure drug was dissolved in 100 ml of methanol to prepare the standard solution and it was then suitably diluted with distilled water (1:10). Equivalent to 20 mg of drug, each film was dissolved, diluted suitably with distilled water and filtrated. The standard and sample solutions were then analyzed using UV Spectrophotometer at 222 nm wavelength [5]. The amount of drug loading was then calculated by comparing the absorbance of standard and test solution. The concentration of the drug was calculated. Each sample was assayed in triplicate and an average, SD of three determinations was calculated.

2.5.3 *In-vitro* dissolution studies

In-vitro dissolution studies of the different prepared films were performed adopting the USP XXII dissolution method type V paddle over disk apparatus method [15]. A disk assembly holding the film was located in the bottom of the vessel. Five hundred mL of phosphate buffer (pH 5.5) was used as dissolution media at 32±0.5℃ maintaining stirring speed at 50 rpm. The samples were withdrawn at specified time intervals and replaced with an equivalent volume of fresh dissolution medium at different time intervals to keep the volume constant and estimated spectrophotometrically at λ max 222 nm for dissolving drug using phosphate buffer (pH 5.5) as blank [16]. All dissolution tests were performed in triplicate and an average ± SD of the three determinations was calculated.

2.5.4 Permeation studies

Permeation studies were done for best three films showing higher dissolution using Franz cell apparatus. Franz cell consists of an upper donor compartment and the lower receptor compartment surrounded by water jacket to maintain the temperature of receptor phase at 37±1℃. Films coated with artificial membrane (membrane-cell, Serva) presoaked in buffer solution for 24 hours were placed in upper donor compartments. A three mL phosphate buffer (pH 5.5) was filled in each receptor compartments. The uniformity of the solution in the receptor phase was maintained by stirring at a speed of 600 rpm using a tiny Teflon coated magnetic bead. From each receptor compartment of Franz cell, samples of 3 mL from each compartment were withdrawn at the specific time intervals for estimation of drug content. The receptor phase was immediately replaced with fresh receptor solvent stored at 37±1℃ [17]. The collected samples were filtered through membrane filter, diluted 1:5 with distilled water and were analyzed by UV spectrophotometer at a detection wavelength 222 nm using phosphate buffer (pH 5.5) as blank. All tests were performed in triplicate and an average ± SD of the three determinations was calculated.

2.5.5 Bioavailability study

2.5.5.1 Study design

Study was carried out to compare the absorption of dexibuprofen from the prepared film showing higher release from Franz diffusion cell (treatment A) to commercial tablets, Dexa-ibufen 400 product of Hochster Pharmaceutical Industries, Egypt (treatment B) following administration of a single dose each using randomized cross over design.

A total number of twelve white male rabbits (Boskat breed) weighing from 2-2.5 kg were used as a model animals for determining the bioavailability of dexibuprofen. They were divided into two groups of six rabbits each. Animals were obtained from the animal house of the NODCAR; the ethical protocol for this study was approved by the head of NODCAR and the manager of the Animal House. Animals were kept individually in cages with wire-mesh bases constructed of galvanized steel for two weeks before treatment for acclimatization in a room with controlled lighting (14 h/day), constant temperature (16-20℃) and relative humidity (55-65%). Sick, injured and abnormal animals were eliminated. Rabbits were fed a commercial pellet diet and water *ad libitum*.

Six films were applied on the rabbits' back after removal of the hair (treatment A) and five tablets were well pulverized and suspended in 500 mL distilled water. Five mL from each treatment were given orally to each rabbit with oral cannula (treatment B). Blood samples (2 mL) were collected prior to administration and after 0.25, 0.5, 0.75, 1, 1.5, 2, 4, 6 and 8 hours of drug administration. Blood samples were transferred to a series of graduated centrifuge tubes containing EDTA.

Samples were centrifuged at 2,500 rpm for 5 min. Plasma was separated and transferred into another set of sample tubes and frozen until assay. The dexibuprofen concentration in blood samples was analyzed using the modified HPLC method [18].

2.5.5.2 Chromatographic conditions

The mobile phase was composed of acetonitrile (HPLCgrade): acetate buffer: acetic acid 0.1M (65:35:0.3 v/v/v) with the pH adjusted if required to 5.5±0.1 using acetic acid 0.1 M. The mobile phase was degassed for 20 min in an ultrasonic bath prior to use. HPLC system was equipped with a column (Phenomenex, Synergi, 4 µm polar-RP 80A, 100 × 4.6 mm, USA). Chromatography was performed at a flow rate of 2 mL/min at 25℃ [18]. All solutions were filtered through a 0.45 µm membrane prior to use. The channel on the diode-array detector was configurated to acquire data at 222 nm. The injection volume was 20 µL. The column was equilibrated for a minimum of 30 min with the mobile phase flowing through the system before injection of the drug standards. The run time was set at 5 min with the system operating at an air-conditioned temperature of 25℃.

2.5.5.3 Preparation of stock and standard working solutions

Stock solutions of dexibuprofen (1 mg/mL) were freshly prepared by dissolving 100 mg of dexibuprofen standard in 100 mL acetonitrile. The standard stock solutions were stored at 4℃ in a clear glass volumetric flask and light protected with aluminum foil. Dexibuprofen concentrations in the working solutions used for the calibration curve were 10, 20, 40, 60, 80 and 100 µg/mL. Quality control (QC) samples (of low, medium, and high concentrations) at 25, 50, and 90 µg/mL were prepared in the same way as the calibration standards. These working solutions were prepared fresh daily by making dilutions of the stock solution in acetonitrile.

2.5.5.4 Calibration curve

Blank plasma samples were spiked with working standard solutions to obtain final concentrations in the range of 10-100 µg/mL.

2.5.5.5 Method validation

Plasma calibration curves were prepared and assayed in triplicate on three different days. Inter-day assays were determined by analyzing QC samples in triplicate and were analyzed on three different days. Intra-day assays were determined for each QC sample in plasma, each in triplicate on one day so as to evaluate linearity, precision, accuracy, recovery, limit of quantification (LOQ), limit of detection (LOD), and stability.

2.5.5.6 Preparation of test solution and extraction procedure

Test solution was prepared by addition of acetonitrile to the plasma samples (90:10 v/v) and centrifuged at 10,000 rpm for 10min to deprotonate it. The supernatant obtained was filtered through 0.45um membrane filter and injected into the HPLC system.

2.5.5.7 Pharmacokinetic analysis

The maximum plasma concentration C_{max} was obtained directly from the experimental data; T_{max} was defined as the first occurrence of C_{max}. The terminal elimination rate constant (K_{el}) was estimated using least squares regression analysis of plasma concentration-time data obtained during the terminal log-linear elimination phase. Individual half-lives ($t½$) were calculated as 0.693/K_{el} and mean half-lives were defined as 0.693/mean K_{el}. The area under the plasma concentration-time curve (AUC) from 0–time t (AUC_{0-t}) was estimated by linear trapezoidal approximation [19,20]. The AUC from t to infinity ($AUC_{t-\infty}$) were estimated as *ct, est* K_{el}, where *ct, est* represents the estimated concentration at time t based on the regression analysis. The total area under the curve ($AUC_{0-\infty}$) was estimated as the sum of (AUC_t) plus ($AUC_{t-\infty}$).

2.6 Statistical Analysis

The pharmacokinetic parameters for both treatments A and B were analyzed using one way analysis of variance using the Graphpad Prism 6 computer program.

3. RESULTS AND DISCUSSION

3.1 Physical Properties

Physical properties of the prepared films are shown in Table 2. The prepared films were off-white color, opaque, smooth, moist and non-sticky. The uniformity of weight test indicates that increasing the amount of HPMC and PVP K30 leads to increasing weight of transdermal film. Folding endurance test results indicate that all the patches will withstand to rupture and would maintain their integrity with general skin folding, when used. The folding endurance was measured manually and it lied in between 145.67±5.03 to 224±7.81. It was found to be higher in patches containing higher amount of the HPMC. Strength of the film and the risk of film cracking were indicated by its tensile strength. The prepared transdermal films showed good tensile strength and there were no signs of cracking in the prepared transdermal film. This might be attributed to the addition of the plasticizer, DBP. Plasticizers are generally used to improve the mechanical properties of a polymer matrix [11]. Plasticizer embeds between the chains of polymers, spacing them apart and making the polymeric patch more flexible [21]. Tensile strength was found in between 10.14±0.94 to 67.16±1.43 g/cm^2, the difference depends on the amount of polymer used. There was increase in tensile strength with increase in the polymer blend. All the patches showed near to hundred percent flatness, which indicates negligible amount of constriction of the prepared transdermal patches. Thus, patches do not constrict, when it is applied on the skin. Moisture content and moisture absorption studies indicates that, the increase in the concentration of hydrophilic polymer i.e. HPMC and PVP was directly proportional to the increase in moisture content and moisture absorption of the patches. Due to moisture uptake from the atmosphere, significant changes in properties like increased porosity, increased pore diameter and reduced crushing strength has been reported for matrix film containing hydrophilic polymers [11].

3.2 Determination of Loading Efficacy

Table 3 shows the loading efficacy of the prepared films indicating that drug content of all batches were within the range between 97.49±1.04 to 99.64±0.97%. As shown in the table results were much closed to 100%, indicating that there is no any loss of drug during the preparation of the transdermal patches and also there was homogeneous mixture of drug in polymer matrix.

3.3 *In-vitro* Dissolution Studies

The dissolution profiles of dexibuprofen from the prepared films were done and graphically represented in Figs. 1-3. Table 4 shows the percent dexibuprofen released from different formulae. Release of drug from a transdermal drug delivery system mainly involves diffusion factors [22]. One such factor is the amount of hydrophilic polymer. As the amount of hydrophilic polymer (PVP) increases the amount of drug released and dissolution increase so that drug release from F3>F2>F1, also F6>F5>F4 and F9>F8>F7. PVP has been shown to enhance dissolution of poorly soluble drug from solid dosage form [23] that dissolution of more and more PVP in the diffusion medium forms pores which increase the rate of diffusion [21]. The amount and rate of drug released after 30 minutes from F3 was 99.84±0.42% which is higher than that released from F6; 45.09±1.32% and F9; 40.14±0.61% although they contain the same concentration of PVP, this is due to the different concentration of HPMC in these formulae which is lower in F3 than F6 and F9, higher concentration of HPMC leads to increasing viscosity which retards the drug release.

3.4 Permeation Studies

This study was done for F1, F2 and F3 formulae because they showed higher dissolution rate and amount of drug release. The release profiles of dexibuprofen from the prepared films were graphically represented in Fig. 4. Table 5 shows the cumulative percent dexibuprofen released from different formulae. The amount and rate of drug released after 150 minutes from F3 was 97.09±0.47% and from F2, F3 were 71.6±0.54%, 59.12±0.57% respectively. The amount of PVPK30 in F1, F2, F3 formulae is 25, 50, 75 mg respectively, F3 formula that containing higher amount of PVPK30 showed higher release because it forms pores which increase the rate of diffusion [21].

Table 2. Physical properties of the prepared films

Formulae	Weight uniformity (mg/cm^2)	Folding endurance	Tensile strength (g/cm^2)	%Flatness	% Moisture content	% Moisture absorption
F1	30.44±1.43	145.67±5.03	10.14±0.94	99.41±0.76	6.83±0.15	16.03±0.56
F2	34.07±2.23	147.33±5.69	11.10±1.83	99.83±0.16	9.37±0.61	19.05±0.64
F3	34.62±1.70	154.33±2.08	12.75±1.16	99.49±0.89	9.89±0.69	20.78±0.95
F4	35.41±2.67	174.67±3.21	23.24±0.50	99.92±0.14	10.55±1.35	21.76±1.11
F5	36.18±1.05	176.00±6.24	24.18±0.86	98.81±1.17	12.01±0.68	26.68±1.09
F6	36.41±1.29	184.00±3.61	52.68±1.20	99.89±0.20	13.41±0.56	32.30±1.66
F7	36.50±1.00	208.33±5.51	52.09±0.56	98.24±1.60	16.89±0.83	32.78±0.89
F8	40.10±0.95	216.33±8.96	59.86±1.53	97.89±1.67	17.81±0.84	34.18±0.44
F9	41.79±0.97	224.00±7.81	67.16±1.43	98.01±1.89	18.19±0.74	36.17±1.13

Table 3. Loading efficacy of the prepared films

Formulae	Theoretical content	Loading efficacy (%)
F1	20	99.31±0.35
F2	20	99.26±0.52
F3	20	99.30±0.55
F4	20	97.49±1.03
F5	20	99.63±1.00
F6	20	99.20±0.74
F7	20	98.30±0.64
F8	20	98.64±0.97
F9	20	99.30±0.57

Table 4. *In vitro* release of dexibuprofen from the prepared formulae in dissolution study

	Percentage (%w/w) of dexibuprofen after the following time intervals in minutes					
Time / Formulae	5	10	15	20	25	30
F1	16.15±0.4	20.27±0.44	28.21±0.52	36.87±0.88	46.09±0.63	59.47±0.78
F2	16.39±0.45	23.73±0.08	35.1±0.66	44.09±0.90	51.98±0.65	72.11±0.88
F3	23.62±1.16	29.73±0.94	39.51±1.26	66.47±1.22	80.11±0.4	99.84±0.21
F4	7.72±0.67	8.64±0.76	17.98±0.72	18.85±0.60	21.05±0.52	22.69±0.93
F5	12.1±0.47	19.56±1.13	23.01±1.47	23.74±1.18	33.53±0.57	38.95±1.20
F6	16.01±1.59	21.07±0.6	27.2±0.502	32.10±0.54	36.99±1.05	45.09±1.32
F7	9.38±1.15	10.87±0.57	16.83±0.52	28.24±0.33	31.2±1.16	34.79±0.50
F8	11.16±0.83	24.01±0.52	26.99±0.26	30.70±1.32	34.19±0.3	36.81±0.61
F9	25.18±1.20	33.94±0.54	34.89±1.35	37.98±0.54	38.86±0.68	40.14±0.60

3.5 Bioavailability Study

3.5.1 Calibration curves, precision, accuracy and linearity

The calibration curve for dexibuprofen was linear in the concentration range of 10-100 ug/mL in rabbit plasma. The correlation coefficient of the line was 0.999. The precision and accuracy of the assay were determined from the low (40 μg/mL), medium (80 μg/mL), and high (100 μg/mL) QC plasma samples. Intra and inter-day precision in this study was expressed as percent of coefficient of variation (CV). Accuracy was expressed as the mean percentage of analyte recovered in the assay [24]. According to Center for Drug Evaluation Research (CDER) [25], the precision determined at each concentration should not exceed 15% of CV except for LOQ, where it should not exceed 20% of the CV. The results of the precision and accuracy determined by the intra- and inter-day method are shown in Table 6.

Table 5. Release of dexibuprofen from F1, F2 and F3 formulae during permeation study

	Cumulative Percent (%w/w) of dexibuprofen after the following time intervals in minutes								
Time / Formulae	5	15	30	45	60	75	90	120	150
F1	19.65±0.25	31.97±0.8	40.79±0.23	44.79±1.13	50.24±0.53	53.85±1.01	57.19±0.46	58.24±0.49	59.12±0.57
F2	20.31±0.56	36.95±0.88	46.16±0.72	57.13±0.46	59.58±1.97	67.64±1.05	69.47±0.61	71.34±0.5	71.6±0.54
F3	26.57±0.32	53.55±0.73	69.18±0.3	77.46±0.45	82.57±0.47	86.13±0.47	89.54±0.45	94.03±0.43	97.09±0.47

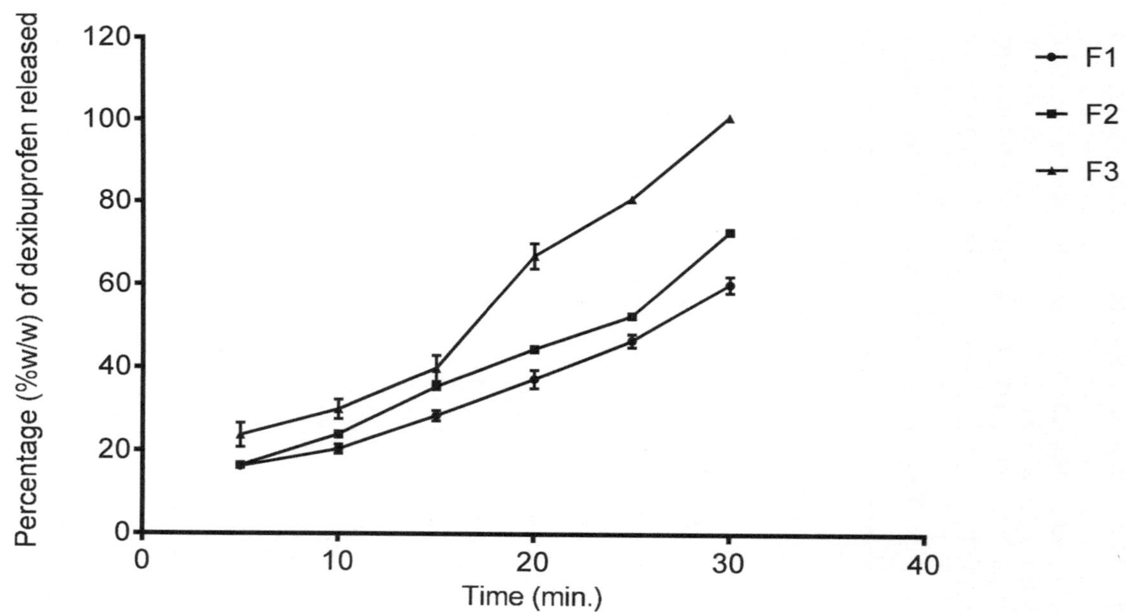

Fig. 1. ***In vitro*** **release profile of dexibuprofen from F1. F2 and F3 formulae**

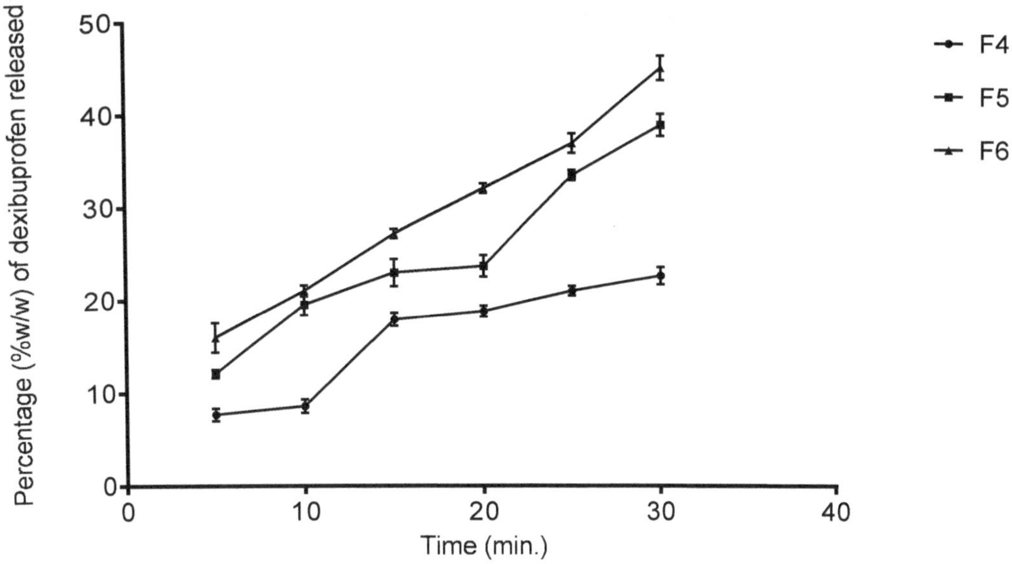

Fig. 2. ***In vitro*** **release profile of dexibuprofen from F4. F5 and F6 formulae**

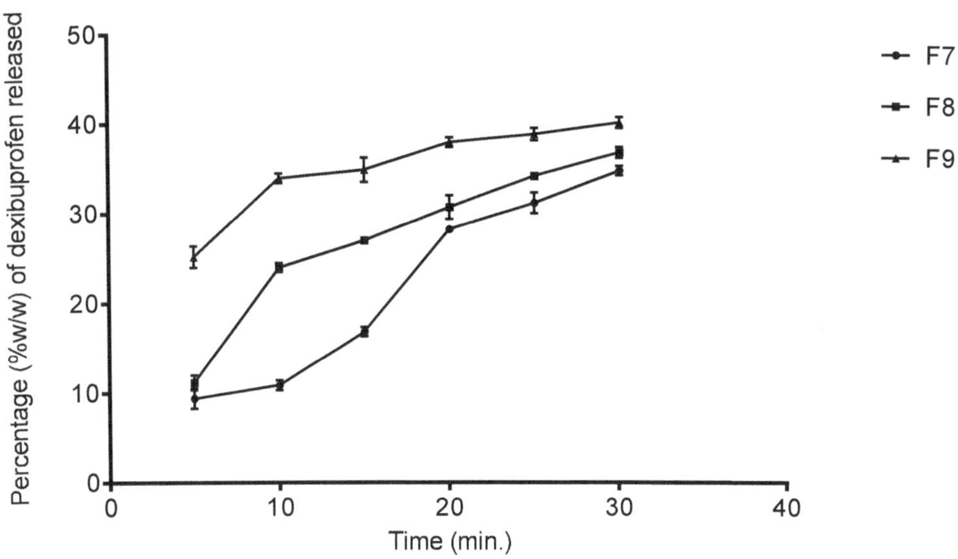

Fig. 3. ***In vitro*** **release profile of dexibuprofen from F7. F8 and F9 formulae**

Table 6. Intra-and inter-day accuracy and precision of the assay method

	Nominal concentrations (µg/mL)	Mean concentrations observed (µg/mL)	Accuracy (%)	Precision (%)
Inter-day	40	39.60	99.00	0.264
	80	81.00	101.25	0.928
	100	101.58	101.58	0.604
Intra-day	40	40.09	100.07	0.52
	80	80.62	100.77	1.65
	100	102.07	102.07	1.02

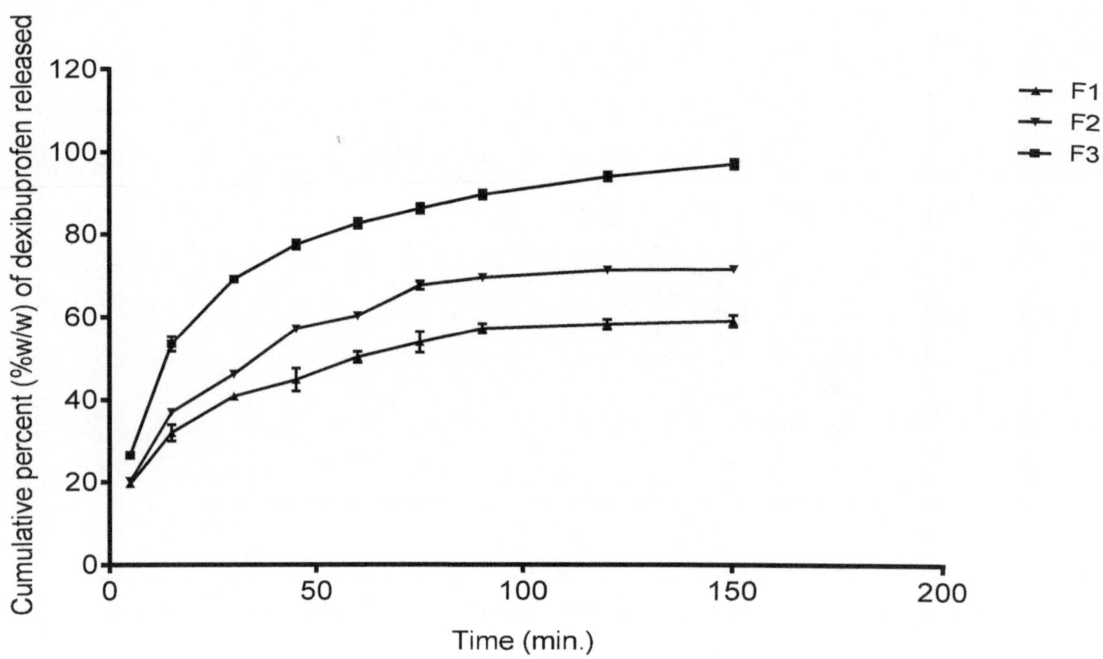

Fig. 4. Release profile of dexibuprofen from F1. F2 and F3 formulae during permeation study

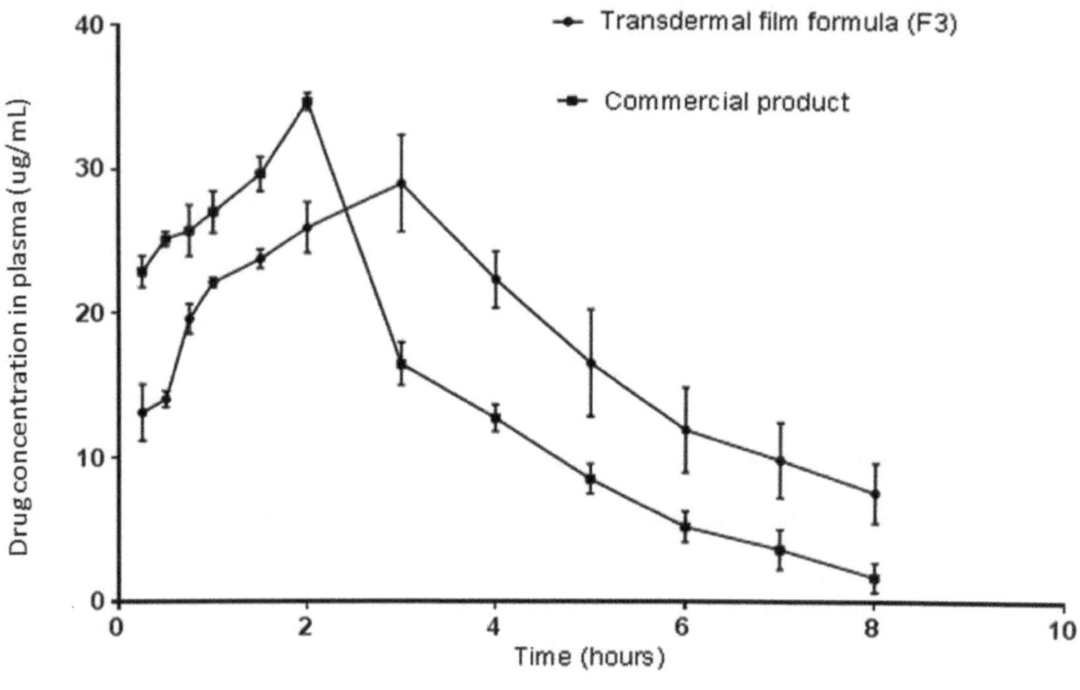

Fig. 5. Mean plasma level of dexibuprofen in rabbits following application of transdermal film (F3) and commercial product. Each value represents the mean ± SD (n = 6)

Table 7. Comparison of pharmacokinetic parameters between transdermal film formula (F3) (Treatment A) and commercial product of dexibuprofen (Treatment B), (*t*-test for independent data)

Items	Transdermal film (F3) (Treatment A)			Commercial product (Treatment B)			*p*
	Mean	SD	SE	Mean	SD	SE	
C_{max}(μg/mL)	28.98	3.36	1.37	34.67	0.61	0.25	0.0022
T_{max}(h)	3.00	0.00	0.00	2.00	0.00	0.00	-
K_{ab}(h^{-1})	0.89	0.06	0.02	2.10	1.39	0.57	0.0572
$T_{(1/2)}ab$ (h)	0.78	0.05	0.02	0.43	0.21	0.08	0.0022
K_{el}(h^{-1})	0.28	0.06	0.02	0.49	0.17	0.07	0.0177
$T_{(1/2)el}$ (h)	2.63	0.64	0.26	1.56	0.47	0.19	0.0078
TCR(mL/min)	10.29	1.62	0.66	3.02	0.25	0.10	<0.0001
AUC_{0-8}(μg·h /mL)	144.68	12.86	5.25	116.76	3.13	1.28	0.0004
$AUC_{0-\infty}$(μg·h/mL)	145.82	13.09	5.34	117.44	3.15	1.28	<0.0001
$AUMC_{0-8}$(μg·h^2/mL)	500.64	64.90	26.50	299.95	15.49	6.33	<0.0001
$AUMC_{0-\infty}$(μg·h^2/mL)	528.01	70.95	28.97	305.35	16.50	6.74	<0.0001
MRT(h)	3.61	0.17	0.07	2.60	0.10	0.04	<0.0001
Cmax/AUC_{0-8}(h^{-1})	0.20	0.01	0.01	0.30	0.01	0.00	<0.0001

3.5.2 Pharmacokinetic study

Mean plasma concentration-time profiles in treatments A and B are presented in above Table 7 and Fig. 5. The peak time (T_{max}) in treatments A and B is 3 hours and 2 hours respectively. The average peak plasma concentration values (C_{max}) were 28.98±3.356 and 34.67±0.606 μg/mL, respectively. The mean area under the plasma concentration-time curve (AUC_{0-8}) values were 144.68±12.86 and 116.76±3.13 μg·h/mL and $AUC_{0-\infty}$ values were 145.82±13.09 and 117.44±3.15 μg·h/mL respectively. Statistical analysis of the pharmacokinetic data revealed that there were significant differences between treatments A and B in C_{max}, $t_{(1/2)}ab$ K_{el}, $t_{(1/2)}el$, *TCR*, AUC_{0-8}, $AUC_{0-\infty}$, $AUMC_{0-8}$, $AUMC_{0-\infty}$, and *MRT*. Also, there was a not significant difference in K_{ab}, while there was a significant difference in C_{max} /AUC_{0-8}.

4. CONCLUSION

Transdermal film containing soluble form of dexibuprofen can be applied instead of oral tablets. Increasing the amounts of HPMC and PVP K30 leads to increasing weight, folding endurance, tensile strength, moisture content and moisture absorption. F9 formula containing 75 mg PVP K30 and 100 mg HPMC shows higher rate, amount of dexibuprofen released from dissolution medium and Franz cell. The bioavailability study shows that there were significant differences between treatments A and B in most of the pharmacokinetic parameters.

CONSENT

It is not applicable.

ACKNOWLEDGEMENTS

This work was supported by a grant from Department of Pharmaceutical Technology, Faculty of Pharmacy, Tanta University and Dr. Ola EL-Houssini, Researcher in National Organization for Drug Control and Research.

COMPETING INTERESTS

Authors have declared that no competing interests exist.

REFERENCES

1. Jannat S, Masum AA, Sharmin F, Islam A and Reza S. Formulation and evaluation of sustained release matrix type transdermal film of ibuprofen. Bangladesh Pharmaceutical Journal. 2012;15(1):17-21.
2. Joseph R, Robinson, Vincent HL. Controlled drug delivery fundamentals and

applications. Revised and Expanded: Lee. Marcel Dekker, Inc. 2005;524.

3. Adams SS, Bresloff P, Mason CG. Pharmacological differences between the optical isomers of ibuprofen evidence for metabolic inversion of the (-) isomer. J Pharm Pharmacol. 2004;28:256-257.
4. Bomabello A, Galmozzi MR, Canaparo R, Isaia GC, Serepe L, Muntoni E. Dexibuprofen (S(+)-Isomer Ibuprofen) reduces gastric damage and improves analgesic anti-inflammatory effects in rodents. Anesth Analg. 2003;97:402-408.
5. El-Houssieny BM, El-Dein EZ, El-Messiry HM. Enhancement of solubility of dexibuprofen applying mixed hydrotropic solubilization technique. Drug Dis. and Ther. 2014;8(4):178-184.
6. Hussain A, Khan GM, Shah SU, Shah KU, Rahim N, Wahab R, Rehman AU. Development of a novel ketoprofen transdermal patch: Effect of almond oil as penetration enhancers on in-vitro and ex-vivo penetration of ketoprofen through rabbit skin, Pak. J. Pharm. Sci. 2012;25(1):227-232.
7. Saroha K, Yadav B, Sharma B. Transdermal Patch: A Discrete Dosage Form. Inter. J. of Curr. Pharm. Res. 2011;3(3).
8. Pachisia N, Agrawal SS. Formulation, development and evaluation of transdermal drug delivery system of Glimepiride. Inter J of Pharm and Pharm Res. 2012;2(1):1-8.
9. Saroha K, Yadav B, Sharma B. Transdermal patch: A discrete dosage form. Inter J of Curr Pharm Res. 2011;3(3):98-108.
10. Tanwar YS. Development and evaluation of carvedilol transdermal patches. Acta Pharm. 2007;57:151-159.
11. Shinde AJ, Shinde AL, Paithane MB, More HN. Design and evaluation of gliclazide transdermal patch containing film former. Int J of Pharm and Tech. 2010;2(3):792-809.
12. Jannat S, Abdullah Al Masum MD, Sharmin F, Islam A, Reza S. Formulation and evaluation of sustained release matrix type transdermal film of ibuprofen. Ban Pharm J. 2012;15(1):17-21.
13. Mukherjee B. Sorbitan monolaurate 20 as a potential skin permeation enhancer in transdermal patches. The J of App Res. 2005;51:96-108.
14. Pillai SS, Senthil Kumar KL, Panneerselvam T, Shabaraya AR, Muneer TK. Effect of polymeric activity on transdermal patches of Glipizide. Res in Pharm. 2011;1(2):1-5.
15. The United States Pharmacopeia 37th Revision. The National Formulary 32nd Edition. 12601 Twinbrook Parkway, Rockville, MD 20852. 2014;352.
16. Rajesh K, Rahul Nair, Rajalakshmi R, Latha P, Arun kumar KS, Nama V. Inclusion complex of dexibuprofen and its in-vitro and *In-vivo* evaluation. Int Bio Pharm Res. 2011;2:34-38.
17. Hussain A, Khan GM, Jan SU, Shah SU, Shah KU, Akhlaq M, Rahim N, Nawaz A, Wahab A. Effect of olive oil on transdermal penetration of Flurbiprofen from topical gel as enhancer. Pak. J. Pharm. Sci. 2012;25(2):365-369.
18. Hasan N, Chaiharn M, Mirani ZA, Qambrani NA. Validated RP-HPLC method for determination of dexibuprofen: Application in pharmaceutical dosage and human serum. ACAIJ. 2013;12(8) 283-290.
19. Weiner DL. Design and analysis of bioavailability studies. Marcel Dekker, Inc., New York, NY, USA. 1981;205-229.
20. Shargel L, Yu ABC. Applied Biopharmacetics and Pharmacokinetics, 3rd ed. Prentice-Hall, New York, NY, USA. 1993;47-76.
21. Ghosal K, Rajabalaya R, Maiti AK, Chowdhury B, Nanda A. Evaluation of physicochemical properties and in-vitro release profile of glipizide-matrix patch. Bra J of Pharm Sci. 2010;46(2):213-218.
22. Tojo K, Valia KH, Chotani G, Chien YW. Long-term permeation kinetics of estradiol IV: A theoretical approach to simultaneous skin permeation and bioconversion of estradiol esters. Drug Dev Ind Pharm. 1985;11(6):1175-1193.
23. Rowe RC. Handbook of Pharmaceutical Excipient. (Sheskey PJ, Cook WG, Fenton ME, ed.). Pharmaceutical Press, London SE1 7JN, UK. 2012;661.
24. Gan SH, Ismail R. Validation of high performance liquid chromatography method for tramadol and O-desmethyl tramadol in human plasma using solid-phase extraction. J Chromatogr B. 2001;759:325-335.

25. Guidance for Industry, Bioanalytical Method validation, U.S. Department of Health and Human Services. Food and Drug Administration. Centre for Drug Evaluation and Research (CDER). Center for Veterinary Medicine (CVM); 2001.

9

Study of Acid-base Indicator Property of Ethanolic Extract of *Nerium indicum* Flower

Khalid Da'u Khalid[1*], Mustapha Balarabe Idris[1], Naziru Alhassan Muhammad[1] and Ahmad Bala[1]

[1]Department of Chemistry, Jodhpur National University, Narnadi, Jhanwar Road, Boranada, Rajasthan, India.

Authors' contributions

This work was carried out in collaboration between all authors. All authors read and approved the final manuscript.

Article Information

Editor(s):
(1) Nawal Kishore Dubey, Centre for advanced studies in Botany, Banaras Hindu University, India.
Reviewers:
(1) Daniel A. Abugri, Tuskegee University, USA.
(2) Anonymous, HNB Garhwal central University Campus, India.
(3) Tulay Aşkin Çelik, Adnan Menderes University, Turkey.
(4) Anthony Cemaluk C. Egbuonu, Michael Okpara University of Agriculture Umudike, Nigeria.

ABSTRACT

A study has been done to investigate the indicator property of ethanolic extract of *Nerium indicum*. The commonly used synthetics indicators cause environmental pollution and pose hazardous effects in human body. Natural pigments in plants are highly coloured substance and may change with pH variation. The equivalence points of the titrations using flower extract is almost close or coincide with that of phenolphthalein (synthetic indicator). Therefore, use of ethanolic extract of *Nerium indicum* as an indicator for acid-base titration could be effectively employed as a substitute to the synthetic acid-base indicators.

Keywords: Equivalence point; ethanol; indicator; Nerium indicum; pH and titration.

1. INTRODUCTION

In spite of the numerous instrumental techniques currently available for the chemical analyses of various samples, conventional methods of analysis such as gravimetry and titrimetry are still relevant. The end point in traditional titrimetry is usually indicated by some substances added into

**Corresponding author: Email: khalid126dkhalid@yahoo.com*

the analyte solution, which change colour immediately after the equivalence point has been attained [1]. The substances that change colour when the acidity of the solution changes are known as acid-base indicators [2]. Acidimetry and alkalimetry include the titration of free bases with a standard acid and the titration of free acids with a standard base respectively. The reactions involve the combination of hydrogen and hydroxyl ions to form water [3]. This can only be identified by the use of colourant called indicator. A pH indicator is a halochromic chemical compound that is added in small amounts to a solution so that the pH (acidity or alkalinity) of the solution can be determined easily [4]. For simplicity, we represent a general indicator by the formula HIn for acidic indicators and InOH for basic indicator. The ionization of acidic indicator in a solution is represented by the equilibrium [5].

$$HIn \rightarrow H^{+} + In^{-}$$

Commercial indicators are expensive and some of them have toxic effects on users and can also cause environmental pollution [6]. For these reasons there has been an increasing interest in searching for alternative sources indicators from natural origins, these alternatives would be cheaper, more available, simple to extract, less toxic to users and environmentally friendly [4]. Almost any flowers such as blue, purple or red in colour contain a class of organic pigment called anthocyanins that change colour with pH [7]. Several authors have reported on the effectiveness of indicators extracted from natural sources in acid base-titration. Some of these were *Dianthus plumarius* and *Antirrhium majus [8], Nerium odoratum* [9], *Ipomoea biloba* [10], *Jacaranda acutifolia* flower [11], pride of barbados [12], *Morus alba linn* fruit [6].

Nerium indicum belongs to the family Apocynaceace; the plant is commonly known as "Kaner" [13]. It is widely distributed in Mediterranean region and subtropical Asia but is native of Indian subcontinent and cultivated elsewhere [14]. In Northern regions it may be grown as an indoor or patio plant; oleander has flexible branches with green, smooth bark eventually turning to dark-grey [14].

2. MATERIALS AND METHODS

All reagents and chemicals used in this study were of analytical grade.

2.1 Flower Collection and Identification

The flower *Nerium indicum* was collected from the plants grown at college compound of Jodhpur National University, India and authenticated by a botanist; Dean Faculty of Science Dr. N. L. Vyas. The flower was then kept in laboratory.

2.2 Extraction of *Nerium indicum* Flower

Any extract from either plant leaves or flowers that have a pH different from neutral and can change colour in acidic and basic medium can be used as indicator. The collected flowers were cleaned with distilled water, cut into small pieces and 5.0g was weighed using analytical weighing balance. It is then soaked into 30 mL of 90% ethanol and allowed to stand for 48hrs for complete extraction of colourant present. pH of the extract was determined to be slightly acid in the range of 6-6.5.

2.3 Titrations

0.1 ml of the extract was added as an indicator for each titration type: Strong acid-strong base (HCl versus NaOH), strong acid-weak base (HCl versus $NaHCO_3$), weak acid-strong base (CH_3COOH versus NaOH) and weak acid-weak base (CH_3COOH versus $NaHCO_3$) of 1M, 2M and 3M respectively. The trials were repeated 3 times to check the precision. The titrations were again performed using phenolphthalein indicator as standard and the results obtained were compared with the results of titrations using the flower extract indicator. The end points of the titrations using the extract were reached when colour changed from yellow to light pink. The results for titrations were shown in the Table 1.

3. RESULTS AND DISCUSSION

The extract from *Nerium indicum* flower was tested for its use as an acid-base indicator and the results was compared with that obtained using phenolphthalein for strong acid-strong base (HCl and NaOH), strong acid-weak base (HCl and $NaHCO_3$), weak acid-strong base (CH_3COOH and NaOH) and weak acid-weak base (CH_3COOH and $NaHCO_3$) titrations. The equivalence point of the titrations using flower extract is almost close or coincides with that of phenolphthalein for all the titrations as shown in Table 1.

The result obtained in the presence study is in cognomen with those in related literature using

Table 1. Parametric result screening of acid base titration

Titrant/Titrand	Indicator	Mean value of titration ±SD
	Phenolphthalein	
1M HCl / NaOH		9.67±0.06
2M HCl / NaOH		9.60±0.15
3M HCl / NaOH		10.10±0.02
1M HCl / $NaHCO_3$		9.77±0.01
2M HCl / $NaHCO_3$		10.20±0.07
3M HCl / $NaHCO_3$		9.86±0.14
1M CH3COOH / NaOH		10.03±0.06
2M CH3COOH / NaOH		10.10±0.04
3M CH3COOH / NaOH		9.53±0.05
1M CH3COOH / $NaHCO_3$		10.03±0.12
2M CH3COOH / $NaHCO_3$		10.10±0.16
3M CH3COOH / $NaHCO_3$		10.20±0.12
	***Neriun indicum* (extract)**	
1M HCl / NaOH		9.83±0.06
2M HCl / NaOH		9.45±0.11
3M HCl / NaOH		10.40±0.13
1M HCl / $NaHCO_3$		10.03±0.12
2M HCl / $NaHCO_3$		10.10±0.21
3M HCl / $NaHCO_3$		9.97±0.13
1M CH3COOH / NaOH		10.0±0.06
2M CH3COOH / NaOH		9.70±0.05
3M CH3COOH / NaOH		9.50±0.05
1M CH3COOH / $NaHCO_3$		10.70±0.04
2M CH3COOH / $NaHCO_3$		9.90±0.12
3M CH3COOH / $NaHCO_3$		10.70±0.11

different plant extract [7,10], however there was slight difference in the result as compared with the one obtained in [15]. This show usefulness of flower extracts as an indicator in acid- base titration and its use in weak acid-strong base was found to be more significant over standard indicator as it gives sharp colour change.

4. CONCLUSION

The results obtained in all the types of acid-base titrations in the present study revealed that the *Nerium indicum* extract could effectively be used as acid-base indicator (and subsequently substitute phenolphthalein synthetic) indicator owing to the factors like wild availability of the flower, simple preparation, and good performance, precise and accurate results.

CONSENT

It is not applicable.

ETHICAL APPROVAL

It is not applicable.

ACKNOWLEDGEMENT

The authors wishes to acknowledge Dr. N. L. Vyas and Dr. Kamlesh Gautam; faculty of applied science, Jodhpur National University India, for their immense contribution toward the completion of this research work.

COMPETING INTERESTS

Authors have declared that no competing interests exist.

REFERENCES

1. Izonfuo WAL, Fekarurhobo GK, Obomanu FG, Daworiye LT. Acid-base indicator properties of Dyes from local Plants I: Dyes from *Basella alba*. (Indian spinach) and *Hibiscus sabdariffa* (Zobo). J. Appl. Sci. Environ. Mgt. 2006;10(1):5-8.
2. Pimpodkar NV, Shikalgar S, Shinde N, Bhise S, Surve B. *Rhoeo syathacea* and *Allamanda cathartic* extract as a natural indicator in Acidimetry-Alkalimetry. Asian. J. Pharm. Ana. 2014;4(2):82-84.

3. Abugri1 DA, Apea OB, Pritchett G. Investigation of a simple and cheap source of a natural indicator for acid-base titration: Effects of system conditions on natural indicators. Green Sustainable Chem. 2012; 2:117-122.
4. Eze SO, Ogbuefi RA. Analytical potentials of dye extracts from *Aspilia africana* (Oramejula) flowers. Asian J. Nat. Appl. Sci. 2014;3(1):54-60.
5. Pimpodkar NV, Surve BS, Bhise SH. Use of *Argyreia cuneata* flower extract as a natural indicator in acid base titration. J. Curr. Pharma. Res. 2014;4(2):1124-1127.
6. Pathade SK, Patil SB, Konda-war N, Magdum CS. Morus alba fruit-herbal alternative to synthetic acid base indicators. Int. J. Chem. Tech. Res. 2009; 3(1):549-551.
7. Bhise SH, Shinde NG, Surve BS, Pimpodkar NV, Shikalgar SS. *Acalypha wilkesiana* as natural pH indicator . Int. J. Nat. Prod. Res. 2014;4(1):33-35.
8. Jaspreet S, Kanika A, Parminder N, Geeta D. Herbal indicators as an upcoming trend in titrimetric analysis. Int. J. Pharma. 2011; 2(4):177-179.
9. Vaibhav GN, Vishal BK, Prashant DN, Ganpatrao NM, Suresh TS, Ashish SS. Study of *Nerium odoratum* as natural, economical and effective alternative to synthetic indicator and litmus paper. Intl. J. Pharm. Chem. Sci. 2014;3(2):440.
10. Abbas SK. Study of acid-base indicator property of flowers of *Ipomoea biloba*. Int. Curr. Pharm. J. 2012;1(12):420-422.
11. Eze SO, Ogbuefi RA. Analytical potentials of dye extracts from *Aspilia africana* (Oramejula) flowers. Asian J. Nat. Appl. Sci. 2014;3(1):54-60.
12. Gupta P, Jain P, Jain PK. Dahalia flower sap a natural resource as indicator in Acidimetry and alkalimetry. Int. J. Pharm. Tech. 2013;4(4):5038-5045.
13. Patrakar R, Gond N, Jadge D. Flower extract of *Jacaranda acutifolia* used as a natural indicator in acid base titration. Int. J. Pharmtech Res. 2012;2(3):1954-1957.
14. Nwosu FO, Adekola FA, Ihedioha KC. Simple titrimetric colour indicators from some natural flower petals. Centre Point (science edition). 2004;12(1):74-89.
15. Saini P, Kannapan N, Kumar P, Diwan A, Antil V, Sharma S, Singh S. CNS activity of *Nerium indicum* flower part. Res. J. Pharm. Bio. Chem. Sci. 2010;1(3):546 -550.

10

Assessment of the Hematological Parameters of Albino Rats Fed on High Dose of whole Wheat

Anaka Ogochukwu Ngozi[1], Omoti Caroline Edijana[2], Owolabi Omonkhelin Josephine[3*], O. Innih Silvanus[4] and Nwagwu Chinonye Sophia[1]

[1]Department of Pharmacology and Toxicology, Faculty of Pharmacy, Igbinedion University, Okada, Nigeria.
[2]Department of Haematology, University of Benin Teaching Hospital, Benin, Nigeria.
[3]Department of Pharmacology and Toxicology, Faculty of Pharmacy, University of Benin, Benin, Nigeria.
[4]Department of Anatomy, School of Basic Medical Sciences, College of Medical Sciences, University of Benin, Nigeria.

Authors' contributions

This work was carried out in collaboration between all authors. Authors AON and OCE conceived and designed the study, authors OOJ, AON, OIS and NCS collected, analysed the data and assisted in the writing of manuscript. All authors read and approved the final manuscript.

Article Information

Editor(s):
(1) Edward G Rowan, Strathclyde Institute of Pharmacy and Biomedical Sciences, University of Strathclyde, Glasgow, UK.
(2) Othman Ghribi, Department of Pharmacology, Physiology & Therapeutics, University of North Dakota, USA.
(3) Alyautdin Renad N, Chair of The Department of Pharmacology (Pharmaceutical Faculty), I. M. Sechenov MSMU, Moscow, Russia.
Reviewers:
(1) Anthony Cemaluk C. Egbuonu, Michael Okpara University of Agriculture, Umudike, Nigeria.
(2) Barnabe Lucien Nkono Ya Nkono, University of Yaounde 1, Cameroon.
(3) Carmen Lizette Del Toro Sanchez, Universidad De Sonora, Mexico.
(4) Md. Golam Hafiz, Bangabandhu Sheikh Mujib Medical University, Bangladesh.

ABSTRACT

Aim: The aim of this study was to investigate the hematological profile of albino rats fed on whole wheat based on its widespread use. Whole wheat grain (*Triticum aestivum*) is a cereal regularly consumed and also used for various medicinal purposes.
Study Design: Laboratory based work with the use of rodents.
Place and Duration of Study: Department of Haematology, University of Benin Teaching Hospital

**Corresponding author: Email: owolabi@uniben.edu*

and Department of Anatomy, College of Basic Medical Sciences, University of Benin, Nigeria, between April 2013 and April 2014.

Methodology: In the experiment a total of sixty (60) albino rats were used. The rats were divided into five (5) groups of 12 rats each. Group I served as a control and received distilled water (2 ml/kg), while groups II, III, IV and V were orally administered whole wheat at 1, 2, 4 and 8 g/kg doses respectively. The administration of wheat and distilled water were done daily while the rats were weighed weekly for 30 days, after which the rats were sacrificed. Blood samples were collected via the abdominal aorta, the plasma was then analyzed for various hematological parameters.

Results: The rats treated with whole wheat had significantly ($p<0.05$) increased levels of red blood cells, hemoglobin, mean corpuscular hemoglobin concentration and red blood cell distribution width when compared to the control group. Though the white blood cells were increased, the values were not significantly different from the control. However the mean corpuscular volume was significantly ($p<0.05$) reduced in the experimental groups.

This result indicates the potentials of wheat as a functional food for therapeutic effect against abnormal hematological changes associated with diabetes mellitus, atherosclerosis, hyperlipidemia and other CVS problems. Consequently, wheat could serve as an adjunct to dietary therapy especially for diabetes mellitus and hyperlipidemia.

Conclusion: In conclusion a hematological protective effect as seen from the increase in the red blood cells and hemoglobin is an excellent discovery from our study.

Keywords: Wheat; red blood cells; white blood cells; haematology.

1. INTRODUCTION

Herbal medicine is the use of medicinal plants for prevention and treatment of diseases: it ranges from traditional and popular medicines of every country to the use of standardized and titrated herbal extracts [1].

Whole Wheat (*Triticum aestivum*) is a cereal [2]. The grain is grown on more land area than any other commercial food. World trade in wheat is greater than for all other crops combined [3]. Globally wheat is the leading protein in human food having a higher protein than any other cereals, maize, rice (Nutrient data laboratory' The United State Depart of Agriculture). Wheat grain is a staple food used to make flour for leavened bread, flat and steamed or bread, biscuit, pasta, noodles, couscous [4] and for fermentation to make beer [5]. Wheat is planted to a limited extent as a forage crop for livestock, and its straw can be used as a construction material for roofing thatch [6,7]. The whole grain can be milled to leave just the endosperm for white flour and is a concentrated source of vitamins, minerals, and protein, while the refined grain is mostly starch [3].

Whole wheat bran is used as a supplemental source of dietary fiber for preventing colon diseases (including cancer), preventing gastric cancer, treating Irritable Bowel Syndrome (IBS), reducing the risk of hemorrhoids and hernia, hypercholesterolemia, hypertension, reducing the risk of breast cancer and gallbladder disease, and type 2 diabetes [8].

The seeds are used in folk remedies for cancers, corns, tumors, warts, whitlow and reported to be antivinous, bilious, demulcent, discutient, diuretic, emollient, excipient, intoxicant and laxative.

Common whole wheat is a folk remedy for burns, cancer, diarrhea, dysentery, ecchymosis, epistaxis, fertility, fever, flux, gravel, hematuria, hemoptysis, hemorrhage, incontinence, leprosy, leucorrhea, menorrhagia, neurasthenia, nightsweat, perspiration, scald, tumor, warts, whitlow, and wounds [8].

The consumption of the plant *Triticum aestivum,* has increased due to its use as a herbal medicine in different parts of the World, especially as dietary adjunct in diabetes, hypertension and obesity. There is no known scientific report, to the best of our knowledge on the safety of this plant on haematological parameters considering its wide spread use. This study therefore focused on investigating the effects of *Triticum aestivum* on hematological parameters to validate its safety.

2. METHODOLOGY

2.1 Plant Material

The whole wheat grain used for the study was purchased from one of our local Markets, Benin

City, Edo State, Nigeria. Impurities which may consist of stones, dirt were removed before passing through the milling machine; the process of grinding was done repeatedly so as to get a fine powder flour.

2.2 Experimental Animals

Albino rat (both sexes) which weighed between 120-270 g purchased and were bred in the animal house of the department of Anatomy University of Benin, Benin City, Nigeria. They were housed in standard cages, fed rat chow and drinking water *ad libitum*. The rats were exposed to natural lightening condition, room temperature and were handled according to the international protocols [9].

2.3 Experimental Design

The animals were divided into (5) groups of 12 rats each. Group I served as control and received distilled water at the dose of 2 ml/kg then groups II, III, IV and V were given the wheat orally at the dose of 1, 2, 4, and 8 g/kg respectively through the use of an oro-gastric tube. The administration of the whole wheat flour and distilled water was done every day while the rats were weighed weekly for 30 days.

2.3.1 Collection of blood

At the end of the 30 days, blood was collected from each of the rat with a 5 ml syringe and needle through the abdominal aorta under chloroform anesthesia. The blood samples were transferred immediately into EDTA bottles and then centrifuged for 5 mins at 4000 rev/min. The supernatant clear plasma thus obtained was transferred carefully with the aid of micropipette into plain test tubes for estimation. The clear supernatant from the EDTA bottles was collected and used for heamatological analysis as described below.

2.3.2 Determination of hematological parameters

This was done using the automated blood cell counter (Erma Inc. Hematology Analyzer. PCE. 2010). The basic principles underlying this technique is electronic impedance and light scatter. The blood counts estimated are hematocrit (Hct), hemoglobin (Hb), red blood count (RBCC), white blood cell count (WBCC), and their differential platelet count, red cell indices, red cell distribution, width etc. Estimation of blood count was done.

2.4 Drugs and Chemicals

Sodium nitroprusside, phenol concentrate, hypochloride concentrate, glycerol-3– phosphate oxidase, glycerol kinase, 2-4 dinitrophenohydrazine, ammonium fe (1) sulphate, L-aspartate, L-alanine, pitric acid, sodium hydroxide, sulphoric acid, 4-amino-phenazine,urease, phosphate buffer, ammonium hepatomolybate; all from Randox, UK. Sodium thymolpthalein, magnesium chloride (TECO diagnostic, USA)], 2-amino-2 methyl propanol buffer (TECO diagnostic, USA), methanol, chloroform, concentrated H_2SO_4 (Sigma, UK).

2.5 Statistical Analysis

Data was expressed as mean±SEM. Where applicable, the data were analyzed statistically by student-test using Graph pad instat version 2.05a. $P < .01$ and $P < .05$ were considered as significant.

3. RESULTS AND DISCUSSION

3.1 The Effect of Treatment with Different Doses *Triticum aestivum* on Some Hematological Parameters

Fig. 1 shows the effect of the treatment with different doses of whole wheat on mean corpuscular volume (MCV), mean platelet volume (MPV) and platelet distribution width (PDW). No significant effect was seen on the MCV except at the 4 g/kg where a reduction was observed, meanwhile no effect on the MPV at all doses used. Although an increase in the level of PDW was seen at the 1 and 8 g/kg, and a decrease seen at 2 and 4 g/kg, none of these effects was significant.

Platelet distribution width is a simple, practical and specific marker of activation of coagulation. Increase PDW is an indication for anisocytosis of platelet. The study shows that the level of PDW was not significantly affected at all doses.

The MPV for the wheat treated groups were not significantly different from the control.

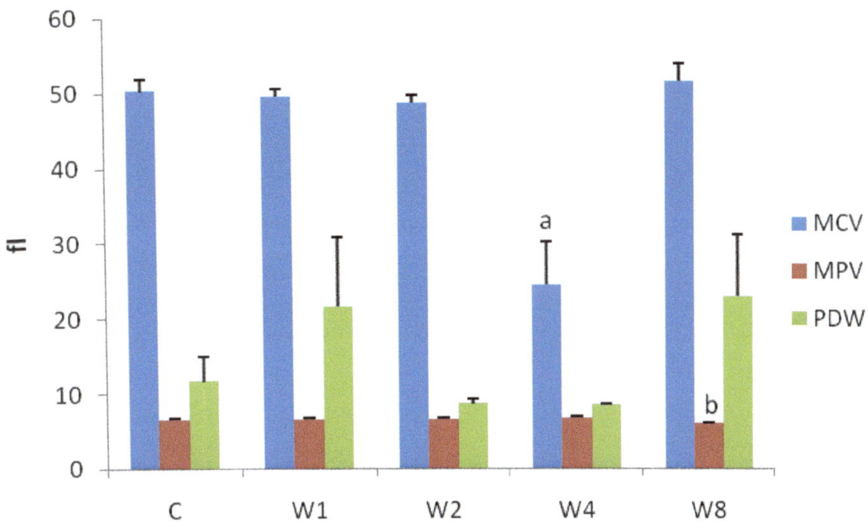

Fig. 1. The effect of the different doses of wheat on some hematological parameters in albino rat

Values are presented as mean±SEM, [a]P<0.0002,[b]P<0.02 significantly reduced when compared to the control, C: control group treated with 2 ml/kg of distilled water, W1: the group treated with 1 g/kg of whole wheat, W2: the group treated with 2 g/kg of whole wheat, W4: the group treated with 4 g/kg of whole wheat, W8: the group treated with 8 g/kg of whole wheat, MCV: mean corpuscular volume, MPV: mean platelet volume, PDW: platelet distribution width; fl: femtoliters (10^{-15})

3.2 The Effect of Treatment with Different Doses of *Triticum aestivum* on the White Blood Cells, Lymphocytes, Monocytes and Granulocytes in Albino Rats

Table 2 shows the effect of the treatment with different doses of whole wheat on white blood cells (WBC), lymphocytes (LYM), monocytes (MO) and granulocytes (GR). The WBC was increased at 1 ($p<0.05$), 2 and 8 g/kg, though not significantly at 2 and 8 g/kg doses. LYM was also increased at 1, 2 and 4 g/kg doses and decreased at 8 g/kg, but none of these effects was significant.

The monocytes were insignificantly decreased at 1, 2, 4 and 8 g/kg doses and finally the granulocytes was significantly ($P<0.05$) increased at 1 g/kg and insignificantly decreased at 2, 4 and 8 g/kg doses.

An increase in the WBC indicates a boosting of the immune system and the reverse in cases of decrease [10]. The cells identify and eliminate pathogens, either by attacking larger pathogens through contact or by phagocytosis [10]. They form part of the innate immune system, which is also an important mediator in the activation of the adaptive immune system [11]. The reduced immunity can contribute to the various complication associated with diabetes mellitus, hyperlipidemia, atherosclerosis and other health problems. In this study, there was an increase in the WBC at all doses except at 4 g/kg though not significant.

The result obtained showed a significant increase at 1 g/kg of granulocytes levels in the rat. Increase in granulocyte levels indicates anti-infective effect [12] which suggests the ability of arresting allergy and bacterial infection.

Monocyte is a type of white blood cell and is part of the immune response system. Increase in monocyte prevents the attack by harmful pathogens [13]. The treatment with whole wheat showed a decrease in monocyte level although non-significant.

3.3 The Effect of Treatment with Different Doses of Aqueous Extract of *Triticum aestivum* on the Mean Corpuscular Hemoglobin Concentration and Hemoglobin

The results on the mean corpuscular hemoglobin concentration (MCHC) and hemoglobin (HGB) of albino rats fed whole wheat at different doses are presented in Table 2. The hemoglobin was significantly increased $P<0.05$ at 8 g/kg dose.

Table 1. The effect of different doses of whole wheat on some hematological parameters

	x10^3/µl			
	WBC	**LYM**	**MO**	**GR**
C	5.80±1.5	3.10±1.0	1.80±0.5	1.80±0.5
W1	9.80±2.0[a]	5.00±0.8[a]	1.50±0.2	3.60±0.5[a]
W2	6.00±1.3	4.10±0.9	1.30±0.3	1.80±0.5
W4	5.50±2.0	3.50± 1.0	1.20±0.5	2.00±0.8
W8	6.20±1.8	2.80±0.6	1.20 ±0.5	1.80±1.5

Values are presented as mean± SEM, n= 8 , [a]P<0.05 is significantly different from the control, C: control group treated with 2 ml/kg of distilled water, W1: the group treated with 1 g/kg of whole wheat, W2: the group treated with 2 g/kg of whole wheat, W4: the group treated with 4 g/kg of whole wheat, W8:the group treated with 8 g/kg of whole wheat, WBC: white blood, cell, LYM: lymphocyte, MO: monocyte, GR: granulocyte

Hemoglobin content helps to stimulate erythropoietin release in the kidney which is the humoral regulator of RBC production [14]. Hemoglobin concentration also reveals the degree of anaemia. Therefore the significant increase of hemoglobin at 8 g/kg may help prevent anaemia.

Our study showed no significant changes in the lymphocyte level at all doses tested in comparison with the control. Lymphocyte is a small white blood cell that plays a role in defending the body against disease; they are cells that determine the specificity of the immune response to infectious microorganisms and other foreign substances [15].

Table 2. The effect of different doses of whole wheat on MCH and HGB

	MCHC (g/dl)	HGB (g/dl)
C	35.00±3.0	12.00±2.0
W1	33.00±5.0	12.50±1.5
W2	36.05±2.0	12.00±1.0
W4	38.50±3.0	11.80±2.0
W8	38.20±2.0	18.00±5.0[a]

Values are presented as mean±SEM, n= 8, [a]P< 0.05, significantly different from the control ,C: control group treated with 2 ml/kg of distilled water, W1: the group treated with 1 g/kg of whole wheat, W2: the group treated with 2 g/kg of whole wheat, W4: the group treated with 4 g/kg of whole wheat, W8: the group treated with 8 g/kg of whole wheat, MCHC: mean corpuscular hemoglobin concentration, HGB: Hemoglobin

The MCHC is an index of the size of the RBCs, and when RBCs are of normal size are they are termed normocytic [16]. The RBC size categories are used to classify anemias. Failure to produce hemoglobin results in cells smaller than normal. This occurs in many diseases, including iron deficiency anemia, thalassemia (an inherited disease in which globin chain production is deficient), and anemias associated with chronic infection or disease. Iron is an essential component of many enzymes in cells and is also part of the haem group in hemoglobin (which consists of a porphyrin ring containing iron). Much of the body's iron stores are within red blood cells where iron is critical for hemoglobin synthesis. Iron deficiency could be due to inadequate intake or absorption of iron, excessive loss with external hemorrhage, or interference with iron metabolism [16]. In this study, there was a significant reduction in the mean corpuscular volume at the dose of 4 g/kg when compared with the control suggesting an interference with iron uptake into hemoglobin.

Molecular Corpuscular Hemoglobin Concentration (MCHC) and Molecular Corpuscular Hemoglobin (MCH) are useful indices in detecting the average hemoglobin concentration of the cell and to suggest the oxygen carrying capacity of the blood. The rapid synthesis of RBC is improved by the level of MCHC and MCH [17]. In our study, a significant increase at 4 and 8 g/kg dose was produced by whole wheat, thus suggesting prevention of anaemia with oral intake of whole wheat probably because of the presence of flavonoid and tannis in wheat.

3.4 The Effect of Treatment with Different Doses of *Triticum aestivum* on the Hematocrit and Red Blood Cells Distribution Width

Table 3 shows the effect of the treatment with different doses of whole wheat on hematocrit (HCT) and red cell distribution (RDW). HCT was significantly increased at 1 g/kg (*P<0.05).*

The red blood cell distribution width (RDW) is a measure of the variation of red blood cell volume; it is also used to determine the possible cause of anaemia. The result showed an insignificant increase in RDW at 1 and 4 g/kg which may indicate the production of individual red blood cell thereby preventing anemia, as was also seen in the significant increase in hemoglobin.

Table 3. The effect of different doses of whole wheat on HCT and RDW

	HCT (%)	RDW (%)
C	32.50±2.0	15.00±0.5
W1	42.20±3.0[a]	15.50±1.0
W2	35.00±1.5	15.80±0.5
W4	31.00±3.0	16.00±0.2
W8	25.50±4.0	16.10±0.10

Values are presented as mean±SEM, n= 8, [a]P<0.05, significantly different from the control, C: control group treated with 2 ml/kg of water, W1: the group treated with 1 g/kg of whole wheat, W2: the group treated with 2 g/kg of whole wheat, W4: the group treated with 4 g/kg of whole wheat, W8:the group treated with 8 g/kg of whole wheat, RDW: Red blood cell distribution width, HCT: Hematocrit

3.5 The Effect of Different Doses of *Triticum aestivum* on the RBC, MCH, PLT and PCT

Table 4 shows the effect of the treatment with different doses of whole wheat on RBC, MCH, PLT and PCT.

The red blood cells were significantly (*P<0.01*) increased at 1, 2, 4 and 8 g/kg although just the effect of 4 g/kg was insignificant as seen from 6.50±0.42 in the control group to 8.42±0.63, 8.65±1.44 and 14.61±4.61 in the groups given 1, 2 and 8 g/kg doses.

The Mean corpuscular hemoglobin was increased at 2, 4, 8 g/kg and decreased at 1 g/kg but none of these was significant. The platelets were also insignificantly increased at 1 and 8 g/kg but lowered at 2 and 4 g/kg but not significantly. The effect of wheat on the PCT was not significant at all doses despite increase observed by some doses.

It was interesting to note that whole wheat produced a significant increase in RBC count particularly with the 1 g/kg dose. A decrease in the RBC can lead to anaemia [18]. Therefore whole wheat can also be of benefit in some anaemic conditions characterized by decreased RBC count.

Platelets are fragment of cells that participates in blood clotting, they initiate repair of blood vessel walls and are also considered as an acute phase reactant to infection or inflammation [19]. Platelets play a major role in the development as well as in the stability of atherosclerotic plaques and as a consequence, anti-platelet agents have been used clinically in patients at risk for myocardial ischemia, unstable angina and acute myocardial infarction. A decrease in the PLT levels is useful in reducing the incidence of cardiovascular diseases as some studies have suggested various mechanisms by which flavonoids exert their anti platelet property by lowering intracellular Ca^{2+} levels, altering the metabolism of cyclic AMP, and thromboxane A_2 [20,21]. In this study the platelet level was not significantly changed at all doses tested.

Platelet crits showcases the precise method of determining the degree of acute blood loss [19]. Decrease can be associated with inflammatory status and increase may be due to the overproduction of hematopoietic regulatory elements such as colony stimulating factors, erythropoietin and thrombopoietin by the stromal cells and macrophages in the bone marrow [22] thus providing the local environment for hematopoiesis [23]. The study shows that platelet crits was not significantly affected at any dose.

Table 4. The effect of different doses of whole wheat on some hematological parameters

	RBC (x10^6/µl)	MCH (pg)	PLT (x10^3/µl)	PCT (%)
C	6.50±0.42	17.76±0.73	491.13±63.60	0.32±0.04
W1	8.42±0.63[a]	16.07±1.58	533.13±57.54	0.34±0.05
W2	8.65±1.44[a]	17.58±0.38	426.86±57.45	0.25±0.04
W4	6.71±0.86	18.98±0.40	309.00±97.84	0.20±0.06
W8	14.61±4.61[a]	22.79±3.21	525.50 ±11.93	0.32±0.00

Values are presented as mean±SEM, n=8 ,[a]P<0.01, significantly different from the control, C: control group treated with 2 ml/kg of distilled water, W1: the group treated with 1 g/kg of whole wheat, W2: the group treated with 2 g/kg of whole wheat, W4: the group treated with 4 g/kg of whole wheat, W8:the group treated with 8 g/kg of whole wheat, RBC: Red blood cells, MCH: mean corpuscular hemoglobin, PLT: Platelets, PCT: Platelet crit

Previous studies has shown that some phytochemical constituent such as flavonoids, and alkaloids have hematological and immunological properties [24], tannins possesses strong antioxidant capacity [25], and therefore could inhibit peroxidation of polyunsaturated fatty acid in the cell and hemolysis of red blood cell [26] and wheat have been shown to be rich in flavonoids and alkaloids.

It was observed that the effect of wheat on MCV, GR, RDW and RBC were not dose dependent, in that a better response was not obtained at higher doses. Possibly as earlier stated the phytochemical constituents in wheat responsible for these effects may not have increased in concentration with increasing dose, hence higher doses gave no better effect than the lower dose.

4. CONCLUSION

The study shows that whole wheat could improve some haematological parameters as evident from the increase in the RBC, MCH, MCHC and HGB levels and thus could be a remedy in various anaemic conditions. Further work is encouraged to ascertain and isolate the exact biochemical components responsible for these notable effects of whole wheat and its consumption is encouraged.

CONSENT

It is not applicable.

ETHICAL APPROVAL

All authors hereby declare that "Principles of laboratory animal care" (NIH publication No. 85-23, revised 1985) were followed, as well as specific national laws where applicable. All experiments have been examined and approved by the appropriate ethics committee.

COMPETING INTERESTS

Authors have declared that no competing interests exist.

REFERENCES

1. Firenzuoli F, Gori L. Herbal medicine to day: Clinical and research issues. Evid Based comple alt Med. 2007;4:37-40.
2. Belderok R, Mesdag H, Donner, Dingena A. Bread-making quality of wheat. Springer. 2000;3:54-58.
3. Curtis M, Rajaraman A, Mac Pherson A. Bread wheat. Food and Agriculture Organization of the United Nations. 2002;234–342.
4. Cauvain C, Stanley P, Cauvain P. Bread making. CRC Press. 2003;540.
5. Palmer A, John J. How to brew. Defenestrative Pub Co. 2001;233.
6. Smith A, Albert O. Handbook of weed management systems. Marcel Dekker. 1995;411.
7. Bridgwater W, Beatrice A. The columbia-viking desk encyclopedia. Columbia University. 19-59.
8. Hadjivassiliou M, Grunewald A, Sharrack B, Sanders D, Lobo A, Williamson C, et al. Gluten ataxia in perspective: Epidemiology, genetic susceptibility and clinical characteristics. Brain. 2003;126:685–691.
9. National Institute of Health USA: Public Health Service Policy on Humane Care and Use of Laboratory; 2002.
10. Egunyomi A, Moddy J, Eletu O. Antisickling activities of two ethnomedicinal plant recipes for the management of sickle cell anemia in Ibadan, Nigeria. Afri J Biotechnol. 2009;8:20-25.
11. Bruce A, Alexander J, Julian L, Martin R, Keith R, Peter W. Leukocyte functions and percentage breakdown. Molecular Biology of the Cell (4th ed.). New York: Garland Science. 2002;41-56.
12. Tanko Y, Mabrouk B, Adelaiye Y, Fatihu, Musa K. Antidiabetic and some hematologicasl effect of ethyl acetate and n-butanol fraction of *Indigofera pulchra* extract on alloxan-induced diabetic wistar rats. J. Diab. Endocrin. 2011;2(1):1-7.
13. Swirski F, Nahrendorf M, Etzrodt M, Wildgruber M, Cortez-Retamozo V, Panizzi P, et al. Identification of splenic reservoir monocytes and their deployment to inflammatory sites. Science. 2009;325:612-616.
14. Polenakovic M, Sikole A. Is erythropoietin a survival factor for red blood cells? J. Am Soc. Ephrology. 1996;7(8):1178-1182.
15. Albers G. Antithrombotic agents in cerebral ischemia. Am. J. Cardiol. 1995;75:34-38.
16. Chernecky C, Barbara J, Berger A. Laboratory tests and diagnostic procedures, 3rd ed. Philadelphia, PA: W. B. Saunders Company. 2001;78-98.
17. Abu-Zalton A. Antidiabetic activity of *Ferula asafetida* extract in normal and alloxan

induced diabetic rats. Pak J Biol Sci. 2010;13:97-100.

18. Marieb R. Essentials of humany anatomy and physiology. 4th ed, California: The Bejamin/Cummings Publishing Co. In. 1994;34.
19. Ganong T. A review of medical physiology. 19th Edn. Appleton and Lange, Stanford, USA. 1999;187–241.
20. Roy A, Gordon M, Kelly C, Hunter K, Carpentar T, Williams. Inhibitory effect of *Ginkgo biloba* extract on human platelet aggregation. Platelets. 1999;10:298-305.
21. Kang S, Chung H, Lee Y, Park B, Zhang H, Yoo H, Yun YP. Antiplatelet activity of green tea catechins is mediated by inhibition of cytoplasmic calcium increase. J. Cardiovasc. Pharmacol. 2001;38:875-884.
22. Chang-Gue S, Seung-Hyun H, Jung-Hyo C, Jang-Woo S, Chin-Ho C, Yeon-Weol L, Chong-Kwan C. Induction of hemopoiesis by saenghyuldan, a mixture of Ginseng radix, Paeoniae radix alba, and Hominis placenta extracts. Acta Pharmacol. Sin. 2003;24:120-126.
23. Udut E, Zhdanov V, Gur'iantseva L, Minakova M, Dygai A. Mechanisms of the erythropoiesis-stimulating effect of skull cap (*Scutellaria baicalensis*) extract. Experimental' naiai Klinicheskaia Farmakologiia. 2005;68:43-45.
24. Iwu M, Igboko O, Okunji C, Tempesta M. Antidiabetic and aldose reductase activities of Biflavanones of *Garcinia kola*. J. Pharm. Pharmacol. 1999;42:290–292.
25. Akah O, Okpi O, Okoli A. Evaluation of the anti inflammatory, analgesic and antimicrobial activities of *Afzelia africana*. Niger. J Nat Prod.Med 2007;11:48-52.
26. Torrell A, Chillard T. Antioxidant activity of flavonoid and reactivity with peroxy radical. Phytochemistry. 1986;2:383-385.

Assessment of Analgesic and Neuropharmacological Activity of Different Extracts of *Euphorbia hirta* (Linn.) Leaf

Md. Razibul Habib[1], Mohammad Mustakim Billah[2*], Kashfia Nawrin[2], Md. Rakibul Hasan[3], Md. Ibrahim Khalil[2] and Md. Mominur Rahman[4]

[1]Directorate General of Drug Administration, Bangladesh.
[2]Department of Pharmacy, East West University, Dhaka, Bangladesh.
[3]Department of Pharmacy, North South University, Dhaka, Bangladesh.
[4]Department of Pharmacy, International Islamic University Chittagong, Bangladesh.

Authors' contributions

This work was carried out in collaboration between all authors. Author Md. Razibul Habib designed the methodology and coordinated the project. Authors MMB and KN performed the neuropharmacological investigation of the extracts and prepared the manuscript. Authors Md. Rakibul Hasan and MIK provided assistance to perform the analgesic activity tests of the extracts. Author MMR helped in the preparation of the extracts and experiments. Author MMB acted as the author of correspondence for this manuscript. All of the authors have read and approved the manuscript.

Article Information

Editor(s):
(1) Othman Ghribi, Department of Pharmacology, Physiology & Therapeutics, University of North Dakota, USA.
Reviewers:
(1) Ayona Jayadev, All Saints' College, Trivandrum, Kerala, India.
(2) Bhaskar Sharma, Suresh Gyan Vihar University, Jaipur, Rajasthan, India.

ABSTRACT

Aims: The present study was carried out to investigate the possible analgesic and neuropharmacological activities of the aqueous, ethanol and ethyl acetate extracts of *Euphorbia hirta* (Linn.) leaves.
Methods: The analgesic and neuropharmacological potential was studied at the dose of 400 mg/kg of body weight in mice. Analgesic potential of the extracts was evaluated using mice writhing method and formalin induced pain tests. In addition, neuropharmacological property of extracts was carried out by hole cross, open field and elevated plus maze tests.

**Corresponding author: Email: mustakimbillah@hotmail.com*

Results: In writhing test, the aqueous extract significantly (89.51%) inhibited the peripheral nociception while in formalin test the ethyl acetate extract significantly (p>0.001) inhibited the licking time in both phases. The ethanolic extract exhibited convincing reduction of exploratory behavior in hole cross and open field tests. Furthermore, an increase in the frequency and duration in the open arm of EPM displayed by all three extracts indicates the evidence of their anxiolytic activity.

Conclusion: These results may rationalize the scientific basis for use of this plant in traditional medicine for treatment of analgesia and anxiety related disorders.

Keywords: E. hirta; writhing; locomotor; formalin; anxiety.

1. INTRODUCTION

Euphorbia hirta (Linn.), belonging to the spurge family of Euphorbiaceae, is an herbaceous plant and very common in tropical countries like Bangladesh. It is a small, erect or ascending annual herb (50 cm high) with hairy stems. The leaves are opposite, elliptical, oblong or oblong-lanceolate with a faintly toothed margin and darker on the upper surface [1]. The leaves produces white or milky juice when cut [2].

E. hirta is being used as a traditional source of medicine for many years in Bangladesh. The Tripura tribe in Chittagong hill tracts of Bangladesh uses this plant for increasing lactation after childbirth and to treat body sores, asthma and chronic bronchitis [3]. The Plant is used for the treatment of cough, asthma, chronic bronchitis, bowel complaints, worm infestation, kidney stones, bronchial affections, conjunctivitis. The crude extract is used as Analgesic, Anti–pyretic, Anxiolytic, Sedative, and Anti–inflammatory and also as Anti–coagulant [4]. Though the aqueous extract has been reported to have central analgesic activity in low dose [5], there was hardly any experimental data found to support the peripheral analgesic properties; alongside no investigation was done for this property with the other two extracts at 400 mg/kg dose. These well-established traditional uses of this plant acted as the driving force to conduct the present study. Again, many studies have been done on *E. hirta,* none of them compared aqueous, ethanol and ethyl acetate extracts of leaf for sedative-anxiolytic activities. The reason that these three extracts had been chosen was due to the extraction capacity of the solvents; aqueous (polar compounds), ethanol (slightly polar to non-polar compounds) and ethyl acetate (highly non-polar compounds) and thereby it can be hypothesized that these three extracts retained maximum number of compounds that can be responsible for the activities observed.

2. MATERIALS AND METHODS

2.1 Collection and Identification of Plant Material

The plant was collected from Chittagong Hill Tracts (between 21°25' N to 23°45' N latitude and 91°25' E to 92°50' E longitude) of Bangladesh in October 2011 when leaves were in their maximum densities (Accession number DACB 39517).

2.2 Preparation of Extracts

The shade dried leaf was coarsely powdered and 500 g extracted with 0.5 L each of water (EHAQ), ethanol (EHET) and ethyl acetate (EHEA) by maceration method at room temperature for a period of 7 days with occasional shaking and stirring. The extracts were filtered and concentrated on rotary evaporator and further dried and weighed about 10% of viscous mass [6].

2.3 Animals

Swiss Albino mice (20-25 g) of either sex were procured from International Centre for Diarrheal Disease Research, Bangladesh (ICDDR, B). The animals were housed under standard conditions of temperature (22±1°C), relative humidity (55±10%), 12 hr light/dark cycles and supplied with food and water *ad libitum* at the Laboratory Animal House, Department of Pharmacy, East West University, Bangladesh. The animals were divided into five groups (N=4) designated as Control (water), EHAQ (400 mg/kg), EHET (400 mg/kg), EHEA (400 mg/kg) and standard for all experiments.

2.4 Drugs and Chemicals

Diclofenac Sodium and Diazepam were obtained from Square Pharmaceuticals Ltd., Bangladesh. Acetic Acid were obtained from Mark, Germany.

Formalin was purchased from CDH, India. All chemicals used were of analytical reagent grade.

2.5 Acute Toxicity Test

Randomly grouped (n = 5) mice separately received the aqueous, ethanol and ethyl acetate extracts orally at doses of 500, 1000, 1500 mg/kg. The control group received the vehicle. The animals were observed for possible allergic reactions, and mortality for the next 72 h and extended up to 14 days.

2.6 Sedative Activity

2.6.1 Hole cross test

The test was performed for screening sedative activity in mice. A steel partition was fixed in the middle of a cage having a size of 30×20×14 cm with A hole of 3 cm diameter at height 7.5 cm in the partition. The number of crossing from one chamber to other was counted for a period of 3 min on 0, 30, 60, 90 and 120 min after the oral gavage with test drugs. Diazepam was used in the positive control group as reference standard at the dose of 1 mg/kg [7].

2.6.2 Open field test

The experiment was carried out according to the methods described by Nyeem et al. [8]. The floor of the open field of a square meter was divided into several squares. The apparatus was enclosed with 40 cm high wall. The number of squares visited by the mice was counted for 3 min, on 0, 30, 60, 90 and 120 min immediately after the oral test drug treatment.

2.7 Anxiolytic Activity

2.7.1 Elevated Plus-Maze (EPM) test

The method initially suggested by Handley and Mithani was employed with minor modifications [9]. The procedure was conducted in a sound attenuated room. Sixty minutes after administration of the test drugs, each animal was placed at the center of the maze. During the 5-min test period, the number of open arms entries and duration were recorded. An Entry was defined when the animal places all four paws onto the arm.

2.8 Analgesic Activity

2.8.1 Mouse writhing test

This was based on the method described by Meera et al. [10]. Diclofenac sodium (10 mg/kg, i.p.) was administered as positive control. 30 minutes later all groups received intraperitoneal injection of 0.7%, 0.1 ml/10 gm acetic acid solution. Mouse were observed and the number of writhing or stretches were counted for 20 min immediately after administering acetic acid. Reduction in the number of writhes compared to the control groups was considered as evidence of analgesic effect.

2.8.2 Formalin test

The method was done according to the method described Sharma et al. [11]. 30 minutes after the groups received their respective treatments, 20 μl of 5% formalin was injected subcutaneously into the right hind paw of mice. The time (in sec) spent in licking and biting the injected paw for next 30 min (0-5 and 16-30 min) were taken as an indicator of pain response.

2.9 Statistical Analysis

Statistical analysis for animal experiments was carried out using one-way analysis of variance (ANOVA) followed by Dunnett's multiple comparison tests using SPSS 20 for windows. The results obtained were compared with the vehicle control group. *P* values < 0.05, 0.01 and 0.001 were considered to be statistically significant.

3. RESULTS

3.1 Acute Toxicity Test

Observations of all three extracts dosing from 500–1500 mg/kg, did not produce any mortality in mice within 72 h and further observation period, suggesting that these extracts of leaves of *E. hirta* have low toxicity profile with LD50 greater than 1500 mg/kg.

3.2 Hole Cross Test

The number of hole crossed by the mice was moderately reduced by the ethanolic extract. The inhibition was observed from the 2nd to the 5th observation period (Fig. 1).

3.3 Open Field Test

The ethanolic extract significantly suppressed the number of square travelled by the mice (Fig. 2). Maximum suppression was observed from the 3rd observation period and was comparable with the reference drug. The data of ethyl acetate extract was also convincing. The data were statistically significant.

3.4 Elevated Plus Maze

Table 1 shows that all extracts effectively increased the percent number of entry into the open arm which indicates its anxiolytic potential.

3.5 Writhing Test

All three extracts significantly (*P>0.001*) inhibited the nociception induced by acetic acid on mice (Table 2). But the aqueous extract showed maximum inhibition (89.51%) which was comparable with the reference drug (92.30%).

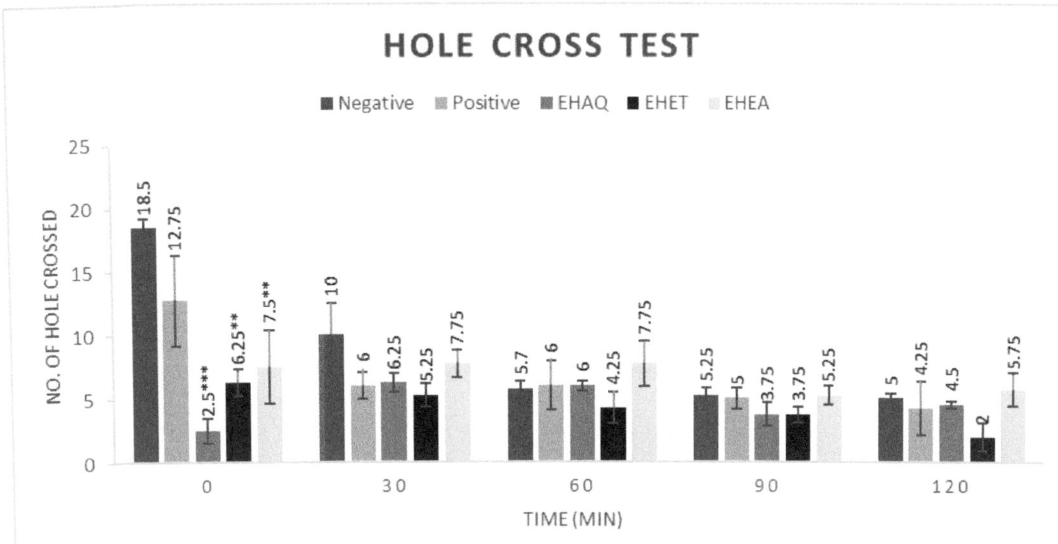

Fig. 1. Effect of the aqueous, ethanol and ethyl acetate extracts of leaves of *E. hirta* on hole cross test in mice

*Values are mean ± S.E.M., (n = 4); ** P < 0.01, *** P < 0.001 Dunnet test as compared to control (Vehicle = 0.5 mL/mouse)*

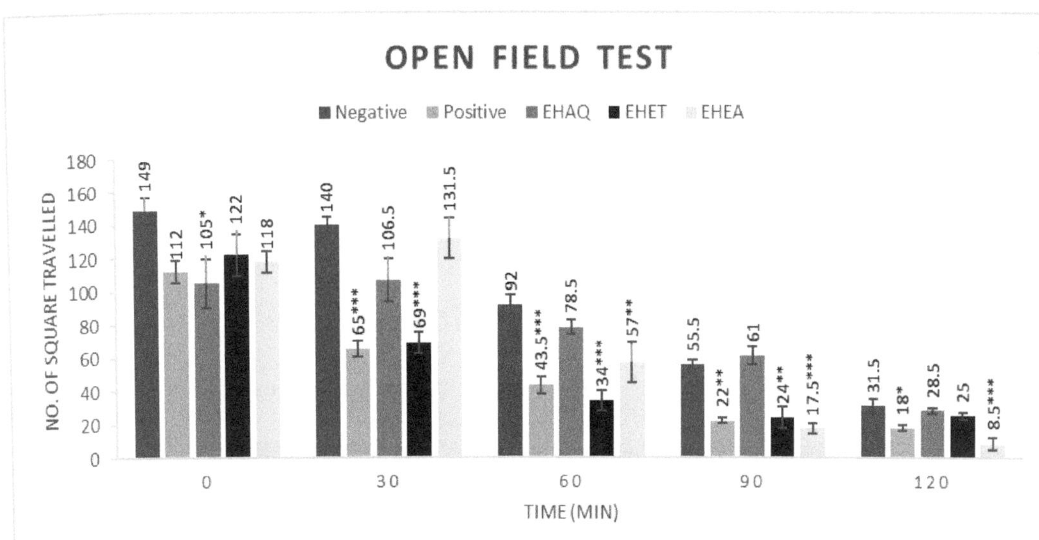

Fig. 2. Effect of the aqueous, ethanol and ethyl acetate extracts of leaves of *E. hirta* on open field test in mice

*Values are mean ± S.E.M., (n = 4); * P < 0.05, ** P < 0.01, *** P < 0.001 Dunnet test as compared to control (Vehicle = 0.5 mL/mouse)*

3.6 Formalin Test

Table 3 shows the effect of extracts on formalin induced persistent pain on two phases. EHEA significantly (*P>0.001*) inhibited the licking time in either of the phases.

4. DISCUSSION

In vivo screening of locomotor activities is considered an effective method to investigate the sedative potential. The ethanol extract significantly decreased the locomotor activity as shown by the results of the open field and hole cross tests. The locomotor activity lowering effect was evident at the 2nd observation (30 min) and continued up to 5th observation period (120 min) (Figs. 1 & 2). As the major inhibitory neurotransmitter in CNS is the Gamma-amino-butyric acid (GABA) and different anxiolytic, muscle relaxant, sedative-hypnotic drugs showed their action through GABAA, it can be hypothesized that ethanol extract of *E. hirta* also act by membrane hyperpolarization which potentiates GABA-ergic inhibition in the CNS that leads to either decrease in the firing rate of critical neurons in the brain or direct activation of GABA receptor [12]. Thus decreased spontaneous motor activity could be attributed to the CNS depressant activity of the extracts. Moreover, elevated plus-maze test validates psychomotor performance and emotional aspects of rodents. The results showed that extracts of *E. hirta* leaf increased the time spent in open arms to little extent. This effect can be attributed to the action on GABA

Table 1. EPM test of *E. hirta* Dunnett t (2-sided)[a]

Group (N=5)	% no. of entry into the open arm	% time spent in the open arms
Positive	77.47±3.037***	79.21±2.789**
Negative	55.71±2.221	51.93±2.080
EHAQ	60.62±0.599	30.77±0.582*
EHET	56.73±1.609	28.95±5.601**
EHEA	59.30±2.061	33.74±5.837*

*Each value is presented as the mean ± SEM (n = 5). ***P < 0.001, **P < 0.01, *P < 0.05*
a. Dunnett t-test treats one group as control and compares all other groups against it.

Table 2. Acetic acid induced writhing test of *E. hirta* Dunnett t (2-sided)[a]

Group (N=5)	No. of writhing (Average ± S.E.M)	% inhibition
Positive	2.75±0.478***	92.30
Negative	35.75±3.099	0
EHAQ	3.75±0.478***	89.51
EHET	9.25±0.661***	74.12
EHEA	10.25±1.089***	71.32

****the mean difference is significant at the 0.001 level.*
a. Dunnett t-test treats one group as control and compares all other groups against it.

Table 3. Formalin test of *E. hirta* Dunnett t (2-sided)[a]

Group (N=5)	Early phase licking time (Average ± S.E.M)	% inhibition	Late phase licking time (Average ± S.E.M)	% inhibition
Positive	41.5±2.397***	62.94	26.25±1.931***	62.76
Negative	112±6.770	0	70.50±1.707	0
EHAQ	109±4.778	2.67	62.75±2.529	10.99
EHET	94.25±5.344	15.84	61.50±3.476	12.76
EHEA	49.25±1.931***	56.02	34.5±3.926***	51.06

****the mean difference is significant at the 0.001 level.*
a. Dunnett t-test treats one group as control and compares all other groups against it.

benzodiazepine receptor complex, stimulation of glucocorticoid production and release in the adrenal cortex [13], after administration of 5-HT1B receptor antagonists and 5- HT1A agonists [14]. Therefore with the present data, it is difficult to predict the precise mechanism for the anxiolytic activity of the *E. hirta* leaf.

These three extracts were also evaluated in the formalin and acetic acid-induced writhing test for their analgesic activity. The acetic acid induced writhing response is an established procedure to evaluate peripheral analgesics. The response is thought to be mediated by the prostaglandin pathways, peritoneal mast cells and acid sensing ion channels [15-17]. Therefore, the significant pain reduction of the plant extracts may be due to acting with the prostaglandin pathways or interfering with other mediators responsible for peripheral pain.

The formalin test is another reliable model of analgesic which is better correlated with clinical pain [18,19]. This method elucidates central and peripheral activities. The response of early phase is believed to represent a direct chemical stimulation of pain, due to the irritant effect of formalin on sensory C fibers [19]. The late phase response is most likely secondary to the development of an inflammatory response and the release of allergic mediators [20]. Inhibition of licking response of the extracts in the early phase and late phase signifies the analgesic effect of the extracts.

The medicinal potential of *Euphorbia hirta* (Linn.) is believed to be due to the presence of alkaloids, flavonoids, tannins, saponins, cardiac and cyanogenic glycosides in its crude extract [21]. However, phytochemical screening of each of the crude extract is necessary to attribute to the compound responsible for specific activity.

5. CONCLUSION

In vivo study showed that all three extracts possess analgesic or neuropharmacological activity which supports the traditional use of this plant leaf for medical ailments. Though, studies are required on higher animal model and subsequently on human subjects to prove its clinical efficacy as an analgesic and CNS depressant agent. This study provides a scientific acknowledgement of its use and concludes that oral preparation of this plant extract for human use is safe and beneficial.

CONSENT

It is not applicable.

ETHICAL APPROVAL

It is not applicable.

COMPETING INTERESTS

Authors have declared that no competing interests exist.

REFERENCES

1. Patil SB, Naikwade NS, Magdum CS. Review on phytochemistry and pharmacological aspects of *Euphorbia hirta* (Linn.) linn. Journal of Pharmaceutical Research and Health Care. 2009;1(1): 113-133.
2. Rao KV, Karthik L, Elumalai EK, Srinivasan K, Kumar G. Antibacterial and antifungal activity of *Euphorbia hirta* (Linn.) l. leaves: A comparative study. Journal of Pharmacy Research. 2010;3(3):548-549.
3. Hossan MS, Hanif A, Khan M, Bari S, Jahan R, Rahmatullah M. Ethnobotanical survey of the Tripura tribe of Bangladesh. American-Eurasian Journal of Sustainable Agriculture. 2009;3(2):253-261.
4. Nagori BP, Solanki R. Role of medicinal plants in wound healing. Research Journal of Medicinal Plants. 2011;5(4):392-405.
5. Lanhers MC, Fleurentin J, Dorfman P, Mortier F, Pelt JM. Analgesic, antipyretic and anti-inflammatory properties of *Euphorbia hirta*. Planta Med. 1991;57(3): 225-231.
6. Raihan MO, Habib MR, Brishti A, Rahman MM, Saleheen MM, Manna M. Sedative and anxiolytic effects of the methanolic extract of *Leea indica* (Burm. f.) Merr. leaf. Drug Discov Ther. 2011;5(4):185-189. DOI: 10.5582/ddt.2011.v5.4.185
7. Subhan N, Alam MA, Ahmed F, Shahid IJ, Nahar L, Sarker SD. Bioactivity of *Excoecaria agallocha*. Braz J Pharmacogn. 2008;18:521–526. DOI: 10.1590/S0102695X2008000400004
8. Nyeem MAB, Alam MA, Awal MA, Mostofa M, Uddin SJ, Islam N, et al. CNS depressant effect of the crude ethanolic extract of the flowering tops of rosa damascena. Iranian J. Pharmacol Ther. 2006;5:171-174.

9. Braida D, CapurroV, Zani A, Rubino T, Viganò D, Parolaro D, et al. Potential anxiolytic- and antidepressant-like effects of salvinorin A, the main active ingredient of Salvia divinorum, in rodents. British J Pharmacol. 2009;157:844-853. DOI: 10.1111/j.1476-5381.2009.00230.x
10. Meera S, Kumar NS, Guptatyam VSSS. Screening of anti-arthritic, antiinflmmatory and analgesic activity of a polyherbal formulation. Int J Pharmacol. 2008;4(5): 398-402. DOI: 10.3923/ijp.2008.398.402
11. Sharma A, Bhatial S, Kharyaz MD, Gajbhiye V, Ganesh N, Namdeo AG, Mahadik KR: Anti-inflammatory and analgesic activity of different fractions of Boswellia serrata. International Journal of Phytomedicine. 2010;2:94-99.
12. Khatun MH, Islam MR, Mamun A, Nahar L, Luth F, Islam MAU: *In Vivo* evalu atio n of CNS dep ressant and antinociceptive activities of methanol extract of *Hibiscus sabdariffa* fruit. J of Appli Scie Rese. 2011; 7(6):798-804.
13. Nishikava H, Hata T, Funakami Y. A role for corticotropin-releasing factor in repeated cold stress-in duced anxiety-like behavior during forced swimming and elevated plu s-maze test in mice. Biol Pharm Bull. 2004;27(3):352-356.
14. Millan MJ, Hjo rth S, Samanin R, Schreiber R, Jaffard R, De Ladonchamps: B. S1553 5, A novel benzodioxopiperazine ligand of serotonin (%-5HT) 1A receptor: II. Modulation of hippocampal serotonin release in relation to p otential an xiolytic properties. J Pharmacol Exp Ther. 1997;282:148-161.
15. Hossain MM, Ali MS, Saha A, Alimuzzaman M: Antinociceptive activity of whole plant extracts of *Paederia foetida*. Dhaka University Journal of Pharmaceutical Science. 2006;5:67-69.
16. Ronaldo AR, Mariana LV, Sara MT, Adriana BPP, Steve P, Ferreira SH, Fernando QC. Involvement of resident macrophages and mast cells in the writhing nociceptive response induced by zymosan and acetic acid in mice. European Journal Pharmacology. 2000; 387:111-118.
17. Voilley N: Acid-Sensing Ion Channels (ASICs): New targets for the analgesic effects of Non-Steroid Anti-inflammatory Drugs (NSAIDs). Current Drug Targets-Inflammation an Allergy. 2004;3:71-79.
18. Ghannadi A, Hajhashemi V, Jafarabadi H: An investigation of the analgesic and antiinflammatory effects of Nigella sativa seed polyphenols. Journal of Medicinal Food. 2005;8:488-493.
19. Sandra D, Susana A, Domingo MH. Peripheral analgesic and anti-inflammatory effects of smilax canariensis in an animal model. Pharmacology & Pharmacy. 2015; 6:391-400. DOI: doi.org/10.4236/pp.2015.68040
20. Hunskaar S, Hole K. The formalin test in mice: dissociation between inflammatory and noninflammatory pain. Pain. 1987;30: 103-114.
21. Ogbulie JN, Ogueke CC, Okoli IC, Anyanwu BN. Antibacterial activities and toxicological potentials of crude ethanolic extracts of *Euphorbia hirta* (Linn.). African Journal of Biotechnology. 2007;6(13): 1544-1548.

12

Free Radical Scavenging Activity and Protein Concentration and Profile of the Blowfly Maggot (*Lucilia robineau*) Excretion/Saliva Extract

I. C. J. Omalu[1*], E. C. Egwim[2], K. Abdulraman[1], S. Ibrahim[1], C. Hassan[1], S. S. Eke[1], E. D. Ubanwa[1], A. Aliyu[3] and A. A. Boyi[1]

[1]*Department of Biological Sciences, Federal University of Technology Minna, Nigeria.*
[2]*Global Institute for Biotechnology and Exploration, Federal University of Technology Minna, Nigeria.*
[3]*Ministry of Livestock and Fisheries, Niger State, Nigeria.*

Authors' contributions

This work was carried out in collaboration between all authors. Authors ICJO and ECE designed the study. Authors ICJO, KA and SI wrote the protocol. Authors CH, SSE and EDU performed the laboratory analysis. Authors AA and AAB wrote the first draft of the manuscript. All authors read and approved the final manuscript.

Article Information

Editor(s):
(1) Vasudevan Mani, Universiti Teknologi MARA (UiTM), Selangor, Malaysia.
Reviewers:
(1) Daniela Hanganu, Iuliu Hatieganu University of Medicine and Pharmacy Cluj-Napoca, Romania.
(2) Fai-Chu Wong, Universiti Tunku Abdul Rahman, Malaysia.
(3) Anonymous, University of Lisbon, Portugal.

ABSTRACT

Aim: The aim of this study was to determine the free radical scavenging activity, Protein concentration and profile of Blowfly maggot (*Lucilia robineau*) excretion/secretion (ES).

Place and Duration of Study: Maggot samples were collected from first generation of blowflies reared between June 2014 and July 2015.

Introduction: Maggots of the blowfly have been successfully used as a debridement agent for chronic and infected wounds through history.

Methodology: Antioxidant activity, protein concentration and profiles of the maggot ES of *Lucilia robineau* was determined using DPPH free radical scavenging activity and Bradford methods

Results: Results showed that maggot ES expressed a free radical scavenging activity with IC_{50} of 152.66 μg/ml compared with L-ascorbic acid with IC_{50} of 108.99 μg/ml as a positive control while

Corresponding author: Email: omaluicj@futminna.edu.ng

total protein concentration was 430.51 mg/ml. Protease and specific activities are $1.5x10^{-2}$ mg/ml and 28,700.67 IU while the protein fractions are Albumins 36.96%, Alpha Globulins 21.32%, Beta Globulins 31.69% and Gamma Globulins 10.02%.

Conclusion: Therefore, this study revealed that the proteomic content of maggot ES of *Lucilia robineau* has promising natural antioxidants. This is the first study on antioxidant properties, protein concentration and profile of Blowfly maggot (*Lucilia robineau*).

Keywords: Antioxidants; DPPH; free radical; maggot ES and protein fractions.

1. INTRODUCTION

Maggots have long been used as a traditional way of cleansing and healing gangrenous wounds. The first modern clinical study of maggot therapy was initiated in 1989, at the University of California. The result of many clinical trials and studies has indicated that maggot therapy is still useful today as a safe and effective treatment tool for some types of wounds. Those studies also demonstrated that there is no reason to withhold maggot therapy until all other modalities has been exhausted, nor use it only as a "last resort". While published accounts of "pre-amputation maggot therapy" show a limb salvage rate of over 40%, the success of maggot debridement therapy MDT when used earlier in the course of treatment (say a 2nd or 3rd or 4th line treatment) is even more dramatic [1].

In recent decades, there has been an increasing world-wide spread of hospital-acquired pathogens exhibiting resistance against one or more of the clinically applied antibiotics. This serious problem attracted renewed attention to the old-fashioned and almost forgotten therapy of Maggot Debridement Therapy (MDT). The use of medicinal maggots in USA was approved by the Food and Drug Administration as a medical device in 2004 [2]. Over the last few years, several comparative clinical trials investigating the efficacy of MDT have been performed [3]. In terms of debridement, MDT is more effective than conventional therapies [4]. On the other hand, in terms of wound healing and remodeling, the outcomes of clinical trials are controversial [5]. MDT has attracted great attention due to its successful application and efficacy in the elimination of multi-drug resistant wound pathogens [6].

Antioxidant is a substance capable of frustrating or restricting the oxidation of other oxidizable molecules by suppressing the free radical caused oxidation chain reaction. Antioxidants exhibit their activities by being involved in the oxidation process themselves rather than the biological targets [7].

Free radical-induced oxidative damage is involved in the pathogenesis of many chronic and degenerative diseases, such as cardio-vascular disease, cancer, diabetes, neuro-degenerative diseases and ageing [8-10]. The harmful action of the free radicals can, however be blocked by antioxidant substances which scavenge the free radicals and detoxify the organism.

The objective of this study was to explore the properties of natural products related to cultural uses and ethnic medicine by determining the free radical scavenging activity of maggot excretion/ saliva extract.

2. MATERIALS AND METHODS

2.1 Blowfly (Maggot) Sampling and Maintenance

Raw meat were exposed to blowflies in Minna Abattoir for a period of one to two hours after which the eggs deposited in meat was placed in a nylon bag usually between 25-34°C and kept till it decayed and maggots emerged. Maggots at the third instar pupated for adult emergence. These new adults were transferred to a fresh meat for egg laying and emergence of second generation maggots for the extraction of excretion/secretion of saliva.

2.2 Extraction of Maggot ES

The method described by Shuchi et al. [11] was used. Live adult specimens collected from the field were anaesthetized by chloroform for a short time for identification. After identification, the species were transferred to new cages for oviposition. Eggs laid on the meat were treated with 70% ethanol and sterile distilled water successively three times. The treated eggs were deposited on fresh meat and allowed to hatch to maggots for 2-3 days in an incubator at 35°C.

Late second or early third instar maggots were aseptically transferred to a flat petri-plate and washed with ethanol and sterile distilled water successively three times and soaked in filter paper. Treated larvae were incubated in sterile distilled water (5 μl/larva) for 60 minutes at ambient temperature in the dark [12]. Resultant Maggot Extract (ME) obtained were transferred to another tube using a pipette and autoclaved for 20 minutes at 121°C. Subsequently, the maggot extract is allowed to cool to room temperature. Any remaining were stored at -20°C for analysis and future use.

2.3 Free Radical Scavenging Activity

Antioxidant activity was measured by the method of Blois (1958) [13] in terms of radical scavenging ability using DPPH method in a methanolic medium [14,15]. The lyophilized maggot ES was dissolved in MeOH yielding a 3-time concentration, and the resultant methanolic solution was termed as 3×m maggot ES. Volumes of 100 μl of serial double-fold dilutions of the 3×m maggot ES were pipetted into 96-well plate. Then, all volumes were brought to a final volume of 300 μl by MeOH. Then, 15 μl of methanol DPPH solution (0.002 M) was added and the A516 were taken after 15 min. The same procedures were performed using serial step-wise dilutions of L-ascorbic acid (50 μg/ml) in methanol as a positive control. The PHS was used as a negative control. Finally, a volume of 15 μl of DPPH was added to 300 μl of MeOH and A516 was measured immediately as a control reading. The free radical scavenging activity (%antiradical activity) was estimated from the equation:

% antiradical activity= control absorbance - Sample absorbance/ control absorbance x 100

2.4 Total Protein Estimation, Profiles and Fractions

Total protein concentration assay was executed as described by Bradford (1976) and the standard protocols of Bradford reagent kit [16] using BSA as a standard protein and the PHS as a blank. Concentration was measured in mg/l.

The different protein fractions were quantified by selective precipitation by passing it through a pH gradient i.e. changing the pH over a range of values [17].

Protease activity was determined by measuring the amount of amino acids released upon hydrolysis proteins using bovine serum albumin as a substrate.

Protease activity = amino acid released / Time

Specific activity = protein conc. / protease activity

2.5 Data Analysis

The collected data were analysed using SPSS version 15.0.

3. RESULTS

Results showed a free radical scavenging activity of maggot excretion/secretion with IC_{50} of 152.66±0.69 μg/ml. Similarly, L-ascorbic acid which is the standard was found to be a free radical scavenger with IC_{50} of 108.99±0.34 ug/ml (Fig. 1).

The protein concentration was 430.51 mg/ml (Fig. 2); protease and specific activities are $1.5x10^{-2}$ mg/ml and 28,700.67 IU. Protein fractions are Albumins 36.96%, Alpha Globulins 21.32%, and Beta globulins and Gamma globulins are 31.69% and 10.02% respectively (Table 1). The major protein was albumin, followed by beta, alpha and gamma globulins.

Table 1. Analysis of blowfly maggot *(Lucilia robineau)* excretion/saliva extract protein

Activity	Unit
Bradford assay	430.51 mg/ml
Protease activity	1.5x10-2 mg/ml
Specific activity	28,700.67 IU
Protein fraction	
Albumins	36.96%
Alpha globulins	21.32%
Beta globulins	31.69%
Gamma globulins	10.02%

4. DISCUSSION

Antioxidants are biochemicals, vitamins and other nutrients that protect our cells from damage caused by free radicals. The result of the antioxidant properties of maggot excretion/secretion was high compared to the standard L-ascorbic acid. This is the first study on the free scavenging activities of maggot ES to the best of our knowledge as such we are unable to compare our result with others studies. Leeches that are also animal products have very high antioxidant properties as seen in Malaysian leeches [18] and Nigeria leeches (*Aliolimnatis michaelseni*) [19].

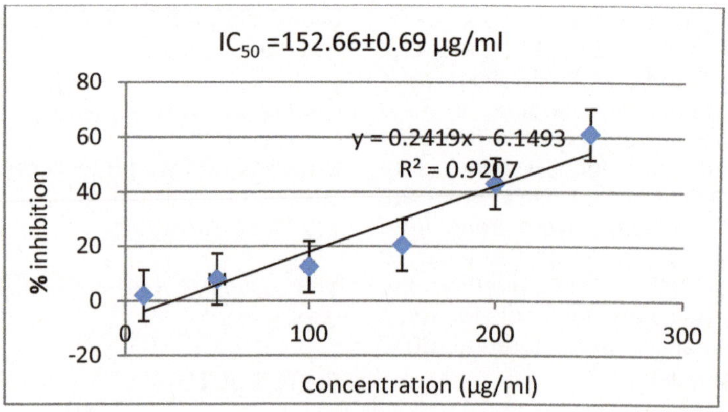

(a)

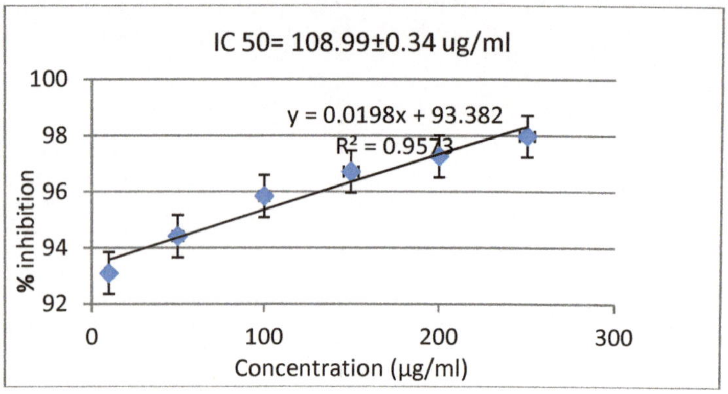

(b)

Fig. 1. DPPH free radical scavenging activity of maggot ES (a) and L-ascorbic acid (b)

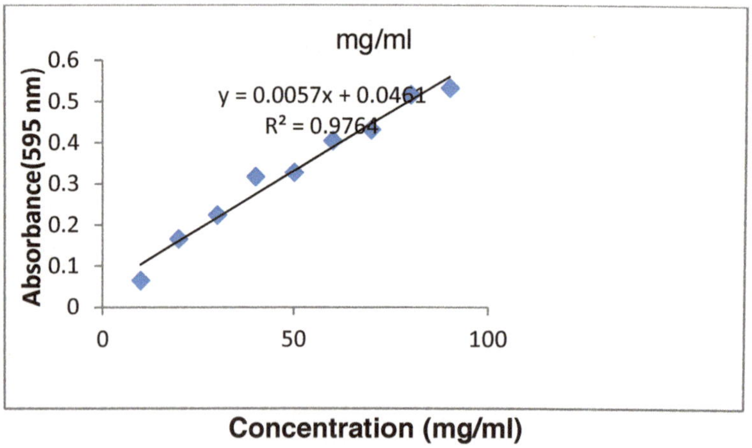

Fig. 2. The standard curve for total protein estimation of maggot ES performed according to Bradford assay

The search for raw materials containing potent antioxidants continues to attract the attention of researchers. Vegetables, fruits and spices are known to be rich sources of natural antioxidants, and medicinal plants and animals are another important source for a wide variety of natural antioxidants. These medicinal plants and animals have high anti-inflammatory activities which could be from, in part, their antioxidant properties.

This result has explored the potentials of natural animal product related to cultural uses and ethnic medicine for the treatment of diseases, since antioxidants have valuable potential applications in medicine and industries. They have very promising applications as prophylactic and therapeutic agents for many life-threatening illnesses [20].

This study also revealed that Maggots ES has a high protein concentration of compared to other animal products like leech saliva [18,19]. Determination of the total protein concentration is an important tool among the procedures used in enzyme and protein characterization and purification. Physiological studies of protein expression and clinical diagnoses of altered protein levels in body fluids, is indicative of a variety of diseases.

Fractionation of proteins is often employed to quantify protein types within food materials. The results of the extracted protein fractions from maggot ES showed that albumin, beta, alpha and gamma globulins were observed and quantified accordingly. The data showed that albumin was the major protein in the maggot ES.

5. CONCLUSION

The excretion/secretion from blowfly maggot, *Lucilia robineau* had a high free radical scavenging activity and a high protein content indicating that it may have some therapeutic properties for the treatment of various diseases.

CONSENT

It is not applicable.

ETHICAL APPROVAL

It is not applicable.

ACKNOWLEDGEMENTS

This study was sponsored by TETFUND/ FUTMINN/2014/08, from the Federal University of Technology Minna.

COMPETING INTERESTS

Authors have declared that no competing interests exist.

REFERENCES

1. Sherman RA, Hall MJR, Thomas S. Medicinal maggots: An ancient remedy for some contemporary afflictions. An. Rev. Entomol. 2000;45: 55–81.
2. Steenvoorde P, Jacobi CE, Van Doorn L, Oskam J. Maggot debridement therapy of infected ulcers: Patient and wound factors influencing outcome – A study on 101 patients with 117 wounds. Annual Royal College Surgeons of England. 2007;89: 596-602.
3. Dumville JC, Worthy G, Bland JM, Cullum N, Dowson C, Iglesias C, Mitchell JL, Nelson EA, Soares MO, Torgerson DJ. Larval therapy for leg ulcers (VenUS II): Randomised controlled trial. Bio Medical Journal. 2009;338:b773.
4. Sherman RA. Maggot versus conservative debridement therapy for the treatment of pressure ulcers. Wound Repair Regeneration. 2002;10:208-214.
5. Huberman L, Gollop N, Mumcuoglu KY, Breuer E, Bhusare SR, Shai Y, Galun R. Antibacterial substances of low molecular weight isolated from the blowfly, *Lucilia sericata*. Med Vet Entomol. 2007;21:127-131.
6. Bello YM, Falabella AF, DeCaralho H, Nayyar G, Kirsner RS. Infection and wound healing. Wounds. 2001;13:127-131.
7. Sies H. Oxidative stress: Oxidants and antioxidants. Exp Physiol. 1997;82: 291-295.
8. Azizova OA. Role of free radical processes in the development of artherosclerosis. Biol. Membrany. 2002;19:457–471.
9. Nagler R, Rezick A, Shafir Y, Shehadeh N. Free radical effects and antioxidants in saliva and serum of adolescents with type 1 diabetes mellitus. Free Radic. Res. 2006;40:5156.
10. Barnham KJ, Masters CI, Bush AI. Neurodegenerative disease and anti-oxidantive stress. Nat. Rev. Drug. Discorv. 2004;3:205–214.
11. Shuchi A, Carl B, Chusing L. Maggot metabolite and combinatory effect with antibiotic *Staphlococcus aureus.* Ann. Clin. Microbiol. Antimicrobes. 2011;10:6.
12. Mariena JA, Cheryl D, Helen CM, Simone K, Jaap T, Peter HN. Combinations of maggot excretions/ secretions and anti-bioticsare effective against *Staphlococcus*

aureus biofilms and bacteria derived fromrhereform. J. Antimicrobialchem. 2010;65(5):917-923.

13. Blois MS. Antioxidant determinations by the use of a stable free radical. Nature. 1958;181:1199-1200.
14. Sanja SD, Sheth NR, Dhaval P, Biraju P. Characterization and evaluation of antioxidant activity of *Portucla oleracea*. Int. J. Pharm. Pharm. Sci. 2009;1:74-83.
15. Althunibat OY, Hashim RB, Taher M, Daud JM, Ikeda MA, et al. *In vitro* antioxidant and antiproliferative activities of three Malaysian sea cucumber species. Europ. J. Sci. Res. 2009;37:376-38.
16. Bradford MM. A rapid and sensitive method for the quantitation of microgram quantities of protein utilizing the principle of protein-dye binding. Anal. Biochem. 1976;72:248-254.
17. Stroev EA, Makarova VG. Laboratory manual in biochemistry. MIR Publishers, Moscow. 1989;158-159.
18. Ghawi AM, Abdualkader AM, Merzouk A, Alaama M. Free radical scavenging activity of the medicinal Malaysian leech saliva extract, *Hirudinaria manillensis*. J. Bioequival. Avail. 2012;S14. DOI: 10.4172/jbb.S14-001
19. Omalu ICJ, Egwim EC, Mgbemena CC, Eke CC, Ubanwa D, Busar MB, Ossai PC. Free radical scavenging activity of the Nigerian leech (*Aliolimnatis michaelseni*) saliva extract. British J. Pharm. Res; 2015. (In press).
20. Bjelakovic G, Nikolova D, Gluud LL, Simonetti RG, Gluud C. Mortality in randomized trials of antioxidant supplements for primary and secondary prevention. JAMA. 2007;297:842-857.

13

Extracts of Eastern Nigeria Mistletoe, *Tapinanthus globiferus* (A. Rich.) Tiegh. Modulate Dexamethasone-induced Insulin Resistance and Exhibit Potent osteogenic Activity in Animal Experimental Model

Omeje Edwin Ogechukwu[1,2,3*], Mohd Parvez Khan[3], Osadebe Patience Ogoamaka[1], Okoye Theophine Chinwuba[4], Ugwoke Christopher Emeka[5], Onugwu Lawrence Ekene[1], Deepshika Tewari[3], Rakesh Maurya[3] and Naibedya Chattopadhyay[3]

[1]Department of Pharmaceutical and Medicinal Chemistry, Faculty of Pharmaceutical Sciences, University of Nigeria, 41001, Nsukka, Nigeria.
[2]Division of Medicinal and Process Chemistry, CSIR-Central Drug Research Institute, Chattar Manzil, P.O.Box 173, 226001, Lucknow, India.
[3]Division of Endocrinology, CSIR-Central Drug Research Institute, Chattar Manzil, P.O.Box 173, 226001, Lucknow, India.
[4]Department of Pharmacology and Toxicology, Faculty of Pharmaceutical Sciences, University of Nigeria, 41001, Nsukka, Nigeria.
[5]Department of Pharmacognosy and Enviromental Medicine, Faculty of Pharmaceutical Sciences, University of Nigeria, 41001, Nsukka, Nigeria.

Authors' contributions

This work was carried out in collaboration between all authors. Author OEO was largely responsible for the design, collection of plant materials and execution of the experiment as well as writing of the initial draft of manuscript. Author MPK contributed largely in the design and execution of the research work. Authors NC and OPO were responsible for the overall supervision of the work and editing of manuscript. Author RM assisted greatly with the extraction process. Authors OTC and OLE assisted with the development of the manuscript. Author DT participated actively in the research design and statistical analysis while author UCE assisted with the plant identification alongside Mr. A. O. Ozioko and also formed part of the editorial team. All authors read and approved the final manuscript.

Article Information

Editor(s):
(1) Syed A. A. Rizvi, Department of Pharmaceutical Sciences, College of Pharmacy, Nova Southeastern University, USA.
Reviewers:
(1) Anna Gumieniczek, Medical University of Lublin, Poland.
(2) Li Yao, Zhejiang Chinese Medical University, China.
(3) Sema Kalkan Ucar, Ege University, Turkey.

**Corresponding author: Email: edwin.omeje@unn.edu.ng*

ABSTRACT

Ethnopharmacological Relevance: Scientific evidence for the traditional use of eastern Nigeria mistletoe as an anti-diabetic and anti-osteoporotic agent has been documented. In our continued efforts to provide further evidence towards eventual approval of the medicinal usage of the eastern Nigeria mistletoes, the present study was undertaken to evaluate its effects on steroid induced insulin-resistance and *in-vivo* bone health parameters in rodent model.

Materials and Methods: Twelve-weeks (12) old Sprague-Dawley (SD) rats of both sexes and weighing 200±20 g were administered with dexamethasone (200 $mgkg^{-1}$) for minimum of 14 days and with or without 100-400 $mgkg^{-1}$ of crude aqueous extract of mistletoe harvested from *Kola acuminata*, in this paper referred to as Kola-mistletoe (KM). The basal glucose levels were established and animals were later exposed to oral glucose tolerance test (OGTT). Blood samples were collected from ketamine-anesthetized animals via cardiac puncture for measurement of biochemical parameters. The femur and vertebrae bones were neatly excised and stored in 70% isopropanol at 4°C until further analysis. µCT determination of excised bones was carried out using the Sky Scan 1076 µCT scanner (Aartselaar, Belgium) as described in our previously published protocols.

Results: The extracts significantly preserved the animals from the effects of dexamethasone mostly at 400 mg/kg dose in terms of weight loss and blood glycaemia. The extract (either alone or in combination with dexamethasone and within the duration of treatments showed better bone quality (higher BV/TV (Bone volume to Trabecular volume ratio), lower Tb.Sp (Trabecular separation) and SMI (Structure model index) indices at the dose of 400 mg/kg compared with vehicle and metformin groups.

Conclusion: The present data show that the Nigeria mistletoes are potent in reversing the adverse effects of prolonged exposure to dexamethasone in rodents and evidently protected the bones from impairment.

Keywords: Dexamethasone; insulin-resistance; Eastern Nigeria mistletoe; osteogenic; Loranthus micranthus; Tapinanthus globiferus.

1. INTRODUCTION

Insulin-resistance induced by prolonged glucocorticoids therapy is an essential metabolic challenge leading to impaired glucose metabolism, diabetes, obesity, osteonecrosis and ultimately osteoporosis usually referred to medically, as glucocorticoid-induced osteoporosis [1,2]. Glucocorticoids are, unavoidably, widely prescribed in several cases of inflammation including but not limited to rheumatoid arthritis, asthma, systemic lupus erythematosus, cancer and organ transplantation [3,4]. Notably, the adverse effect of glucocorticoids on bone growth and metabolism has been recognized for more than six decades [5,6]. This bone effect is characterized by decreased bone formation and *in situ* apoptosis (osteonecrosis) of isolated segments particularly at the trabecular-rich femoral head [6]. Although, postmenopausal osteoporosis, characterized by rapid loss of mineralized bone tissue, disruption of trabecular architecture of the bone and changes in the crystalline properties of mineral deposits with concomitant effect of structural failure (fracture of sites rich in cancellous bone) affects both female and male, the incidence is much higher in women [7]. This obviously, is attributed to the dramatic estrogen withdrawal associated with menopause. Besides this major causative factor promoting osteoporosis, there are avalanche of evidence indicating that most often, more women than men use glucocorticoids for several indirect medical reasons thereby promoting a faster onset of osteoporosis beyond menopause. Hormones such as catecholamine, glucagon, cortisol and thyroxin, either through directly or their influence on other hormones, affect carbohydrate metabolism to elevate blood glucose level leading to insulin resistance [8].

Insulin-resistance has been shown to be present in conditions like type-II diabetes, obesity and dyslipidemia. Thus, interventions to decrease insulin-resistance may postpone the development of type-II diabetes and its complications [9]. Glucocorticoids in excess inhibit insulin secretion from pancreatic beta-cells, decrease glucose utilization, and stimulate glucagon secretion, lipolysis, proteolysis, and hepatic glucose production. Glucocorticoids can modulate the insulin action at both binding sites and post binding sites and cause decreased glucose utilization in muscles. Glucocorticoids also cause insulin resistance by decreasing hepatic glucose utilization, decreasing glycogen synthesis. Free fatty acids may be elevated in insulin resistance because of impaired insulin-dependent down-regulation of lipolysis, hence leading to increase in triglyceride levels in muscles as well as other tissues presumably because of excess of circulating free fatty acids which are then deposited in these organs. The triglycerides are reported to be potent inhibitors of insulin signaling cascade and result in acquired insulin resistance state [10].

The above facts taken together, glucocorticoid-associated insulin resistance is strongly tied with impairment of glucose and bone metabolism. Experimentally, different doses (low to high) of dexamethasone, a common glucocorticoid, have been demonstrated to induce insulin- resistance and diverse metabolic effects in rodents [11,12]. Expectedly, therefore, an ideal antidiabetic agent should in addition to its normal glucose regulatory potentials modulate insulin resistance effectively and reverse the adverse osteonecrotic effects of implicated agents especially antidiabetic patients on prolonged glucocorticoid.

Medicinal plants have formed the basis of health care throughout the world since the earliest days of humanity and have remained relevant in both developing and the developed nations of the world for various chemotherapeutic purposes [13]. The use of plant-derived natural compounds as part of herbal preparations for alternate source of medicament continues to play major roles in chemotherapy especially in third world countries [14,15]. Several studies carried out have shown that traditional medicines could provide better glycaemic control than currently used conventional drugs [16-19]. In fact, the nearest future will witness a fast growing dependence on herbal medicines for the health needs of world's populations, especially with the avalanche of advancing research in science and technology-biotechnology, molecular biology, plant genomics, and fairly recently, metabolomics. In the different geographical regions of Nigeria, several medicinal plants have been evaluated and found to have potent antidiabetic activities. Notable amongst these antidiabetic plants is the Nigeria species of mistletoe [20,21]. We further evaluated the antidiabetic properties of the eastern Nigeria mistletoes and results obtained led credence to the strong claim and ethnomedicinal uses especially as an antidiabetic [19,22]. Recently too and in specific terms, Ogbonnia et al. [23], reported the potent antihyperglycaemic and andtihyperlipidaemic activities of the *Tapinanthus* globiferus, the mistletoe specie commonly available in Nigeria and notably in south eastern region. Mistletoe, a semi-parasitic plant growing on different trees and shrub occurs in all continents of the world and its biological activities have been shown to be influenced mostly by the topography and climate, host tree and season of harvest [21]. In our recent paper, we documented the various traditional uses of the eastern Nigeria mistletoes and isolated some compounds from the eastern Nigeria mistletoes which exhibited potent osteogenic potentials *in vitro* [24]. Currently, mistletoe leaves in different processed forms are not only used traditionally for the numerous clinical conditions, but are also sold in most registered pharmaceutical outlets in Nigeria. This calls for a comprehensive evaluation of the total health benefits of this plant. Our interest to evaluate the effects of mistletoe extracts on dexamethasone-induced insulin resistance and on bone cell parameters was stirred by the strong scientific evidence supporting its potent antidiabetic action [19,21,22] and the folkloric claim of its ability to control postmenopausal syndrome [25]. We hypothesize that mistletoe extract, a known potent antidiabetic agent will reverse insulin-resistance with concomitant mitigation of the deterioration of bone functions occasioned by long therapy with dexamethasone. The present study is therefore, an attempt to test this plausible hypothesis.

2. EXPERIMENTAL

2.1 Materials and Methods

2.1.1 Collection of plant materials

The leaves and twigs of the eastern Nigeria mistletoes; *Tapinanthus globiferus* (A. Rich.) Tiegh. formerly known as *Loranthus micranthus*

Linn. (Loranthaceae) parasitic on the host tree *Kola acuminata* (Linn.), was collected in October 2011, from different locations in Nsukka LGA, Enugu state. The leaves were identified and certified by Mr. A. O. Ozioko, a taxonomist of the Bioresources Development and Conservation Programme, Nsukka, Enugu state. Voucher specimens were kept at the centre with the number BDC-1021-011 for reference purposes and in accordance with rules of the University of Nigeria regarding ethics and preservation of biodiversity.

2.1.2 Reagents and chemicals

All fine chemicals Sigma Aldrich (St. Louis, MO) while methanol was obtained from BDH Ltd., (Poole, England), distilled water. (Science Laboratory Technology Unit, University of Nigeria, Nsukka)

2.1.3 Animals used

All animal experimental procedures were prior approved (Institutional Animal Ethics Committee approval number (CDRI/IAEC/2012/17) and conducted as per the guide lines laid by the Committee for the Purpose of Control and Supervision of Experiments on Animals (CPCSEA 34/199). Sprague-Dawley (SD) rats (10-12 weeks old; 200±20 g each) of both sexes were obtained from the National Laboratory Animal Centre, CSIR-CDRI. Animals were kept in a 12 h light-dark cycle, with controlled temperature (22-24°C) and humidity (50-60%). Standard rodent chow diet and water were provided *ad libitum*.

2.2 Methods

2.2.1 Preparation of crude aqueous extract

The leaves of *Tapinanthus globiferus* (A. Rich.) Tiegh. parasitic on the selected host tree (*Kola acuminata*) were cleansed and dried under shade for 8 days. They were pulverized in mechanized laboratory grinder to fine powder. A total of 2.0 kg of the powdered plant material was macerated repeatedly with distill water (total volume; 6 L) The resulting aqueous extract were lyophilized under vacuum afford dry powdered extract which was weighed and its percentage yield was calculated. The dry extracts were placed in amber-coloured glass bottles and stored in a refrigerator until use. The yield obtained was found to be 24.1%. The extract was completely solubilized in normal saline and diluted accordingly to a chosen regimen.

2.2.2 *In vivo* studies

Seventy-two adult SD rats (60 females and 12 males) were randomly divided into 8 equal groups of 6 animals each and another 2 groups (n=12) as follows: Vehicle group (gum acacia in distilled water p.o.), 100 mg/kg (p.o.) of extract group; 200 mg/kg (p.o.) of extract group; 400 mg/kg (p.o.) of extract group; 100 mg/kg (p.o.) of extract + 200 µg/kg (i.p.) dexamethasone group; 200 mg/kg (p.o.) of extract + 200 µg/kg (i.p.) dexamethasone group; 400 mg/kg (p.o.) of extract + 200 µg/kg (i.p.) dexamethasone group; Metformin 200 mg/kg (p.o.) + 200 µg/kg (i.p.) dexamethasone group; two dexamethasone groups 200 µg/kg (i.p.; female and male; n=12 each). All animals received the above doses daily for 21 days and were closely monitored. The doses were chosen based on our already established protocols [25-27]. Daily weight and any obvious signs (weakness, lethargy, anorexia etc) of each animal were recorded. The animals were fasted for 24 hours and the blood glucose levels were checked at the onset and termination of the study with the Accu-Check® glucometer instrument. Oral Glucose tolerance test (OGTT) was performed on all groups by loading each animal with an oral glucose dose of 2 g/kg following 16-24 hours of fasting and monitoring the glycaemic levels at intervals of 30 minutes for a total period of 2 hours. Finally, all animals were sacrificed on the last day to collect blood (via cardiac puncture), femur, tibia, L5 vertebrae following anesthesia with ketamine. The blood samples centrifuged (7500 rpm; 4°C) to collect serum which was stored at -20°C prior to analysis. Bone samples were stored in 70% isopropanol at 4°C until further analysis. Total triglycerides and cholesterol content of serum (to assess dyslipidemia). All measurements were carried out in at least 5 replicates.

2.2.3 Assessment of various parameters for excised bones

µCT determination of excised bones was carried out using the Sky Scan 1076 µCT scanner (Aartselaar, Belgium) as described in our previously published protocols [28,29]. Femurs, tibias and L5 vertebrae dissected from the animals after sacrifice were cleaned of soft tissue prior to scanning. The samples were scanned in batches of two at a nominal resolution (pixels) of 18 µm. Reconstruction was carried out using a modified Feldkamp algorithm using the Sky Scan Nrecon software, which facilitates network distributed reconstruction carried out on four personal computers running simultaneously. The x-ray source was set at 70 kV and 142 mA, with a pixel size of 18 μm. A hundred projections were acquired over an angular range of 180^0. The trabecular bone of femur head and the callus-dense region of L5 vertebrae were selected by drawing ellipsoid contours with the CT analyzer (CTAn, Skyscan). Micro-architectural parameters including Trabecular bone volume (BV), trabecular numbers (Tb.N), trabecular separation (Tb.sp) and structure model index (SMI) were calculated using the 3D-trabecular analysis software of Skyscan [30,29,31]. The bone mineral density (BMD) of the trabecular bone of femur head and the callus-dense region of L5 vertebrae were computed from their binary images derived from reconstructed volume of interest using CTAn software.

2.2.4 Assessment of mechanical strengths of isolated bones

After μCT measurements, femurs were subjected to three point bending with Bone strength tester Model TK 252C (Muromachi Kikai Co. Ltd., Tokyo, Japan), according to our previously published protocols (Gupta et al. [29]; Siddiqui et al. [28]; Verdelis et al. [30]). Biomechanical parameters of femur including maximum power, stiffness and energy were determined. Taking the mean of control values we derived individual control value as a ratio of the mean ×100 and data expressed as percentage change over the mean value of vehicle group for the various biomechanical parameters. This was also carried out for the L5 vertebrae bones following established protocols.

2.3 Statistical Analysis

Data are expressed as mean ± SEM. The data obtained in experiments with multiple treatments were subjected to one-way ANOVA followed by Turkey's test of significance or Newman-Keuls post-hoc multiple comparism test using Prism 3.0 version software. Where necessary, Student's't' test was used to study statistical significance in experiments with only two treatments.

3. RESULTS

3.1 *In vivo* Studies with Dexamethasone Treated SD Rats of Both Sexes

In order to further strengthen the scientific data supporting the potent antidiabetic activity of the eastern Nigeria mistletoe, we studied it effects in SD rats treated concomitantly with standardized dose of the glucocorticoid, dexamethasone. This was to evaluate the potentiality of the extract preparation in modulating insulin resistance viz-a-viz bone health impairment occasioned by the steroid therapy. The mistletoe harvested from *Kola acuminata* was chosen based on our previous reports and the present data. The results from the *in vivo* studies are shown in Fig. 1 and in Tables 1-3. The effect of extract on the growth rate of SD rats administered with daily dose of 200 μg/kg dexamethasone for 16 days (1A): females, (1B) females and males from independent experiments. Rats treated with extracts alone had comparable growth rate to the vehicle and positive (metformin) controls and at the dose of 400 mg/kg, significantly (**$p<0.01$) reversed severe weight loss caused by dexamethasone administration. 1C: The final (at the end of experiment) fasted plasma glucose level were significantly (***$p<0.001$, **$p<0.01$, *$p<0.05$) higher than the initial (prior to commencement of experiment) in dexamethasone-treated rats when compared to vehicle and positive controls with the 400 mg/kg extract dose being the most potent. 1D: The extract and dexamethasone treated female SD rats showed low sensitivity to OGTT. Evidently, the plasma glycaemic levels of all the animals exposed to 2 g/kg oral glucose normalized within 2 hours. The male SD rats were resistant to OGTT even after 25 days (data not shown). 1E: The extracts either alone or in combination with dexamethasone summarily, did not affect the mean uterine weights of the female animals when compared to vehicle control. Animals with edematous uterus were observed (possibly caused by the significant mineralocorticoid action of dexamethasone) and were as such eliminated from the data. 1F: There was slight but significant (*$p<0.05$) increase in the mean pancreatic weight of animals at the dose 400 mg/kg extract plus dexamethasone and Metformin groups, and very significant (***$p<0.001$) gain in mean pancreatic weight in dexamethasone-alone group compared to the vehicle group. All values are expressed as mean ± SEM (n=6). Table 1 shows that the extract, at the tested doses protected the animals from mortality (100% protection) caused by the adverse effect of the steroid on glucose and energy metabolism compared with the female SD rats treated with dexamethasone alone (50% mortality). In addition, the surviving dexamethasone treated animals were generally weaker, lethargic and anorexic when compared to those receiving extracts simultaneously. The effect of the extract on some serum lipid profile (total triacylglycerides (TG) and cholesterol (TC)) and serum calcium (Ca^{++}) levels of female SD rats is as shown in Table 2. Treatment of animals with dexamethasone significantly (***p<0.001) increased TG levels compared to vehicle group and extract alone (***$p<0.001) treated. The extracts did not cause a significant change in TG ([a]) when compared to vehicle group. However, extracts at 200 and 400 mg/kg in combination with dexamethasone caused a significant (*$$p<0.05) reduction in amount of circulating triglycerides in serum compared to dexamethasone group. Similarly, TC values of extract treated rats alone or in combination with dexamethasone did not vary significantly (NS) from that of vehicle group except for the 100 mg/kg (***p<0.001) extract dose. The extracts at all doses significantly (*p<0.05; **p<0.01; ***p<0.001) preserved serum calcium levels compared to vehicle ad metformin controls and restored serum calcium loss induced by dexamethasone treatment.

Table 1. Mortality rate of animals treated with either extracts or dexamethasone and controls

Group (number)	Death count (number)	Mortality
Vehicle (6)	0	0 %
100 mg Extract (6)	0	0 %
200 mg Extract (6)	0	0 %
400 mg Extract (6)	0	0 %
100 mg Extract + Dexamethasone 200 µg/kg (6)	0	0 %
200 mg Extract + Dexamethasone 200 µg/kg (6)	0	0 %
400 mg Extract + Dexamethasone 200 µg/kg (6)	0	0 %
Metformin 200 mg/kg (6)	0	0 %
Dexamethasone 200 µg/kg (12)	6	50 %
Dexamethasone 200 µg/kg (12; Male SD rats)	0	0 %

Treatment with dexamethasone at 200 µg/kg dose induced severe weight loss, lethargy, weakness and mortality mostly in female SD rats within16 days. The male animals were lethargic but no death occurred in the group. Animals treated with extracts alone or in combination with dexamethasone exhibited a dose dependent resistance of majority of these adverse effects and compared with the controls. The male SD rats were able to survive the treatment period with dexamethasone such that there was zero mortality in the group. However, the animals were generally weak, lethargic and lost substantial weight in the course of the experiment

Table 2. Effect of treatment on some serum lipids and calcium levels after 16 days

Groups	TG	TC	TCa
Vehicle	26.73±2.43	44.20±0.93	8.89±.10
Dexa (200 µg/kg)	51.48±4.96***	52.50±5.93***	8.54±0.27
100 mg/kg extract	30.98±2.17***$, a	51.35±3.26***	9.08±0.10***
200 mg/kg extract	29.03±2.68***$, a	34.98±1.14NS	8.99±0.32***
400 mg/kg extract	30.25±1.91***$, a	35.98±1.61NS	9.13±0.14***
100 mg/kg extract + Dexa	48.35±2.87	37.48±2.09NS	8.72±.10*
200 mg/kg extract + Dexa	40.53±0.48*$$	36.85±2.13NS	8.84±0.18**
400 mg/kg extract + Dexa	39.40±0.47*$$	40.50±3.08NS	8.78±0.10*
Metformin 200 mg/kg + Dexa	52.77±2.86	53.47±7.25	8.98±0.14***

Key: TG (Total triglycerides); TC (Total Cholesterol); TCa (Total calcium)

*Values are expressed as mean ± SEM (n=6ix rats/group). One-way ANOVA was used to compare group means. Treatment of animals with dexamethasone significantly (***p<0.001) increased TG levels compared to vehicle group and extract alone (***$p<0.001) treated. The extracts did not cause a significant change in TG ([a]) when compared to vehicle group. However, extracts at 200 and 400 mg/kg in combination with dexamethasone caused a significant (*$$p<0.05) reduction in amount of circulating triglycerides in serum compared to dexamethasone group. Similarly, TC values of extract treated rats alone or in combination with dexamethasone did not vary significantly (NS) from that of vehicle group except for the 100 mg/kg (***p<0.001) extract dose. The extracts at all doses significantly (*p<0.05; **p<0.01; ***p<0.001) preserved serum calcium levels compared to vehicle ad Metformin controls and restored serum calcium loss induced by dexamethasone treatment.*

Table 3. Effect of extract on the bone mineral density (BMD) of SD rats exposed to prolonged dexamethasone treatment for a period of 16 days

Groups	BMD (%)	
	Trabecular bone	L5 vertebral bone
Vehicle	1.6486 ± 0.0003	1.6060 ± 0.0004
Dexamethasone (200 µg/kg)	1.5235 ± 0.0003	1.5160 ± 0.0004
Metformin 200 mg/kg + Dexamethasone	1.6716 ± 0.0002***a	1.6951 ± 0.0003***a
Extract 100 mg/kg	1.5918 ± 0.0002*b	1.6736 ± 0.0003***b
Extract 100 mg/kg + Dexamethasone	1.6974 ± 0.0002	1.7878 ± 0.0003***
Extract 200 mg/kg	1.6005 ± 0.0002*	1.6335 ± 0.0003**
Extract 200 mg/kg + Dexamethasone	1.6690 ± 0.0002***	1.7117 ± 0.0003***
Extract 400 mg/kg	1.6221 ± 0.0003	1.6999 + 0.0002**
Extract 400 mg/kg + Dexamethasone	1.6662 ± 0.0002**	1.7532 ± 0.0002***

*Mean BMD ± SEM values were computed electronically from binary images of reconstructed volume of interest (VOI) of trabecular and vertebral bone using the CTAn.exe software of the µCT Skyscan equipment. The extract at all doses either alone or in combination with dexamethasone significantly (***p<0.001; **p<0.01; *p<0.05) enhanced BMD in proportion comparable to the positive control, Metformin and very high when compared to untreated vehicle. ***[a](compared to vehicle group); ***[b], *[b](compared to dexamethasone group). Mistletoe extracts therefore enhanced and preserved bone compactness (quality) of SD rats treated alone with extracts or in combination with 200 µg/kg dexamethasone*

A

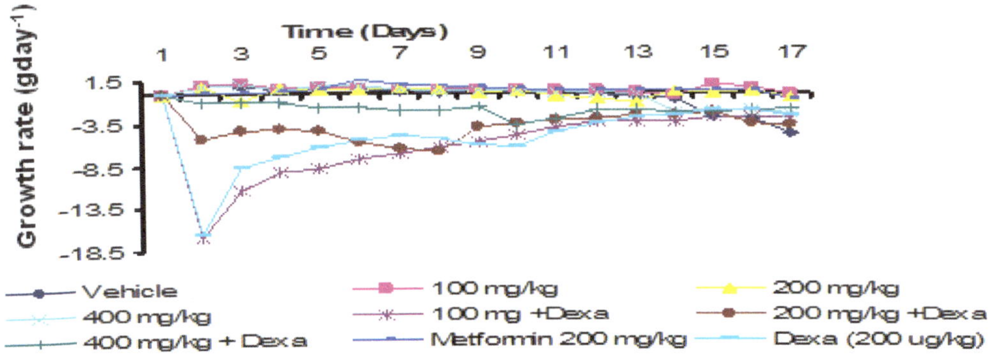

B

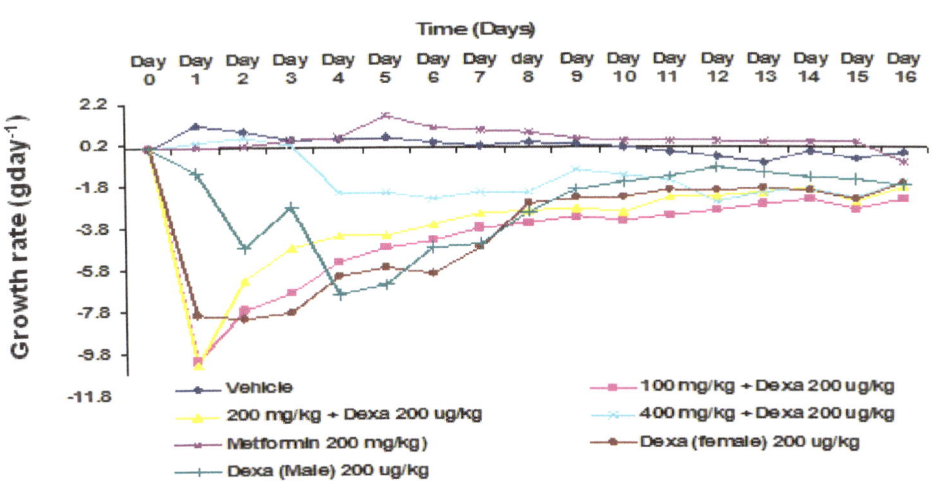

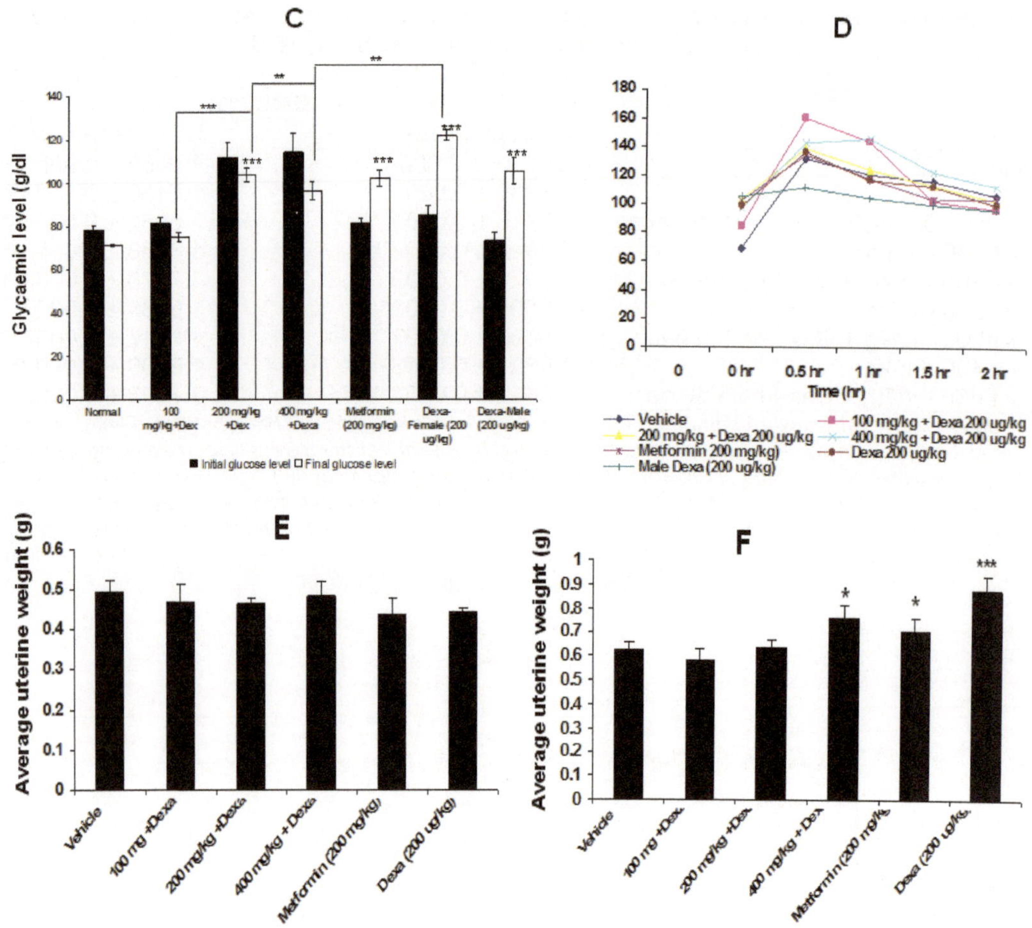

Fig. 1. Effect of extract from mistletoe parasitic on Kola acuminata (KM) on the growth rate of SD rats administered with daily dose of 200 µg/kg dexamethasone for 16 days (1A): females, (1B) females and males from an independent experiment. Rats treated with extracts alone had comparable growth rate to the vehicle and positive (Metformin) controls and at the dose of 400 mg/kg, significantly (p<0.01) reversed severe weight loss caused by dexamethasone administration. 1C: The final (at the end of experiment) fasted plasma glucose level were significantly (***p<0.001, **p<0.01, *p<0.05) higher than the initial (prior to commencement of experiment) in dexamethasone-treated rats when compared to vehicle and positive controls with the 400 mg/kg extract dose being the most potent. 1D: The extract and dexamethasone treated female SD rats showed low sensitivity to OGTT. Evidently, the plasma glycaemic levels of all the animals exposed to 2 g/kg oral glucose normalized within 2 hours. The male SD rats were resistant to OGTT even after 25 days (data not shown). 1E: The extracts either alone or in combination with dexamethasone did not affect the mean uterine weights of the female animals when compared to vehicle control. 1F: There was slight but significant (*p<0.05) increase in the mean pancreatic weight of animals at the dose 400 mg/kg extract +dexamethasone and Metformin groups, and very significant (***p<0.001) gain in mean pancreatic weight in dexamethasone-alone group compared to the vehicle group. All values are expressed as mean ± SEM (n=6)**

3.2 Assessment of Various Parameters for Excised Bones

µCT determination of excised bones was carried out using the Sky Scan 1076 µCT scanner. The result of derived parameters for trabecular and vertebral bones of the animals are shown in Figs. 2A-H and 3A-I. The effect of KM extract on the micro-architectural parameters of trabecular region of SD rats exposed to 16 days dosing with dexamethasone (200 μgkg^{-1}day^{-1}). (A) μCT analysis showing BV/TV, bone volume/tissue volume (%); (B) BS/BV, Bone surface/ Tissue volume; (C) Tb.Th (mm), trabecular (strut) thickness; (D) Tb.Sp., Trabecular (strut) separation (mm); (E) Tb.N., Strut number (1/mm); (F) Tb.Pf., Trabecular pattern factor, (G) Con.D., Connectivity density, and (H) SMI, Structure model index. The extract (either alone or in combination with dexamethasone) and within the duration of treatments showed better bone quality (higher BV/TV, lower Tb.Sp and SMI) parameters indices significantly (***p<0.001; **p<0.01;*p<0.05) at the dose of 400 mg/kg compared with vehicle and metformin groups. The large negative SMI values indicate more plates than rods in new bone formation improving the overall compactness and quality of the trabecular bone region. All values are expressed as mean ± SEM (n=x rats/group). Fig.3: Effect of KM extract on the microarchitectural parameters (A-I) of the load bearing L5 vertebrae trabecular region of SD rats exposed to 16 days dosing with dexamethasone (200 μg.kg-1day-1). The extract similarly (either alone or in combination with dexamethasone and within the duration of treatments showed better bone quality (higher BV/TV, lower Tb.Sp, lower SMI etc) parameters indices significantly (***p<0.001; **p<0.01;*p<0.05) at the dose of 400 mg/kg compared with vehicle and metformin groups. Again, the large negative SMI values indicate more plates than rods in new bone formation improving the overall compactness and quality of the L5 vertebrae. The 100 mg dose of extract failed to lower the SMI in the presence of dexamethasone. All values are expressed as mean ± SEM (n=x rats/group). The computed bone mineral density (BMD) is depicted in Table 3. Mean BMD ± SEM values were computed electronically from binary images of reconstructed volume of interest (VOI) of trabecular and vertebral bone using the CTAn.exe software of the μCT Skyscan equipment. The extract at all doses either alone or in combination with dexamethasone significantly (***p<0.001; **p<0.01; *p<0.05) enhanced BMD in proportion comparable to the positive control, Metformin and very high when compared to untreated vehicle. ***[a](compared to vehicle group); ***[b],*[b](compared to dexamethasone group). Mistletoe extracts therefore enhanced and preserved bone compactness (quality) of SD rats treated alone with extracts or in combination with 200 μg/kg dexamethasone.

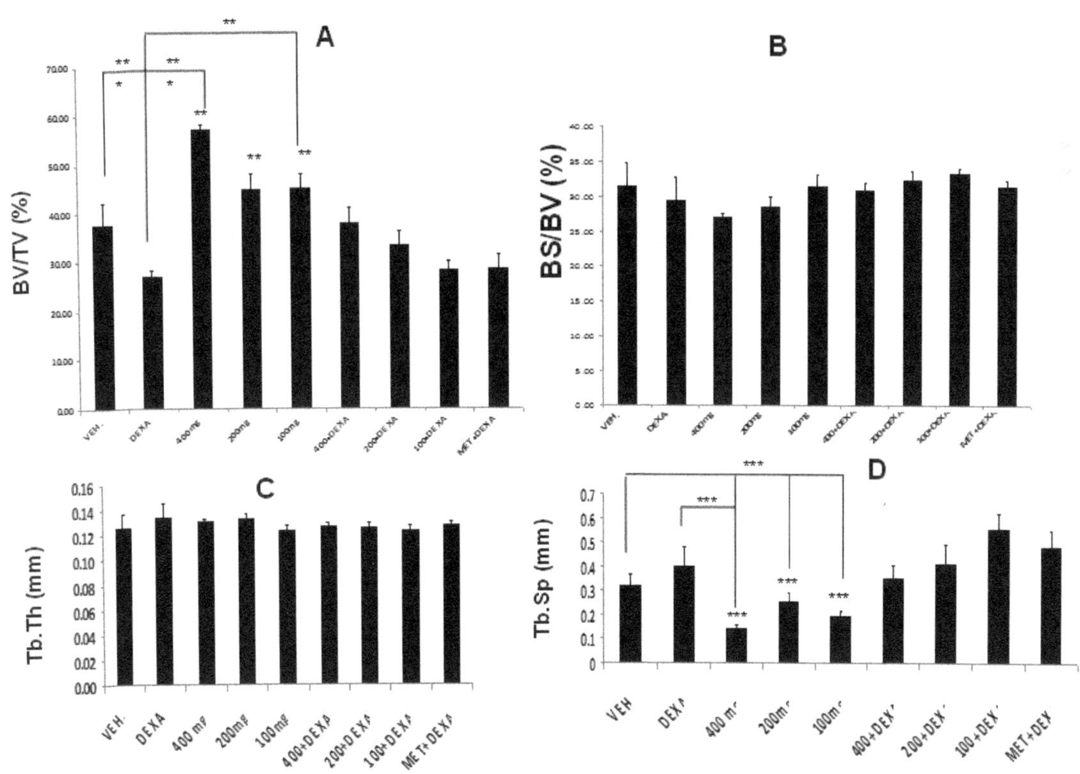

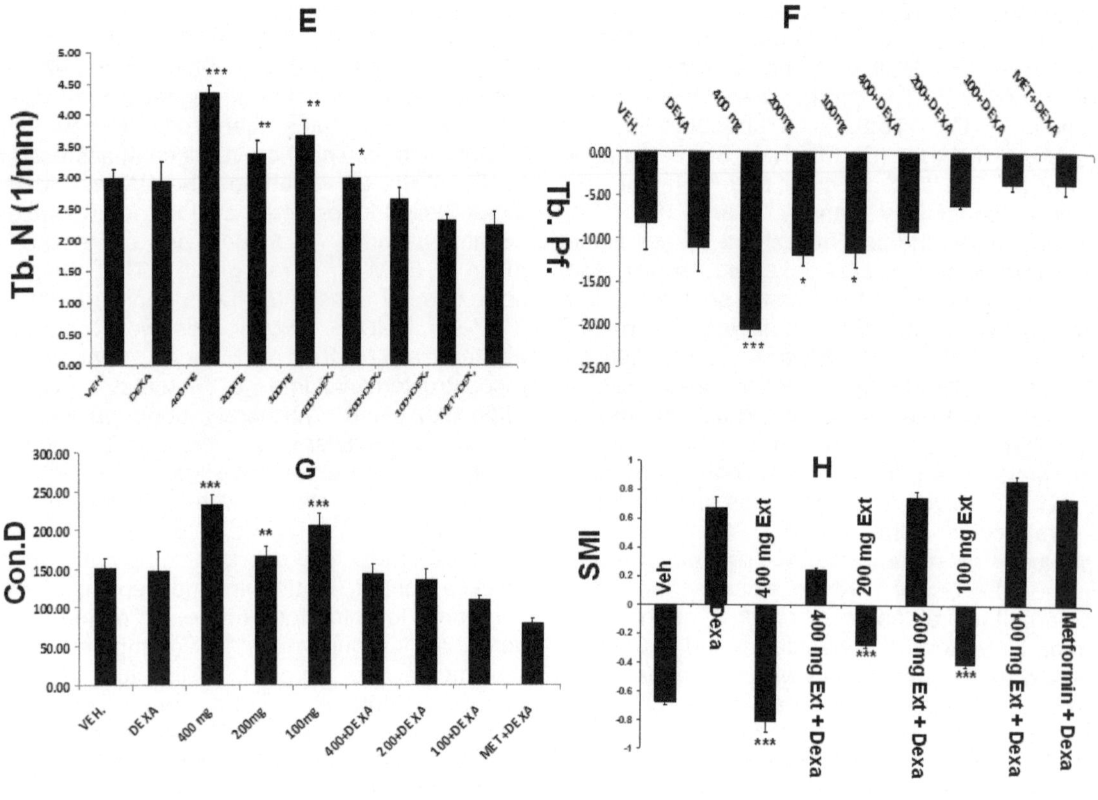

Fig. 2. Effect of treatment with KM extracts on the microarchitectural parameters of trabecular region of SD rats exposed to 16 days dosing with dexamethasone (200 μgkg^{-1}day^{-1}). (A) μCT analysis showing BV/TV, bone volume/tissue volume (%); (B) BS/BV, Bone surface/ Tissue volume; (C) Tb.Th (mm), trabecular (strut) thickness; (D) Tb.Sp. trabecular (strut) separation (mm); (E) Tb.N., Strut number (1/mm); (F) Tb.Pf., Trabecular pattern factor, (G) Con.D., Connectivity density, and (H) SMI, Structure model index. The extract (either alone or in combination with dexamethasone ad within the duration of treatments showed better bone quality (higher BV/TV, lower Tb.Sp and SMI) parameters indices significantly (*p<0.001; **p<0.01;*p<0.05) at the dose of 400 mg/kg compared with vehicle and Metformin groups. All values are expressed as mean ± SEM (n=x rats/group)**

4. DISCUSSION

We recently established the effects of the standardized extracts of eastern Nigeria mistletoe harvested from three host trees (*Kola acuminata, Citrus spp, Garcinia kola*) on the cell viability and ALP activity using cultured rat calvariae osteoblasts [24]. Our findings showed that there was no cytotoxicity at all tested doses (0.2-3.2 μg/ml) compared to control (NS) and at 0.2 μg/ml dose of *Kola acuminata* derived mistletoe extract, there was a significant (**p<0.01) proliferation of the cells. Similarly, ALP activity (a known bone growth biomarker), of treated rat calvariae cells was significantly (*p<0.05, **p<0.01, ***p<0.001) enhanced by all extracts at dose rage of 0.2-1.6 μg/ml compared the vehicle and positive control, BMP2 (100 ng/ml). The doses of the extracts (100-400 mg/kg) and the estimated EC_{50} of the crude extracts were also low which further leads credence to the overall safety of the crude plant extracts. These doses used in the study were extremely low compared to already established LD_{50} of mistletoe extracts in mice (LD_{50} of *Kola acuminata* derived mistletoe extract> 10,000 mg/kg; and an average LD_{50} value > 7500 mg/kg from five different host trees [25]. In addition, some compounds isolated from the leaves of mistletoe demonstrated potent proliferation of C57BL/6 mice splenocytes and significant immunomodulatory potentials [32,33]. These data, taken together imply that the extracts are safe to the bone forming cells and enhance the activity of bone growth biomarker, ALP (positive osteogenic potential). In our continued efforts to completely characterize the biological effects of local mistletoes used in traditional medical practice of eastern Nigeria, we set to study further activities of the extract in relation to its already established anti-diabetic properties. In the present work, our aim was to investigate the effect of *Kola acuminata*-derived mistletoe extract (KM) on SD rats exposed to prolonged high dose of dexamethasone. In addition, we studied the micro-architectures of designate bones from the treated animals and controls. As have been previously reported [4-6], the

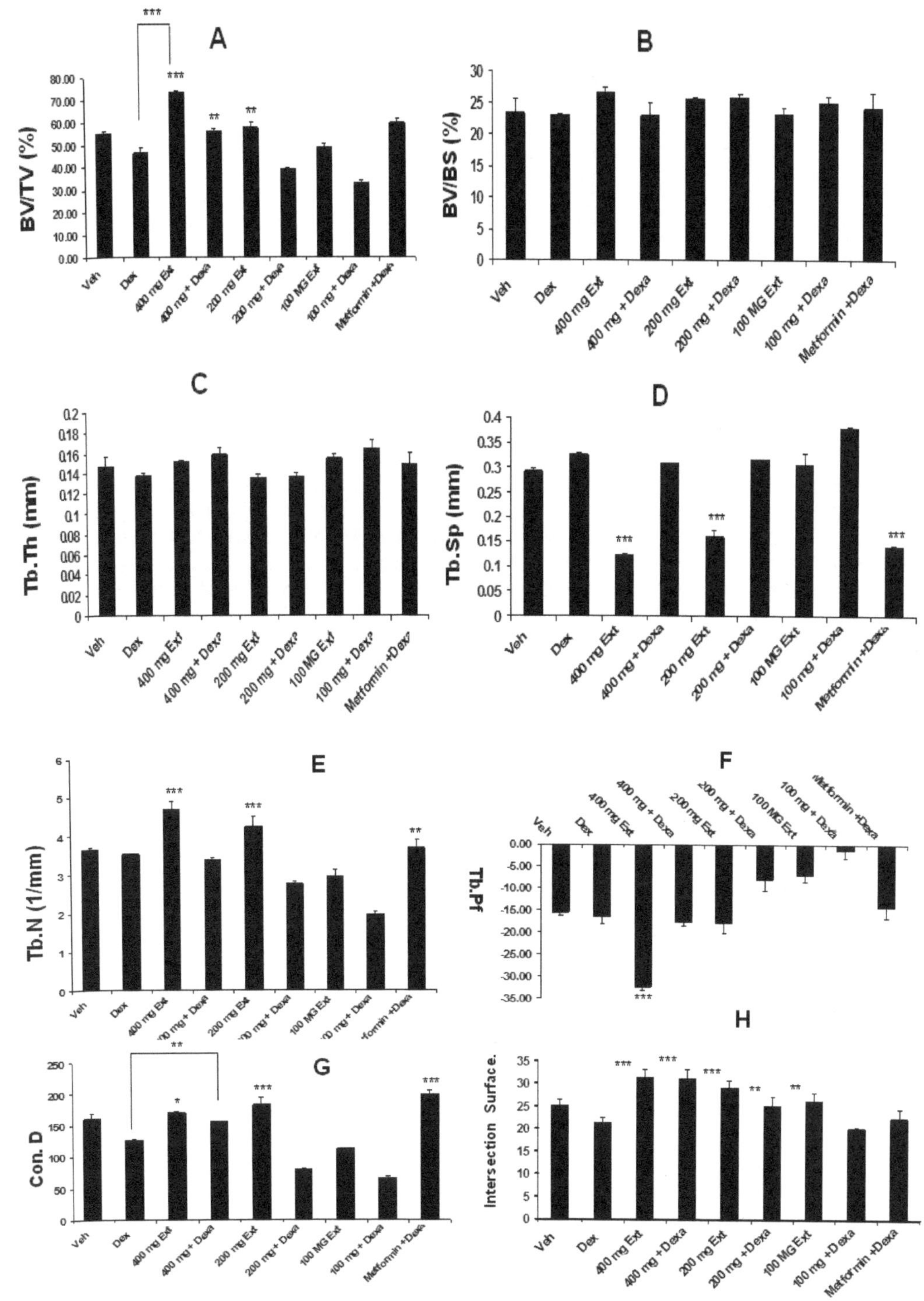

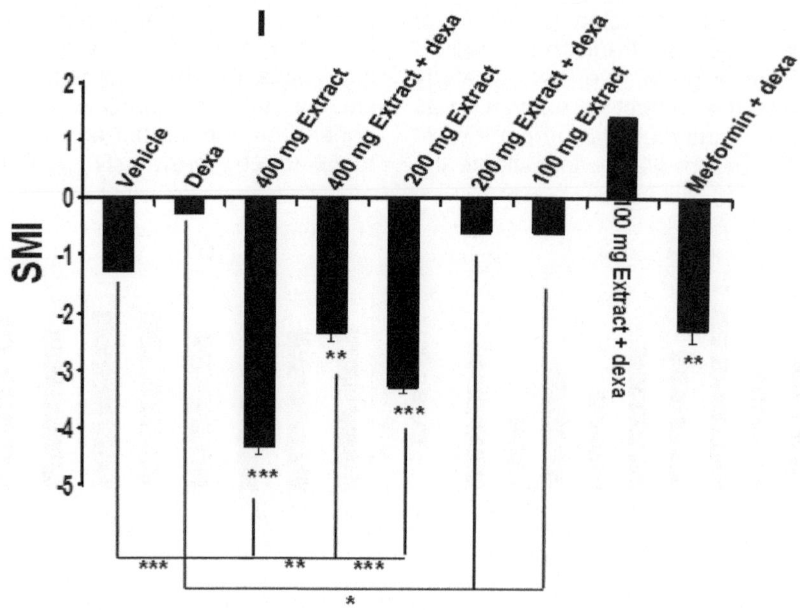

Fig. 3. Effect of treatment with KM extract on the microarchitectural parameters (A-I) of the load bearing L5 vertebrae trabecular region of SD rats exposed to 16 days dosing with dexamethasone (200 µg.kg-1day-1). The extract similarly (either alone or in combination with dexamethasone and within the duration of treatments showed better bone quality (higher BV/TV, lower Tb.Sp, lower SMI etc) parameters indices significantly (*p<0.001; **p<0.01;*p<0.05) at the dose of 400 mg/kg compared with vehicle and Metformin groups. the large negative SMI values indicate more plates than rods in new bone formation improving the overall compactness and quality of the L5 vertebrae. the 100 mg dose of extract failed to lower the SMI I the presence of dexamethasone. All values are expressed as mean ± SEM (n=x rats/group)**

adverse effect of glucocorticoids on bone growth and metabolism is characterized by decreased bone formation and *in situ* apoptosis (osteonecrosis) of isolated segments particularly at the trabecular-rich femoral head [6]. It is expected that the effects of osteogenic extracts or compounds will be manifested more in the female animals because of the interplay between oestrogen and bone metabolism *vi-a-viz,* diabetic syndrome. In the present work, the extract had no significant estrogenic activity which resulted in the non-differentiable action on both sexes in terms of growth rate. More obviously, intake of exogenous steroids like dexamethasone precipitates type-II diabetes which manifests drastic weight loss and increased adipogenesis due to altered glucose metabolism. This results in increased circulating cholesterols, glycaemia and other triglycerides with attendant clinical implications, often insulin resistance. The extract showed a dose dependent reversal effect on weight loss, high glycaemia, high cholesterol and triglycerides in comparison to control groups. Furthermore, the extract at 400 mg/kg body weight dosage was able to protect the loss of calcium ion in the animals dosed with dexamethasone compared with controls. The significance of these findings is that all the effects associated with steroid-induced insulin resistance were either reversed or ameliorated reasonably. This implies that extract of the eastern Nigeria mistletoe used in this study (KM) has added potentials that address the complications of diabetes and insulin resistance. Furthermore, the extract similarly (either alone or in combination with dexamethasone and within the duration of treatments showed better bone quality (higher BV/TV, lower Tb.Sp, lower SMI etc) parameters indices significantly at the dose of 400 mg/kg compared with vehicle and metformin groups. Again, the large negative SMI values indicate more plates than rods in new bone formation improving the overall compactness and quality of the L5 or the load-bearing vertebrae. The 100 mg dose of extract failed to lower the SMI in the presence of dexamethasone. The extract at all doses either alone or in combination with dexamethasone significantly enhanced the bone mineral density (BMD) in proportion comparable to the positive control, Metformin and very high when compared to untreated vehicle and dexamethasone groups. Mistletoe extracts therefore enhanced and preserved bone compactness (quality) of SD rats treated alone with extracts or in combination with 200 μg/kg dexamethasone. This finding is in agreement with our recent report describing the presence of osteogenic compounds in eastern Nigeria mistletoes [24]. Previously, the strong anti-diabetic properties of the crude aqueous methanol extract was established [21] and its relationship with the present findings is clinically relevant. In conclusion, extract of eastern Nigeria mistletoes parasitic on *Kola acuminata* could become a safe and cheaper alternative in the treatment and or management of insulin resistance in diabetic therapy, secondary osteoporosis and related bone diseases.

5. CONCLUSION

The present data show that leave extracts of eastern Nigeria mistletoes are potent in reversing the adverse effects of prolonged exposure to dexamethasone in rodents and evidently protected the bones from impairment. These extracts could therefore be further developed to serve as a cheaper alternative in the management of diabetes and or insulin resistance as well as secondary osteoporosis occasioned by steroid therapy.

CONSENT

It is not applicable.

ACKNOWLEDGEMENTS

The authors wish to acknowledge the support from CV-RAMMAN Post Doctoral Fellowship granted to Dr. E. O. Omeje. Furthermore, we acknowledge the hosting support from Dr. Naibedya Chattopadhyay at CDRI India Mr. Alfred Ozioko, a taxonomist with BDCP, Nsukka is appreciated for identifying the plant material.

COMPETING INTERESTS

Authors have declared that no competing interests exist.

REFERENCES

1. Canalis E, Mazziotti G, Gustiana A, Bilezikian JP. Glucocorticoid-induced osteoporosis: Pathophysiology and therapy. Osteoporosis International. 2007; 18:1319-1328.
2. Michele B, Vanna F, Michela N, Maria B, Pellegrino M, Ettore B, Vincenzo De Tata. Dexamethasone-induced insulin resistance and pancreatic adaptive response in aging rats are not modified by oral vanadyl sulfate treatment. European Journal of Endocrinology. 2001;145:799–806.
3. Silvana MC, Ciomar AB, Ana MK, Adelar B, Emy LI. The metabolic changes caused by dexamethasone in the adjuvant-induced arthritic rat. Mol Cell Biochem. 2007;302: 87-98.
4. Kerachian MA, Harvey EJ, Cournayer D, Chow TY, Nahal A, Seguine C. A Rat model of early stage osteonecrosis induced by glucocorticoids. Journal of Orthopaedic Surgery and Research. 2011; 6:62-67.
5. Cushing H. The basophil adenomas of the pituitary body and their clinical manifestations (pituitary basophilism). 1932. Obes Res. 1994;2:486-508.
6. Kerachian MA, Séguin C, Harvey EJ, Glucocorticoids, in: Osteonecrosis of the femoral head: A new understanding of the mechanisms of action. J Steroid Biochem Mol Biol. 2009;114:121-8.
7. Seo YK, Sebastian S, Jun L, Gregory WD, Chun-Lan C, Katie G, Daniel HS. Risk of osteoporotic fracture in a large population-based cohort of patients with rheumatoid arthritis. Arthritis Res Ther. 2010;12(4): R154.
8. Ghaisas M, Navghare V, Takawale A, Zope V, Tanwar M, Deshpande A. effect of *Tectona grandis* Linn. on dexamethasone induced insulin resistance in mice. J. Ethnopharmacol. 2009;122:304-307.
9. Gholap S, Kar A. Gymnemic acids from *Gymnema sylvestre* potentially regulates dexamethasone-induced hyperglycemia in mice. Pharmaceutical Biology. 2005;43: 192–195.
10. Andrews RC, Walker BR. Glucocorticoids and insulin resistance: Old hormone, new targets. Clinical Science. 1999;96:513–523.
11. Severino C, Brizzi P, Solinas A, Secchi G, Maioli M, Tunolo G. Low-dose Dexamethasone in the rat: A model to study insulin resistance. Am J. Physiol Endocrinol Metab. 2002;283:E367-E373.
12. Rafacho A, Cestari TM, Taboga SR, Boschero AC, Bosqueiro JR. High doses of

dexamethasone induce increased beta-cell proliferation in pancreatic rat islets. Am. J. Physiol Endocrinol Metab. 2009;296:E681-9.
13. Akpaso MI, Atangwho IJ, Akpantah A, Fischer VA, Anozeng O, Igiri OI, Ebong PE. Effect of combined leaf extracts of *Vernonia amygdalina* (Bitter Leaf) and *Gongronema latifolium* (Utazi) on the pancreatic β-Cells of streptozotocin-induced diabetic rats. British Journal of Medicine & Medical Research. 2011;1(1): 24-34.
14. Perry LM. Medicinal plants: Attributed properties and uses. Cambridge: MIT Press. 1980;10-15.
15. Joy PP, Thomas J, Matthew S, Skaria BP. Medicinal Plants. Kerala Agricultural University, Kerala, India. 1998;3-8.
16. Rates SM. Plant as source of drug. Toxicon. 2001;39(5):603-613.
17. Roja G, Rao PS. Anti cancer compounds from tissue cultures of medicinal plants. Journal of Herbs, Spices and Medicinal Plants. 2000;7:71-102.
18. Patel DK, Prasad SK, Kumar R, Hemalatha S. An overview on antidiabetic medicinal plants having insulin mimetic property. Asian Pacific Journal of Tropical Biomedicine. 2012;1:320-330.
19. Osadebe PO, Omeje EO, Uzor PF, David EK, Obum DC. Seasonal variation of the antidiabetic activity of *Loranthus micranthus* methanol extract. Asian Pacific Journal of Tropical Medicine. 2010a; 2010(4):1-5.
20. Obatomi DK, Bikomo EO, Temple VJ. Antidiabetic properties of the African mistletoe in Streptozocin-induced diabetic rats. Journal of Ethnopharmacology. 1994;43(1):13-17.
21. Osadebe PO, Okide GB, Akabogu IC. Study on anti-diabetic of crude methanolic extracts of *Loranthus micranthus* (Linn) sourced from five different host trees. Journal of Ethnopharmacology. 2004;95: 133-138.
22. Osadebe PO, Omeje EO, Nworu CS, Esimone CO, Uzor PF, David KE, Uzoma UU. Antidiabetic principles of *Loranthus micranthus* Linn. parasitic on *Persea americana*. Asian Pacific Journal of Tropical Medicine. 2010b;619-623.
23. Ogbonnia SO, Anyika EN, Mbaka GO, Utah P, Ugwu D, Nwakakwa N, Ota DA. Antihyperglycaemic and andtihyperlipidaemic effects of aqueous ethanol extract of *Tapinanthus globiferus* leaves and *Treculia africana* root bark and their mixture on alloxan diabetic rats. Agriculture and Biology Journal of North America; 2012.
DOI: 10.5251/abjna.2012.3.6.237.246
24. Omeje EO, Mohd PK, Osadebe PO, Deepshika T, Faheem K, Kapil D, Rakesh M, Naibedya C. Analysis of constituents of the eastern Nigeria mistletoe, *Loranthus micranthus* Linn revealed presence of new classes of osteogenic compounds. Journal of Ethnopharmacology. 2014;151:643-651.
25. Osadebe PO, Omeje EO. Comparative toxicities and immunomodulatory potentials of five Eastern Nigeria mistletoes. Journal of Ethnopharmacology. 2009;126:287-293.
26. Sharan K, Siddiqui JA, Swarnkar G, Tyagi AM, Kumar A, Rawat P, et al. Extract and fraction from *Ulmus wallichiana* Planchon promote peak bone achievement and have a nonestrogenic osteoprotective effect. Menopause. 2010a;17:393–402.
27. Sharan K, Swarnkar G, Siddiqui JA, Kumar A, Rawat P, Kumar M. et al. A novel flavonoid, 6-C-beta-d-glucopyranosyl-(2S,3S)- (+)-3′,4′,5,7-tetrahydroxyflavanone, isolated from *Ulmus wallichiana* Planchon mitigates ovariectomy-induced osteoporosis in rats. Menopause. 2010b;17:577–586.
28. Siddiqui JA, Swarnkar G, Sharan K, Chakravarti B, Sharma G, Rawat P, et al. 8,8″-Biapigeninyl stimulates osteoblast functions and inhibits osteoclast and adipocyte functions: Osteoprotective action of 8,8″-biapigeninyl in ovariectomized mice. Mol Cell Endocrinol. 2010;323:256–267.
29. Gupta S, Kuhnisch J, Mustafa A, Lhotak S, Schlachterman A, Slifker MJ, et al. Mouse models of cystathionine beta-synthase deficiency reveal significant threshold effects of hyperhomocysteinemia. FASEB J. 2009;23:883–893.
30. Verdelis K, Lukashova L, Atti E, Mayer-Kuckuk P, Peterson MG, Tetradis S, et al. MicroCT morphometry analysis of mouse cancellous bone: Intra- and inter-system reproducibility. Bone. 2011;49:580–587.
31. Omeje EO, Osadebe PO, Nworu CS, Akira K, Proksch P. Immunomodulatory activity of a lupane triterpenoid ester isolated from the Eastern Nigeria mistletoe, *Loranthus micranthus* (Linn). Asian Pacific Journal of Tropical Medicine. 2011a;4(2):412-420.

32. Omeje EO, Osadebe PO, Akira K, Abdessamad D, Esimone CO, Nworu SC, Proksch P. Steroids and triterpenoids and steroids from the leaves of the Eastern Nigeria mistletoe with immunomodulatory potentials. Phytochemistry Letters; 2011b. DOI: 10.1016/j.phytol.2011.07.011

33. Omeje EO, Osadebe PO, Akira K, Esimone CO, Proksch P, Nwodo NJ. A novel sesquiterpene acid and an alkaloid from leaves of the Eastern Nigeria mistletoe with potent immunostimulatory activity on C57BL6 splenocytes. Pharm Biol; 2011c. DOI: 10.3109/13880209.2011.621129

14

Evaluation of Acute Toxicity and Hypoglycaemic and Hypolipidaemic Effects of *Cyathula prostata* (Linn.) Blume Weeds on Adult Rats

S. O. Ogbonnia[1*], G. O. Mbaka[2], O. E. Akinsande[1], D. A. Otah[3] and T. A. Ayeni[1]

[1]*Department of Pharmacognosy, Faculty of Pharmacy, University of Lagos, Idi-Araba, Lagos, Nigeria.*
[2]*Department of Anatomy, Lagos State University College of Medicine, Ikeja, Lagos, Nigeria.*
[3]*Department of Physiology, College of Medicine of the University of Lagos, Idi-Araba, Lagos, Nigeria.*

Authors' contributions

This work was carried out in collaboration between all authors. Author SOO designed the experiment, the protocol for the study and also partook in the manuscript preparation and statistical analysis. Author GOM undertook the tissue processing and analysis as well as partook in the write up and final editing of the manuscript. Author OEA managed the literature searches. Author DAO perform the spectroscopy analysis. Author TAA managed the experimental process as well as identified the plant species. All authors read and approved the final manuscript.

Article Information

Editor(s):
(1) Wenbin Zeng, School of Pharmaceutical Sciences, Central South University, Hunan, China.
(2) Ke-He Ruan, Director of the Center for Experimental Therapeutics and Pharmacoinformatics (CETP) Professor of Medicinal Chemistry & Pharmacology, Department of Pharmacological and Pharmaceutical Sciences, University of Houston, USA
Reviewers:
(1) Sahar Mohamed Kamal Shams El Dine, Ain Shams University, Cairo, Egypt.
(2) Mario Eduardo Santos Cabral, Federal University of Ceara, Brazil.

ABSTRACT

Objectives: The study aimed at evaluating the acute toxicity and hypoglycaemic and hypolipidaemic effects of *Cyathula prostata* plant used locally in the treatment of various diseases including diabetes.

Materials and Methods: The toxicity of the extract was evaluated in Swiss albino mice by feeding the animals with the graded doses of the extract between 1.0 to 20.0 g/kg body weight (bwt) and continuously observed for the first 4 h, then hourly for the next 12 hand 6 hourly for the next 56 h (72 h, acute toxicity). Diabetes was induced in the male and female Wistar rats with alloxan monohydrate, at the dose of 150 mg/kg, dissolved in normal saline and administered intraperitoneally (i.p). The plasma glucose levels of the induced animals were monitored with a

**Corresponding author: Email: mbaaka2gm@gmail.com*

Glucometer (MERCK) after 72 h. The animals with plasma glucose level ≥200 mg/dl were classified as diabetic and were included in the study. The diabetic animals were randomly distributed into five groups of 5 animals each. The first group was normal not treated but received acacia 2% w/v solution. The second group was induced but not treated while the remaining four groups were treated with the reference drug, glibenclamide, (600 μg-1 kg bwt)/ the extract in graded doses of 75, 150 and 250 mg/kg bwt respectively for 30 days.

Results: The animals that received 20 g/kg bwt of the extract survived beyond 24 hrs, therefore the LD_{50} could be assumed to be above 20 g^{-1} kg bwt. The plasma level of alanine aminotransferase (ALT) was found to have significantly (p≤0.05) increased in the extract treated compared to the negative control whereas aspartate aminotransferase (AST) level showed marked decrease with dose. However, hepatic tissue histology at the highest extract dose treatment showed mild portal hepatitis with hepatocytes vacuolization and sinusoidal congestion. There were no significant changes (p≥0.05) in protein and creatinine levels. There were significant (p≤0.05) reduction in the plasma glucose, cholesterol, triglycerides and LDL levels while a significant increase in HDL levels was observed. The tissue histology of pancreas showed significant survivor of beta cells in the extract treated groups.

Conclusion: The extract was observed to have beneficial effect on alloxan-damaged pancreas as beta cells showed signs of recovery.

Keywords: Acute; toxicity; hypoglycaemic; hypolipidaemic; Cyathula prostata.

1. INTRODUCTION

Diabetes mellitus (DM) is one of the ravaging diseases affecting many lives world over. It is now recognized as one of the leading causes of death in the developing countries where the high prevalence of the disease could be attributed to improved nutritional status coupled with a gross lack of modern facilities for the early diagnosis of the disease [1]. Diabetes, a metabolic disorder of multiple aetiology, is characterised with disturbances of carbohydrate, fat and protein metabolism resulting from absolute or relative lack of insulin or both leading to hyperglycaemia [2], and in general is characterised with some symptoms such as increased thirst, polyuria, blurring of vision and weight loss [3]. They are basically divided into type 1 diabetes resulting from beta-cell destruction, usually leading to absolute insulin deficiency and type 2 also known as Non-Insulin Dependent DM (NIDDM). In type 2 diabetes, insulin is secreted but not being utilized by the tissues or an organ of the body [4].

DM has been conventionally treated with orthodox medicines that function as hypoglycaemic agents and as insulin production modulators or lipoprotein lowering agents [1]. Sulfonylurea and metformin have been invaluable in the management of hyperglycaemia in NIDDM but they are often unable to lower blood glucose concentrations to within the normal range, or to reinstate a normal pattern of glucose homeostasis [5]. Even when effective glycaemic control is achieved, the use of these drugs is restricted by their pharmacokinetic properties, secondary failure rates and accompanied undesirable effects [6,7]. In addition, they are not suitable for use during pregnancy [5,8]. Since the therapy is life long, therapeutic agents devoid of the above side effects would be appreciated and one of such approaches is the use of a popular alternative system of medicine, herbal medicine [9].

Herbal medicine, an oldest mode of therapy, is of great interest as it has been observed to be effective even in small doses for their physiological benefits and is perceived to have minimal side effects. Herbal medicine has been reported to be effective in the treatment of certain diseases such as diabetes where orthodox medicine could only proffer palliative effect. Several herbs have been reported in folk medicine to be successfully employed in the management of DM especially Type 2 diabetes (non-insulin dependent diabetes) [10]. The popularity of herbs and natural products in developing countries could be attributed to their being a cheaper source of healthcare compared to conventional medicines and are also associated with lesser side effects [11].

Cyathula prostata (*C. prostate*) is being used by traditional herbalist in the treatment of diabetes singly or in combination with other herbs. The aim of this study is, therefore, to scientifically evaluate *C. prostata* acute toxicity, hypoglycaemic and hypolipidaemic activity as well as its cardiovascular risk benefits giving credence to its local use.

2. MATERIALS AND METHODS

2.1 Plant Materials

The *C. prostate* (Linn.) Blume (*Amaranthaceae*) plant material was obtained from a traditional herbalist based in Lagos, Nigeria. The plant sample was identified and authenticated by a taxonomist in the Department of Botany of the University of Lagos where the voucher specimen was (LUH 3161) deposited in the Department Herbarium.

The dried powder of *C. prostata* plant (870 g) was soaked in 10 L of boiled (100℃) distilled water over night, with regular stirring. The extract was clarified by filtration with sterilized muslin cloth [12] and lyophilized to yield 122.5 g gel (14.1% yields).

2.2 Acute Toxicity Study

The toxicity study was carried out using twenty-five (25) male and female Swiss albino mice weighing between 20 – 25 g. The animals were randomly distributed into one control group and four treated groups, containing five animals per group. They were maintained on Animal feed, (Livestock feed Nigeria Ltd) provided with water *ad libitum* and were allowed to acclimatize to the laboratory conditions for seven days before the experiment. After overnight fast of the animals received acacia 2% w/v solution orally, while each treated group received orally solution of the extract in the doses of 5 g, 10 g, 15 g and 20 g/kg body weight (bwt) respectively. The stock solution was prepared by dispersing 16 g of the gel with 7 ml of the acacia solution in a 100 ml beaker and then transferred to a 20 mL volumetric flask. The volume was made to mark with the acacia solution to give a stock solution of 800 mg/mL (80% w/v). For mice of average weight of 22.5 g were administered 20,000 mg/kg bwt (20 mg/g), the total volume consumed was 0.56 mL (450÷800 mL) while for 15,000 mg/kg 15 mg bwt (/g) the total volume received was 0.42 mL [13].They were closely observed in the first 4 hours and then hourly for the next 12 hours followed by 6 hourly intervals for the next 56 hours (overall 72 hr) after the drug administration to observe any death or changes in general behaviour and other physiological activities [14,15] (Table 1).

2.3 Determination of LD_{50}

Since all the animals that received 20 g/kg bwt survived beyond 24 hrs, the median lethal dose (LD_{50}) was assumed to be more than 20 g/kg bwt [16]. The results obtained is shown in Table 1.

2.4 Diabetic Study

Healthy Wistar rats of both sexes weighing 120±15 g were used. The animals were fed on Animal feed (Livestock feed, Nigeria Ltd), and provided with water *ad libitum*. Diabetes was experimentally induced after fasting the animals overnight by administering intraperitoneally (i.p) alloxan monohydrate at 150 mg/kg bwt [17] dissolved in normal saline. After 72 hr, the blood sugar levels were monitored with a glucometer (Accu-Chek, Roche Diagnostics) and the rats with plasma glucose ≥ 200 mg/dl were classified as diabetic and were used in the study. A total of six groups containing five animals per group were used. Five groups comprising groups 2-6 were diabetic while group 1 was used as positive control. Treatment was daily for 30 days as follows:

Group 1: Normal rats not induced with diabetes to serve as positive control but received acacia 2% w/v solution.
Group 2: Alloxan-induced diabetic rats not treated, to serve as negative control.
Group 3: Alloxan-induced diabetic rats treated with Glibenclamide 600 μg/kg bwt dissolved in acacia 2% w/v solution [18]
Group 4: Alloxan-induced diabetic rats treated with 250 mg/kg bwt extract
Group 5: Alloxan-induced diabetic rats treated with 150 mg/kg bwt extract
Group 6: Alloxan-induced diabetic rats treated with 75 mg/kg bwt extract

The animals were initially weighed and subsequently weighed every seven days from the beginning to the end of the treatment to observe variations in the body weights. On the 31st day, after overnight fast they were sacrificed under mild diethyl ether and blood was obtained via cardiac puncture and distributed into heparinized, EDTA and fluoride containers respectively for biochemical, haematogical and plasma glucose studies. The blood was centrifuged within 5 min of collection at 4000 rpm for 10 min to obtain plasma which was analysed for glucose level, total cholesterol, total triglycerides, high density lipoprotein (HDL) cholesterol levels by precipitation and modified enzymatic procedures from Sigma Diagnostics [19]. Low density lipoprotein (LDL) and cholesterol levels were calculated using

Friedwald equation [20]. The results are given in Table 2.

Plasma was analysed for alanine aminotransferase (ALT), aspartate aminotransferase (AST), alkaline phosphatase (ALP) and creatinine by standard enzymatic assay analysis and the plasma protein and glucose contents were determined using enzymatic spectroscopic methods [21]. The results are shown in Table 3.

2.5 Phytochemical Evaluation of the Crude Extracts

Phytochemical screening of the extract was performed for the presence of secondary metabolites according to the method of Farnsworth, [22] and Harborne, [23].

2.6 Tissue Histology

The organs were fixed in 10% formal saline for ten days before embedding in paraffin wax. Each organ tissue was sectioned at 5μm and stained with Haematoxylin and Eosin (H and E) stain [24]. The slide specimens were examined under light microscope at high power magnification for changes in organ architecture and photomicrographs were taken.

2.7 Statistical Analysis

Differences in total blood glucose, total plasma cholesterol, total plasma triglyceride, LDL-cholesterol and HDL-cholesterol levels, AST, ALT, creatinine levels and body weight variations for all treated and control rats were determined using an analysis of variance (ANOVA). Significant differences were determined using a Student's t-test and differences were considered significant if $p \leq 0.05$. All data are expressed as mean ± standard error of the mean.

3. RESULTS AND DISCUSSION

Herbal medicines have received greater attention as alternative to clinical therapy in recent times leading to subsequent increase in their demands [8,18]. In rural communities, the exclusive use of herbal drugs in the treatment of various diseases is still very common. Preparations with different parts of *Cyathula prostata* has been used by herbal practitioners in the treatment of various diseases including DM.

The acute toxicity results are shown in Table 1. The median lethal dose (LD_{50}) value of the extract was observed to be higher than 20 g/kg bwt. According to Ghosh [25] and Klaasen et al. [26], the extract can be classified as being non-toxic, since the LD_{50} by oral route was found to be much higher than WHO toxicity index of 2 g/kg.

The postprandial plasma sugar activity is shown in Fig. 1. The extract was observed to demonstrate a significant ($p \leq 0.05$) postprandial plasma sugar lowering effect explaining its' α-glucosidase activities. The weight variations (Fig. 2) results showed the effect of the extract on the body weight of the diabetic and normal rats. Also the effect of the reference drug, glibenclamide, on the diabetic rats was shown. There was a decrease in the weight of the animals treated with the least dose (75 mg/kg) of the extract in the first seven days and subsequently, weight gain was observed compared to the control. The decrease in body weight of the untreated rats was observed throughout the experiment. The body weight of the other treated groups increased marginally but was still lower than those treated with the reference drug at day 7. However, all showed progressive decrease to the last day of the treatment. This showed that the extract might be lacking obesity forming tendency, which is one of the draw backs associated with sulphonylureas.

The result of the biochemical parameters are shown in Table 2. In the extract treated animal groups, the plasma level of ALT was found to have significantly ($p \leq 0.05$) increased compared to the negative control whereas AST level showed marked decrease with dose. An elevation in plasma concentration of ALT is usually due to liver damage while increase in AST level could be linked to damage to either cardiac or hepatic tissues or damage to both [19,20]. The photomicrograph of hepatic tissue at the highest dose of extract treatment showed mild portal hepatitis with hepatocytes vacuolization and sinusoidal congestion while the histology of cardiac tissue treated with the extract indicated no pathological changes. It was therefore obvious from the hepatic tissue morphology that the extract had deleterious effect on the liver at the highest dose of administration. Also, the extract at the highest dose showed significant ($p \leq 0.05$) increase in the ALP levels and the reason for this cannot be readily ascertained.

Table 1. Acute toxicity of aqueous *C. prostata* leaves extract in mice

Doses of the drug (g/kg)	Log dose	Number of mice used	Number of mice dead	%Cumulative number of mice dead
0.50	-0.30103	5	0	0
1.0	0	5	0	0
2.5	0.39794	5	0	0
5	0.69897	5	0	0
10	1.0000	5	0	0
15	1.1761	5	0	0
20	1.3010	5	0	0

Control group received orally 0.3ml acacia solution 2% w/v

Table 2. Plasma glucose level and other biochemical profiles of untreated diabetic rats, diabetic rats treated with the extract and glibenclamide respectively and the normal control rats

Parameters	Group 1	Group 2	Group 3	Group 4	Group 5	Group 6
AST (μ/ mm^3)	115.4±0.62*	178.4±0.14	163.4±0.25*	138.2±0.58*	143.0±0.25*	154.0±0.16*
T.Bil (μmol)	1.3±0.07*	0.6±0.02	0.7±0.03	0.8±0.04	0.4±0.05	0.3±0.02
Creatinine	25.26±0.11*	33.16±0.14	26.72±0.08*	28.90±0.32	28.91±0.34	29.16±0.67
Urea (μmol)	5.6±0.50*	12.6±0.28	6.1±0.24*	7.7±0.40*	8.98±0.42*	9.7±0.16*
ALT (μ/ mm^3)	44.2±0.05	50.2±0.06	42.8±0.62*	66.5±0.36*	59.5±0.15*	59.2±0.67*
Glu (mmol/ mm^3)	3.2±0.16*	13.5±0.14	6.3±0.10*	7.4±0.06*	10.5±0.10*	14.3±0.05
ALB (g/ mm^3)	34.9±0.05	38.6±0.58	35.9±0.45	36.5±0.49	37.2±0.64	37.7±0.30
T.Protein (g/ mm^3)	65.3±0.06*	75.0±0.34	62.8±0.56*	77.9±0.16	67.9±0.29*	71.9±0.31
HDL (mmol/ mm^3)	1.3±0.06	1.5±0.03	1.3±0.02	1.3±0.06	1.5±0.09	1.5±0.09
LDL (mmol/ mm^3)	0.05±0.02	0.41±0.03	0.30±0.02	0.31±0.03	0.34±0.05	0.40±0.01
T.Chol(mmol/ mm^3)	2.03±0.06	2.31±0.06	1.20±0.13	1.40±0.02	1.70±0.12	2.00±0.08
T.G (mmol/ mm^3)	0.72±0.02	1.73±0.02	0.72±0.07	0.88±0.06	0.92±0.05	0.88±0.07
ALP (μmol)	288.6±0.35*	364.3±0.69	415.8±0.29*	434.9±0.28*	377.0±0.24*	470.6±0.26*

Group 1: Normal rats not induced with diabetes to serve as positive control received acacia 2% w/v solution. Group 2: Alloxan-induced diabetic rats not treated, to serve as negative control. Group 3: Alloxan-induced diabetic rats treated with Glibenclamide 600 µg/kg bwt. Group 4: Alloxan-induced diabetic rats treated with 250 mg/kg bwt extract. Group 5: Alloxan-induced diabetic rats treated with 150 mg/kg bwt extract. Group 6:Alloxan-induced diabetic rats treated with 75 mg/kg bwt extract

Table 3. Haematological values of control and diabetic rats treated with the *C. prostata* extract at different doses and the reference drug glibenclamide and normal control rats

Parameters	GRP 1	GRP 2	GRP 3	GRP 4	GRP 5	GRP 6
WBC (10^9/mm^3)	6.1±0.09*	18.4±0.26	8.5±0.12*	10.4±0.20*	11.2±0.21	11.6±0.05
RBC (10^{12}/ mm^3)	7.18±0.06	6.70±0.05	6.47±0.23	7.09±0.10	7.00±0.13	7.94±0.05
HB (g/dl)	12.6±0.10	11.2±0.12	10.8±0.15	13.0±0.10	13.4±0.13	13.7±0.34
PCV (%)	41.5±0.09	13.8±0.35	40.8±0.14*	40.0±0.08*	32.7±0.28*	21.4±0.33*
PLT (10^9/ mm^3)	813±0.18*	116±0.24	802±0.67*	776±0.46*	421±0.32*	255±0.03*
MCV (fL)	57.9±0.57	54.6±0.12	57.9±0.52	56.5±0.75	58.4±0.13	59.1±0.28
MCH(pg)	17.5±0.28	17.1±0.03	17.0±0.21	18.3±0.16	19.1±0.51	19.0±0.46
MCHC (g/dl)	32.8±0.10	29.6±0.38	32.5±0.41	32.4±0.19	31.5±0.53	30.3±0.13
NEU (%)	28.3±0.35*	48.8±0.76	33.1±0.02*	35.5±0.14*	40.6±0.28*	42.0±0.31
LYMPH (%)	32.6±0.10*	71.6±0.39	42.8±0.22*	44.4±0.20*	48.7±0.28*	55.5±0.19*

Group 1: Normal rats not induced with diabetes to serve as positive control received acacia 2% w/v solution. Group 2: Alloxan-induced diabetic rats not treated, to serve as negative control. Group 3: Alloxan-induced diabetic rats treated with Glibenclamide 600 µg/kg bwt. Group 4: Alloxan-induced diabetic rats treated with 250 mg/kg bwt extract. Group 5: Alloxan-induced diabetic rats treated with 150 mg/kg bwt extract. Group 6: Alloxan-induced diabetic rats treated with 75 mg/kg bwt extract

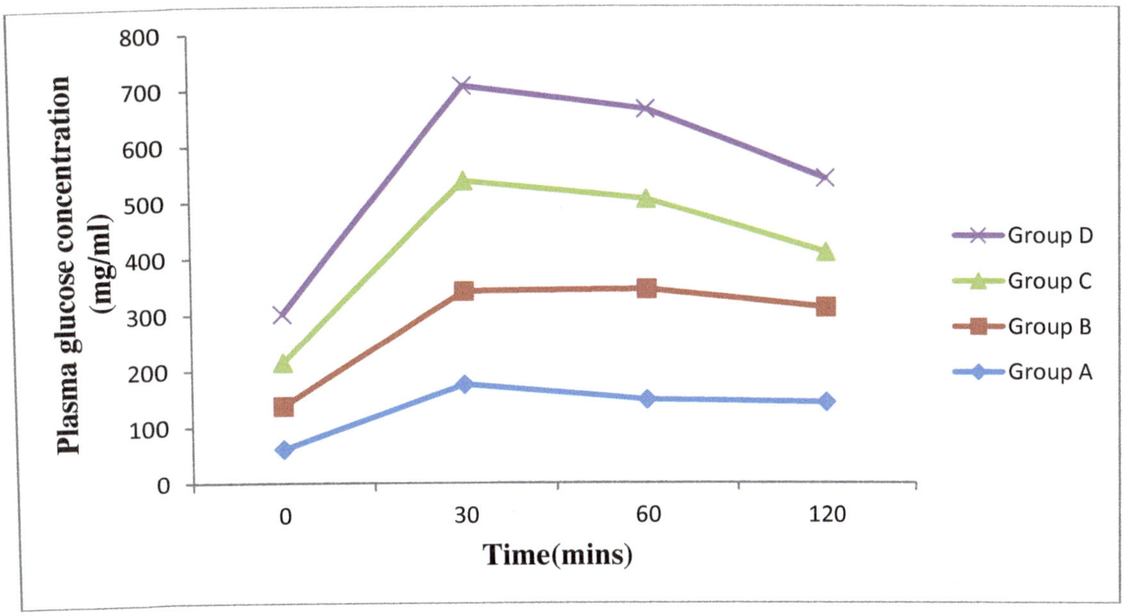

Fig. 1. Evaluation of *Cyathula prostata* extract at different doses and control effects on Post-pandrial glucose level in rats

Group A: Control animals given acacia 2% w/v solution. Group B: Cyathula prostate aqueous extract 140 mg/150g body weight, Group C: Cyathula prostata aqueous extract at 70 mg/150 g body weight, Group D: Cyathula prostata aqueous extract at 7 mg/150 g body weight

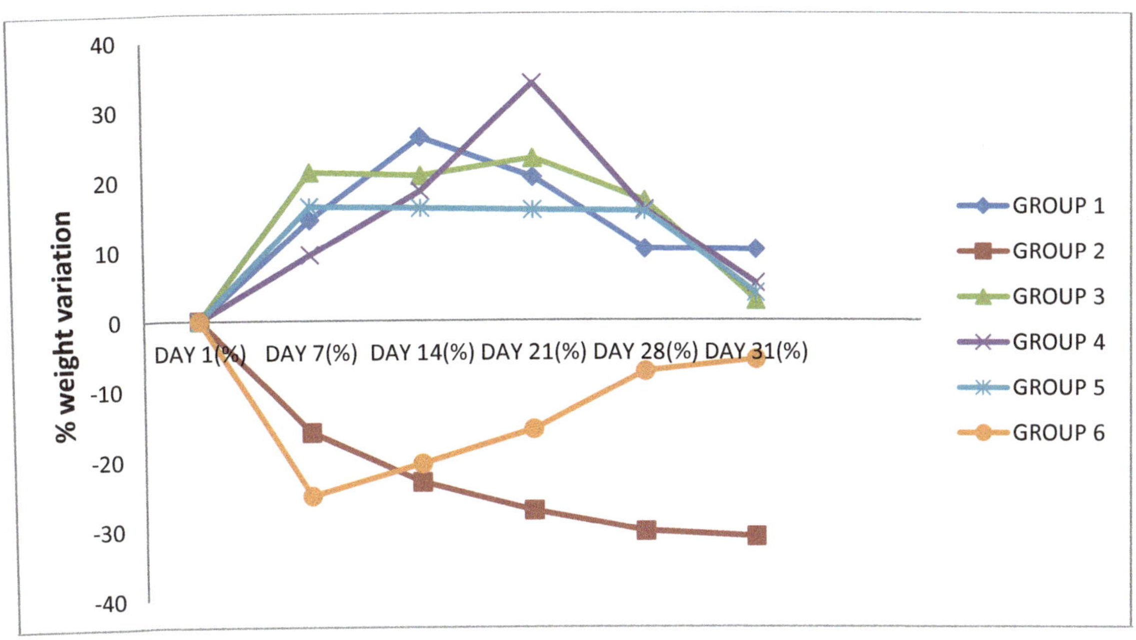

Fig. 2. Percentage weight variations of animals treated with various extract doses

Group 1: Normal rats not induced with diabetes to serve as positive control received acacia 2% w/v solution. Group 2: Alloxan-induced diabetic rats not treated, to serve as negative control. Group 3: Alloxan-induced diabetic rats treated with Glibenclamide 600 µg/kg body weight. Group 4: Alloxan-induced diabetic rats treated with 250 mg/kgbody weight extract. Group 5: Alloxan-induced diabetic rats treated with 150 mg/kg body weight extract. Group 6:Alloxan-induced diabetic rats treated with 75 mg/kg body weight extract

The plasma creatinine and urea levels have been established as markers of glomerular filtration rate (GFR), though plasma creatinine is a more sensitive index of kidney function compared to plasma urea level because creatinine fulfils most of the requirements for a perfect filtration marker [27]. A significant (p≤0.05) decrease in creatinine, urea and protein levels were observed in the treated diabetic animals which showed the extract might not have any damaging effects on the kidney. The tissue histology of kidney indicating no pathological changes was confirmatory to the observation.

Table 4. Phytochemical screening evaluation

Alkaloids	-
Anthraquinones	-
Flavonoids	+
Glycosides	+
Saponins	++
Steroids	+
Tannins	+
Terpenoids	+

The photomicrographs of histological studies (Fig. 3) indicated that the pancreatic beta cells of the diabetic animals treated with the extract exhibited considerable beta cells recovery that was dose depended compared to the diabetic untreated (negative control). The reference drug however exhibited comparably better activity.

There was also observed significant (p≤0.05) decrease in the plasma levels of LDL, triglycerides, total cholesterol and an increase in HDL level. The extract therefore had a reducing effect on the cardiovascular risk factors suggesting good anti-diabetic and anti-atherogenic activities. Many anti-diabetic plants have shown to have beneficial effect on cardiovascular system [16,28,29].

Haematological studies shown in Table 3 indicated increase in Hb and PVC levels. The increase in their levels following extract treatment may be due to changes in the rate of the RBCs production. The calculated RBC indices, MCH, MCV and MCHC were not significantly altered in the extract treated animals which suggested that the activity of the extracts had minimal effect on the size of RBC and therefore did not cause anaemia which might lead to cardiac failure.

The preliminary phytochemical screening result as shown in Table 4 demonstrated the absence of alkaloids and anthraquinones. However, there was presence of tannins, flavonoids, saponins which may occur as glycosides. There was also the presence of polyphenols. These biological active components have been observed in plants with strong hypoglycaemic property [30]. It has been reported that several plant sterols reduce serum cholesterol by the inhibition of intestinal cholesterol absorption [8].

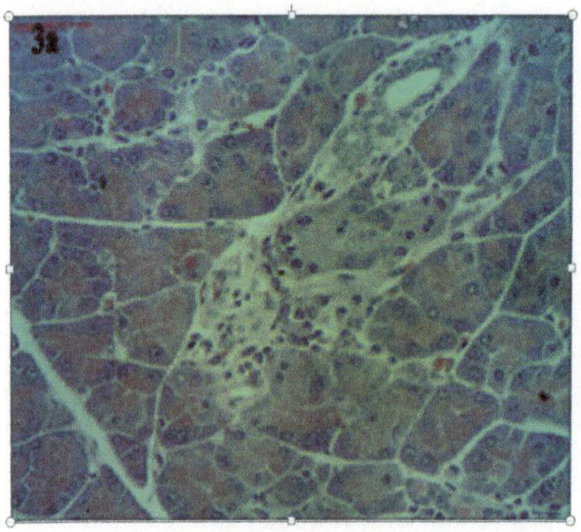

Fig. 3a. Pancreas (diabetic) not treated X400

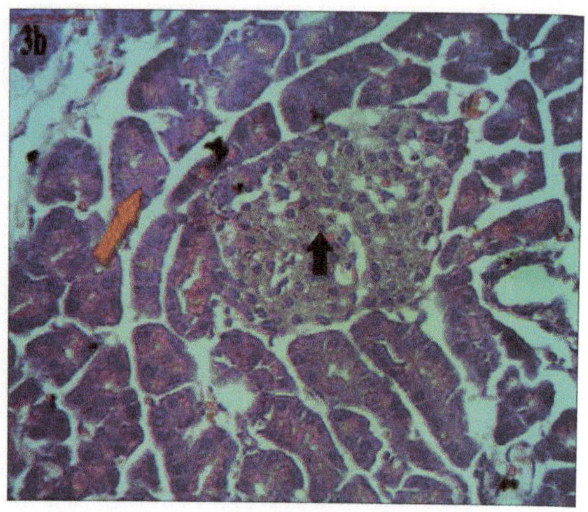

Fig. 3b. Pancreas (diabetic) treated with 250 mg extract X400

Fig. 3. Pancreatic tissue

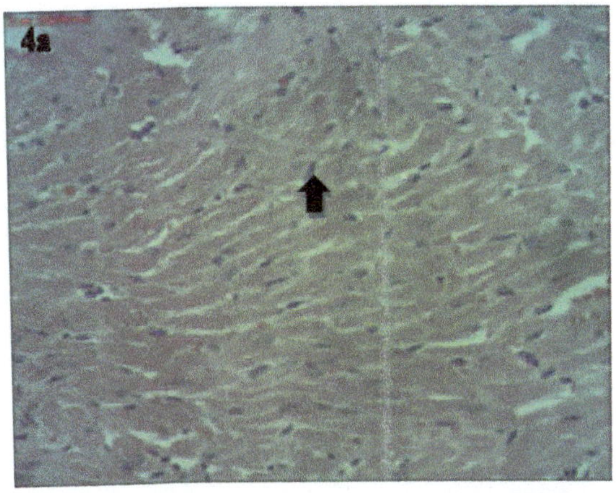

Fig. 4a. Heart (diabetic) not treated X400

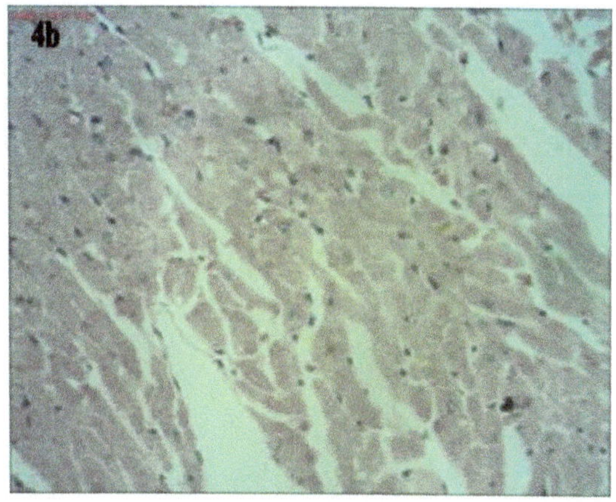

Fig. 4b. X400 Heart (diabetic) treated with 250 mg extract X400

Fig. 4. Cardiac tissue

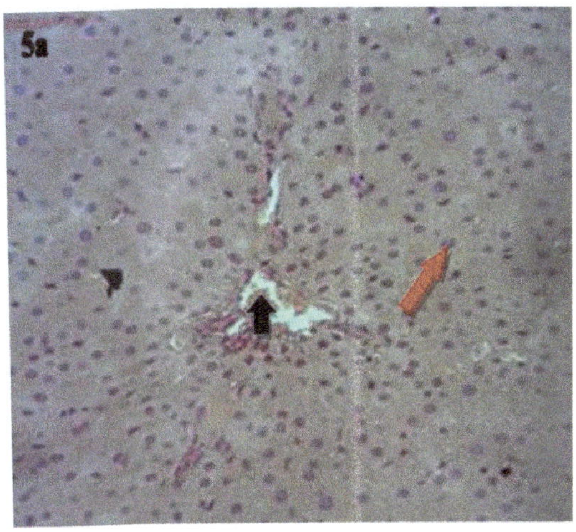

Fig. 5a. Liver (diabetic) not treated X400

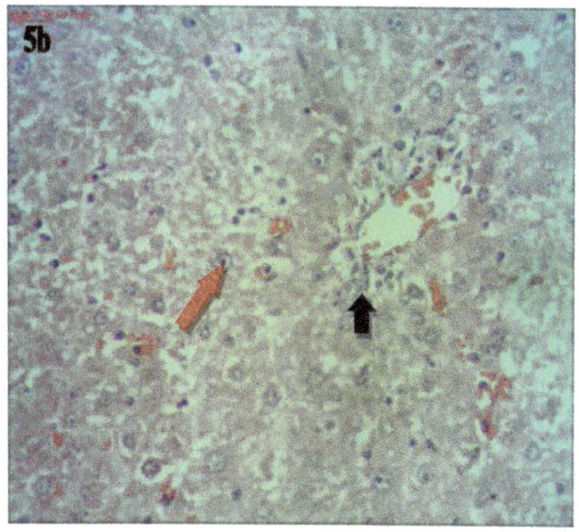

Fig. 5b. Liver (diabetic) treated with 250 mg extract X400

Fig. 5. Hepatic tissue

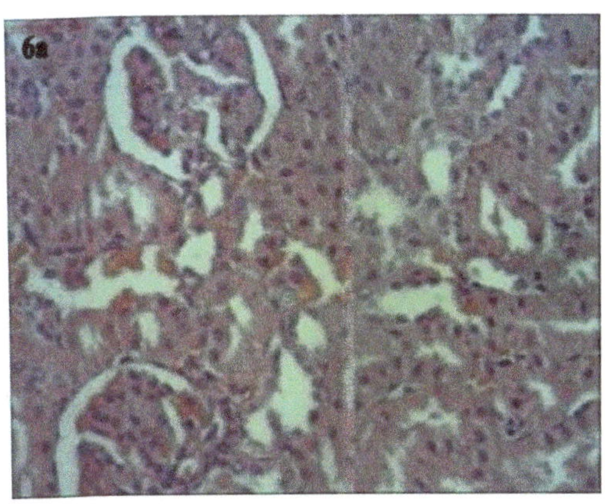

Fig. 6a. Kidney (diabetic) not treated X400

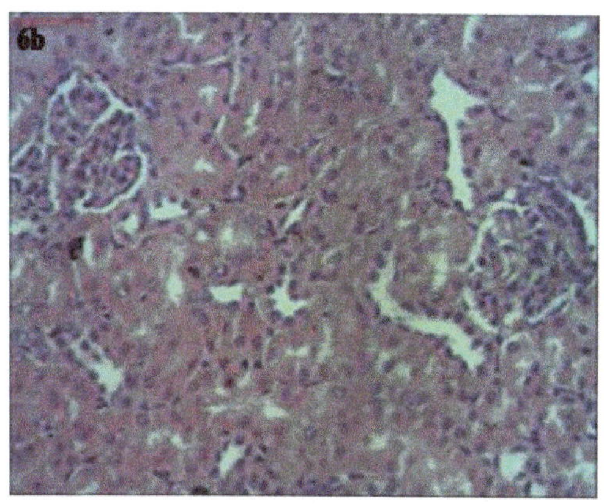

Fig. 6b. Kidney (diabetic) treated with 250 mg extract X400

Fig. 6. Renal tissue

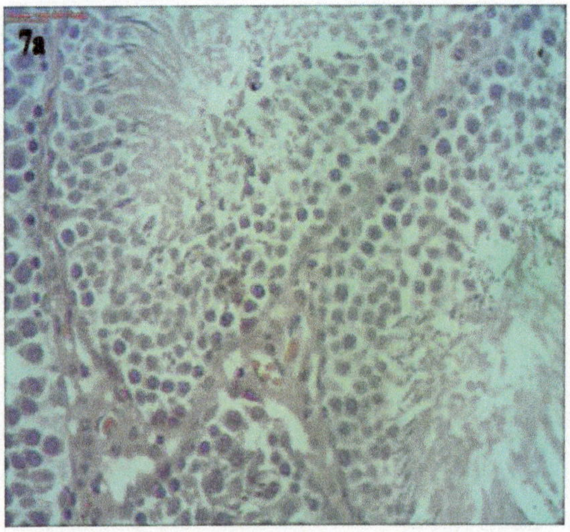

Fig. 7a. Testis (diabetic) not treated X400

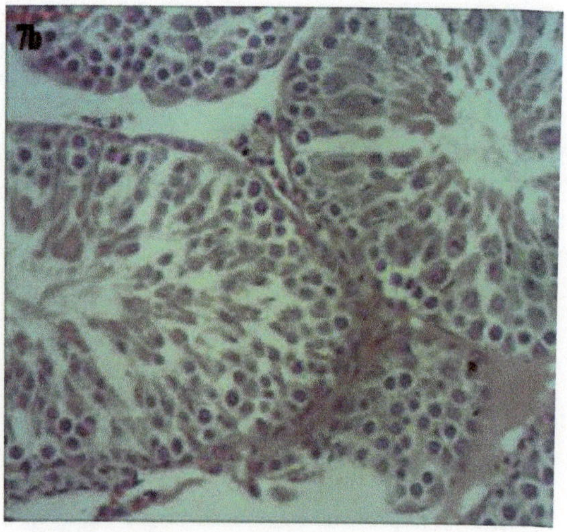

Fig. 7b. Testis (diabetic) treated with 250 mg extract X400

Fig. 7. Testicular tissue

Histological studies of some organs- pancreas, kidney, liver, testes. (3a): the photomicrographs of normal Islet cells, the black arrow points to the beta cell while the red to the pancreatic acni (H & E stain) mag. X400. (3b): Photomicrograph showed scanty survivor beta cells. (4a) Photomicrograph of a cross section of myocardium (heart) showing myocytes (thick arrowed) separated by an unremarkable interstitium. (4b): Photomicrograph of a cross section of myocardium showing no lesion. (5a): Photomicrograph of a cross section of hepatic tissue of the control showing portal tract (thick arrowed) and normal hepatocytes. (5b): The hepatic tissue of animals treated with high dose of the extract exhibited mild portal hepatitis, hepatocytes vacuolization and sinusoidal congestion. (6a): Photomicrograph of a cross section of cortical region of the renal tissue of the control indicating renal corpuscles and convoluted tubules. (6b): The cross section of cortical region of the renal tissue showed no lesion. (7a): The photomicrograph of untreated testicular tissue showed densely packed spermatogenic cells. (7b): Photomicrograph of diabetic animal treated with the extract indicated normal appearance

4. CONCLUSION

The study showed that *C. prostata* extract demonstrated a good hypoglycaemic activity and also had desirable effects on the cardiovascular risk factors. Treatment of the diabetic animals with *C. prostata* extract did not induce weight gain in the animals compared to the reference drug used, glibenclamide, indicating its advantage over synthetic hypoglycaemic agents.

CONSENT

It is not applicable.

ETHICAL APPROVAL

All authors hereby declare that "Principles of laboratory animal care" (NIH publication No. 85-23, revised 1985) were followed, as well as specific national laws where applicable. All experiments have been examined and approved by the appropriate ethics committee of our Institution". All authors hereby declare that all experiments have been examined and approved by the appropriate ethics committee and have therefore been performed in accordance with the ethical standards laid down in the 1964 Declaration of Helsinki.

COMPETING INTERESTS

Authors have declared that no competing interests exist.

REFERENCES

1. Ogbonnia SO, Adekunle AA, Olagbende – Dada SO, Anyika EN, Enwuru VN, Orolepe M. Assessing plasma glucose and lipid levels, bodyweight and acute toxicity following oral administration of an aqueous ethanolic extract of *Parinari curatellifolia* Planch (Chrysobalanceae) seeds in alloxan-induced diabetes in rats. Afr J Biotech. 2008;7(17):2998-3003.
2. Walter BJ. An Introduction to the Principles of Disease. W.B. Saunders Company. Philadelphia USA. 1977;374-377.

3. World Health Organization Department of Non-communicable Disease Surveillance Geneva; Definition, Diagnosis and Classification of Diabetes Mellitus and its Complications. 1999;2.
4. American Diabetes Association Diagnosis and classification of diabetes mellitus. Diabetes Care. 2010;33(Suppl. 1):S62–S69. Bandyopadhyay U, Biswas K, Chattopadhyay I, Banerjee RK, Biological activities and medicinal properties of neem (*Azadiracta indica*). Curr Sci. 2002;82: 1336-1345.
5. Senthilvel G, Jegadeesan M, Austin A, Thirugnanasambathan P, Mayisuvren E, Balasubramanian M, Narayanan N, Viswanathan S. Effect of a poly-herbal formulation (Diarun plus) on Streptozotocin induced experimental diabetes. Int. J. Trop. Med. 2006;2:88-92.
6. El-Nagar BEM, Bartó.Íková L, Îemlâka M, Vajdlenka E, Rabi.ková M, Stranadová V, Neâas J. Antidiabetic effect of Cleome droserifolia aerial parts: Lipid peroxidation–induced oxidative stress in diabetic rats. Acta Vet Brno. 2005;74:347-352.
7. Ogbonnia SO, Mbaka GO, Nkemehule FE, Emordi JE, Okpagu NC, Ota DA. Acute and subchronic evaluation of aqueous extracts of *Newbouldia laevis* (Bignoniaceae) and Nauclea latifolia (Rubiaceae) roots used singly or in combination in Nigerian traditional medicines. Br. J. Pharmacol. Toxicol. 2014;5(1):55-62.
8. Sushruta K, Satyanarayana S, Srinivas N, Sekhar Raja J. Evaluation of the blood–glucose reducing effects of aqueous extracts of the selected Umbellifereous fruits used in culinary practice. Trop. J. Pharm. Res. 2006;5(2):613-617.
9. Pari L, Saravanan R. Antidiabetic effect of Diasulin, an herbal drug, on blood glucose, plasma insulin and hepatic enzymes of glucose metabolism in hyperglycaemic rats. Diabetes, Obesity and Metabolism. 2004;6(4):286-291.
10. Rastigo AK, Chander R, Srivastava KA. Screening of natural products for hypolipidaemic and hypoglycaemic activities. In: Proceedings in International workshop on Medicinal plants their bioactivity, screening and evaluation; 1977.
11. Alzahrani AH, Bakhotmah BA. Top ten natural preparations for the treatment of diabetic foot disorders. Wounds UK. 2010; 6(4):18-26.
12. Sofowora A. Screening plants for bioactive agents. In medicinal plants and traditional in Africa. Spectrum Books Ltd Ibadan, 2ed. 1993;134-156.
13. Ogbonnia SO, Mbaka GO, Nwozor AM, Igbokwe HN, Usman A, Odusanya PA. Evaluation of microbial purity and acute and sub-acute toxicities of a Nigerian commercial polyherbal formulation used in the treatment of diabetes mellitus. Br. J. Pharm. Res. 2013;3(4):948-962.
14. Shah AMA, Garg SK, Garg KM. Subacute toxicity studies on Pendimethalin in rats. Indian J Pharmacol. 1997;29:322-324.
15. Bürger C, Fischer DR, Cordenunzzi DA, Batschauer de Borba AP, Filho VC, Soares dos Santos AR. Acute and subacute toxicity of the hydroalcoholic extract from Wedeliapaludosa (Acmelabrasilinsis) (Asteraceae) in mice. J. Pharmaceut. Sci. (www.cspsCanada.org). 2005;8(2):370-373.
16. Ogbonnia SO, Mbaka GO, Anyika EN, Ladiju O, Igbokwe HN, Emordi JE, Nwakakwa N. Evaluation of anti-diabetics and cardiovascular effects of *Parinari curatellifolia* seed extract and *Anthoclista vogelli* root extract individually and combined on postprandial and alloxan-induced diabetic albino rats. British J. Med. & Med. Res. 2011;1(3):146-162.
17. Mbaka GO, Adeyemi OO, Noronha CC, Anunobi CC, Okanlawon AO. Anti-hyperglycaemic and hypoglycaemic effects of ethanol root extract of *Sphenocentrum jollyanum* in normal and alloxan-induced diabetic rabbits. Braz. J. Morphol. Sc. 2009;26(2):123-127.
18. Ogbonnia SO, Mbaka GO, Adekunle A, Anyika EN, Gbolade OE, Nwakakwa N Effect of a poly-herbal formulation, *Okudiabet,* on alloxan- induced diabetic rats. Agric. Biol. J. N. Am. 2010;1(2):139-145.
19. Wasan KM, Najafi S, Wong J, Kwong M. Assessing plasma lipid levels, body weight, and hepatic and renal toxicity following chronic oral administration of a water soluble phytostanol compound FM-VP4, to gerbils. J. Pharm. Sci. (www.ualberta.ca/~csps). 2001;4(3):228-234.

20. Crook MA. Clinical Chemistry and Metabolic Medicine. 7th Edition. Hodder Arnold, London. 2006;426.
21. Hussain A, Eshrat HM Hypoglycemic, hypolipidemic and antioxidant properties of combination of Curcumin from *Curcuma longa*, Linn and partially purified product from *Abroma augusta*, Linn. instreptozotocin induced diabetes. Indian J. Clin. Biochem. 2002;17(2):33-43.
22. Farnsworth RN. Review on biological and phytochemical screening of plants. J. Pharm. Sci. 1966;55:225-276.
23. Harborne JB. Phytochemical methods: A guide to modern techniques of plant analysis 3 rd Edition. Chapman and Hall, London. 1998;235.
24. Mbaka GO, Ogbonnia SO, Banjo AE. Activity of *Raphia hookeri* root extract on blood glucose, lipid profile and glycosylated haemoglobin on alloxan induced diabetic rats. J. Morphol. Sci. 2012;29(3):1-9.
25. Ghosh MN. Fundamentals of Experimental Pharmacology, 2nd Edition. Scientific Book Agency, Calcutta. 1984;154-157.
26. Klaassen CD, Amdur MO, Doull J. Casarett and Doull's Toxicology: The basic science of poison. 8th Edition. McGraw Hill, USA. 1995;13-33.
27. Perrone RD, Madias NE, Levey AS. Serum creatinine as an index of renal function: New insights into old concepts. Clin Chem. 1992;38:1933-53.
28. Mbaka GO, Ogbonnia SO, Oyeniran KJ, Awopetu PI. Effect of *Raphia hookeri* seed extract on blood glucose, glycosylated haemoglobin and lipid profile of alloxan induced diabetic rats. British J. Med. & Med. Res. 2012;2(4):621-635.
29. Mbaka GO, Ojewale AO, Ogbonnia SO, Ota DA. Antihyperglycaemic and antihyperlipidaemic activities of aqueous ethanol root extract of *Pseudocedrela kotschyi* on alloxan-induced diabetic rats. British J. Med. & Med. Res. 2014;4(36): 5839-5852.
30. Garba R, Saidu AN, Adeyemi HRY, Muhammad HL. Effect of methanolic extract of *Cassia occidentalis* L. root bark on body weight and selected biochemical parameters in alloxan induced diabetic rats. Br. J. Pharmacol. Toxicol. 2015;6(2): 39-49.

15

Inhibition of α-amylase and α-glucosidase by *Acanthus montanus* Leaf Extracts

Akintayo L. Ogundajo[1*], Mutiu I. Kazeem[2], Olamidisun A. Owoyele[1], Abdul Razak O. Ogunmoye[3] and Isiaka A. Ogunwande[1,3*]

[1]Department of Chemistry, Faculty of Science, Natural Products Research Unit, Lagos State University, Badagry Expressway, PMB 0001 LASU Post Office, Ojo, Lagos, Nigeria.
[2]Department of Biochemistry, Faculty of Science, Antidiabetic Drug Discovery Group, Lagos State University, PMB 0001, Ojo, Lagos, Nigeria.
[3]Department of Chemical Sciences, Faculty of Science, Olabisi Onabanjo University, Ago-Iwoye, Ogun State, Nigeria.

Authors' contributions

This work was carried out in collaboration between all authors. Authors ALO and IAO designed the study and supervised the author OAO in the extraction of the plant sample. Author MIK supervised the author OAO in the anti-diabetic analysis, performed the statistical analysis and wrote the initial draft of the manuscript. Authors AROO and IAO managed the literature searches while author IAO wrote the final draft of the manuscript. All authors read and approved the final manuscript.

Article Information

Editor(s):
(1) Elena G. Zavyalova, Chemistry Department, Moscow State University, Russia.
Reviewers:
(1) Mathew Folaranmi Olaniyan, Achievers University, Owo, Nigeria.
(2) Sema Kalkan Uçar, Ege University, Turkey.
(3) Dhastagir sheriff, Benghazi University,Benghazi, Libya.

ABSTRACT

Aim: The aim of this study was to determine the *in-vitro* anti-diabetic potentials of *Acanthus montanus*. This was done by assessing the inhibitory effect of both methanol and ethylacetate extracts of the plant on the activities of α-amylase and α-glucosidase.
Study Design: The design included extraction of *A. montanus* leaves with methanol and ethanol and subsequent evaluation of the extracts for possible hypoglycemic effect.
Place and Duration of Study: The leaves of *A. montanus* were obtained from Badagry Area of

**Corresponding author: Email: ogundajotayo@yahoo.com, isiaka.ogunwande@lasu.edu.ng*

Lagos, Nigeria in December 2012. The plant was identified and authenticated by Dr. S. O. Shosanya of the Forestry Research Institute of Nigeria (FRIN), Ibadan, Nigeria.
Methodology: The powdered leaves were extracted with ethylacetate and methanol separately for 24 h. The resulting infusions were decanted, filtered and evaporated in a rotary evaporator. Dried extracts were weighed and dissolved in dimethylsulphoxide (DMSO) to yield a stock solution from which lower concentrations were prepared. The inhibitory actions of both extracts against α-amylase and α-glucosidase were determined established procedures.
Results: The results showed that of the two extracts, methanol showed more inhibitory action than ethanol against both α-amylase and α-glucosidase. Lineweaver-Burk plot also depicted that the methanol extract inhibited both α-amylase and α-glucosidase in a non-competitive and competitive manner respectively.
Conclusion: It can be concluded that the hypoglycemic effect of extracts of *A. montanus* may be as a result of the inhibition of these enzymes (α-amylase and α-glucosidase). This observation may be elicited by the presence of some phytochemicals present in the extracts.

Keywords: Acanthus montanus; α-amylase;α-glucosidase; antidiabetic.

1. INTRODUCTION

Diabetes is a metabolic disease which is as old as mankind and its incidence is considered to be high (4–5%) all over the world [1]. It is also a major cause of disability and hospitalization and results in significant financial burden [2]. It is considered a "modern day epidemic" and is rightly recognized as a global public health issue. The number of people suffering from the disease worldwide is increasing at an alarming rate with a projected 552 million people likely to be diabetic by the year 2035 as against 382 million estimated in 2014 [3]. There is need for the discovery of anti-diabetic agents from natural sources due to limited efficacy and serious side effects associated with synthetic drugs which include hypoglycaemia, chronic tissue damage and death [4].

Acanthus montanus (Nees) T. Anderson (Acanthaceae) is a small shrub with sparse branches and soft stems. It is commonly known as Mountain Thistle or Bears Breech and is believed to have originated from West Africa [5]. It is used in traditional medicine in the Southern part of Nigeria under the names; 'Mafowokan omomi', 'Agamsoso' and 'Agameru'. It is also used in different parts of Africa in the treatment of various illnesses such as cough, epilepsy, pain, dysmenorrhoea, hypertension, false labour, syphilis, skin infections and diabetes mellitus [6,7]. The pharmacological properties of this plant which include hepatoprotective [8], tocolytic [9], anti-inflammatory, antimicrobial and immunological properties [5] have been reported by several authors. Nana et al. [10] reported the safety of this plant in pregnant rats as well as their offspring while Djami et al. [11] also stated its tolerance in female rats at concentration greater than 1000 mg/kg body weight. Although, there is a study on the hypoglycemic potential of the methanolic extract of this plant [7], there is dirt of information on the possible mechanism by which it elicits its hypoglycemic action.

It is well known that any anti-diabetic agent can act by one or more of the following mechanisms; pancreatic β-cells regeneration, insulin secretion, mimicking the action of insulin, inhibition of carbohydrate metabolizing enzymes as well as slowing down the absorption of sugars from the gut [12]. The aim of this study was to assess the effect of leaf extracts of Nigerian grown *A. montanus* on diabetes-related enzymes (α-amylase and α-glucosidase) as well as its mode of inhibition of these enzymes. In our previously study, the anti-diabetic potentials of some other medicinal plants grown in Nigeria have been reported [13].

2. MATERIALS AND METHODS

2.1 Chemicals and Reagents

Porcine pancreatic α-amylase, rat intestinal α-glucosidase and paranitrophenyl-glucopyranoside were products of Sigma-Adrich Co., St Louis, USA while starch soluble (extra pure) was obtained from J. T. Baker Inc., Phillipsburg, USA. Other chemicals and reagents were of analytical grade and the water used was glass-distilled.

2.2 Plant Sample

The leaves of *Acanthus montanus* were obtained from Badagry Area of Lagos, Nigeria, in December 2012. The plant sample was identified and authenticated by the taxonomist; Dr. S. O.

Shosanya of the Forestry Research Institute of Nigeria (FRIN), Ibadan, Nigeria and voucher specimen (FHI 109720) was deposited in the Institute's herbarium. The leaves were air-dried, pulverized and kept in airtight plastic bags.

2.2.1 Preparation of extracts

The powdered leaves were divided into two portions of 10 g each and these were extracted with ethylacetate and methanol respectively. The mixtures were left to steep in covered conical flasks for 24 h, the flasks were shaken at interval and kept still to allow the plant material to settled at the bottom of the flask. The resulting infusions were decanted, filtered and evaporated in a rotary evaporator (Cole Parmer SB 1100, Shangai, China). Dried extracts were weighed and dissolved in dimethylsulphoxide (DMSO) to yield a stock solution from which lower concentrations were prepared. All extracts were stored at 4°C prior to analysis.

2.3 α-Amylase Inhibitory Assay

This assay was carried out using a modified procedure of McCue and Shetty [14]. A total of 250 µL of extract was placed in a test tube and 250 µL of 0.02 M sodium phosphate buffer (pH 6.9) containing α-amylase solution was added. This solution was pre-incubated at 25°C for 10 min, after which 250 µL of 1% starch solution in 0.02 M sodium phosphate buffer (pH 6.9) was added at timed intervals and then incubated at 25°C for 10 min. The reaction was terminated by adding 500 µL of dinitrosalicylic acid (DNS) reagent. The tubes were then incubated in boiling water for 5 min and cooled to room temperature. The reaction mixture was diluted with 5 mL of distilled water and the absorbance was measured at 540 nm using a spectrophotometer (Spectrumlab S23A, Globe Medical England). The control and blank solutions were prepared using the same procedure by replacing the extract with DMSO and distilled water respectively. The α-amylase inhibitory activity was calculated as percentage inhibition as follows;

$$\% \text{ Inhibition} = [(\Delta A_{control} - \Delta A_{extract})/A\Delta_{control}] \times 100$$

where $\Delta A_{control} = A_{control} - A_{blank}$ and $\Delta A_{extract} = A_{extract} - A_{blank}$

Concentrations of extracts resulting in 50% inhibition of enzyme activity (IC_{50}) were determined graphically.

2.3.1 Mode of α-amylase inhibition

The mode of inhibition of α-amylase by the extract was conducted using the most potent extract according to the modified method described by Ali et al. [15]. Briefly, 250 µL of the (5 mg/mL) extract was pre-incubated with 250 µL of α-amylase solution for 10 min at 25°C in one set of tubes. In another set of tubes α-amylase was pre-incubated with 250 µL of phosphate buffer (pH 6.9). Then, 250 µL of starch solution at increasing concentrations (0.3–5.0 mg/mL) was added to both sets of reaction mixtures to enable the reaction to commenced. The mixture was then incubated for 10 min at 25°C, and then boiled for 5 min after addition of 500 µL of DNS to stop the reaction. The amount of reducing sugars released was determined spectrophotometrically using a maltose standard curve and converted to reaction velocities. A double reciprocal (Lineweaver-Burk) plot (1/v versus 1/[S]) where v is reaction velocity and [S] is substrate concentration was plotted to determine the mode of inhibition.

2.4 α-Glucosidase Inhibitory Assay

The effect of the plant extracts on the activity of α-glucosidase was determined according to the method described previously by Kim et al. [16]. The substrate solution, p-nitropheynyl glucopyranoside (pNPG) was prepared in 20 mM phosphate buffer (pH 6.9). Also, 100 µL of α-glucosidase (E.C. 3.2.1.20) was pre-incubated with 50 µL of the different concentrations of the extracts for 10 min. Then, 50 µL of 3.0 mM pNPG dissolved in 20 mM phosphate buffer (pH 6.9) was added to start the reaction. The reaction mixture was incubated at 37°C for 20 min and stopped by adding 2 mL of 0.1 M Na_2CO_3. The α-glucosidase activity was determined by measuring the yellow coloured para-nitrophenol released from pNPG at 405 nm. The control and blank were prepared using the same procedure by replacing the extract with DMSO and distilled water respectively. Percentage inhibition was calculated thus;

$$\% \text{ Inhibition} = [(\Delta A_{control} - \Delta A_{extract})/A\Delta_{control}] \times 100$$

where $\Delta A_{control} = A_{control} - A_{blank}$ and $\Delta A_{extract} = A_{extract} - A_{blank}$

Concentrations of extracts resulting in 50% inhibition of enzyme activity (IC_{50}) were determined graphically.

2.4.1 Mode of α-glucosidase inhibition

The mode of inhibition of α-glucosidase by the extracts was determined using the extract with the lowest IC_{50} according to the modified method described by Ali et al. [15]. Briefly, 50 μL of the (5 mg/mL) extract was pre-incubated with 100 μL of α-glucosidase solution for 10 min at 25°C in one set of tubes. In another set of tubes, α-glucosidase was pre-incubated with 50 μL of phosphate buffer (pH 6.9). Thereafter 50 μL of pNPG at increasing concentrations (0.63 - 2.0 mg/mL) was added to both sets of reaction mixtures to start the reaction. The mixture was then incubated for 10 min at 25°C after which 500 μL of Na_2CO_3 was added to stop the reaction. The amount of reducing sugars released was determined spectrophotometrically using a para-nitrophenol standard curve and converted to reaction velocities. A double reciprocal (Lineweaver-Burk) plot (1/v versus 1/[S]) where v is reaction velocity and [S] is substrate concentration was plotted to determine the mode of inhibition of the enzyme.

2.5 Statistical Analysis

Statistical analysis was performed using GraphPad Prism 5 statistical package (GraphPad Software, USA). The data were analysed by one way analysis of variance (ANOVA) followed by Bonferroni test. All the results were expressed as mean ± SEM for triplicate determinations.

3. RESULTS AND DISCUSSION

Fig. 1 showed the percentage inhibition of α-amylase by methanol and ethylacetate extracts of *A. montanus*. There were no significant differences between the extracts at low concentrations (0.32 - 0.63 mg/mL). However at higher concentrations, the ethylacetate extract exhibited significantly higher percentage inhibition of the enzyme. The higher percentage inhibition of the enzyme displayed by the ethylacetate extract was corroborated by its lower IC_{50} value compared to that of methanol extract (Table 1).

However, the Lineweaver-Burk plot of the mode of inhibition of α-amylase by the methanol extract of this plant showed that it is a non-competitive inhibitor of the enzyme (Fig. 2).

The percentage of inhibition of α-glucosidase by the extracts of *A. montanus* is shown in Fig 3. At all concentrations tested, methanol extract exhibited significantly higher (P=.05) percentage inhibition of this enzyme compared to ethylacetate extract. However, the inhibition of the enzyme by both extract was dose-dependent. This is supported by the lower IC_{50} value for ethanol extract compared to methanol extract. Kinetic analysis of the mode of inhibition of the enzyme with the aid of Lineweaver-Burk plot showed that the ethanol extract inhibited the enzyme in a competitive manner (Fig. 4).

Table 1. IC_{50} values for α-amylase and α-glucosidase inhibitory potential of *A. montanus* leaf extracts

Extracts	IC_{50} (mg/mL)	
	α-Amylase	α-Glucosidase
Methanol	2.87±0.02[a]	1.65±0.02[a]
Ethylacetate	2.39±0.04[b]	7.10±0.15[b]
Acarbose	2.60±0.01[a]	0.63±0.00[c]

The management of hyperglycemia is the hallmark of treatment in diabetes. A convenient therapeutic approach for decreasing postprandial hyperglycemia is to retard the digestion and absorption of carbohydrates. This is done through the inhibition of carbohydrate hydrolyzing enzymes, α-amylase and α-glucosidase, in the digestive tract [17]. Though, synthetic α-glucosidase inhibitors such as acarbose and voglibose are presently in use but are bedeviled by undesirable side effects such as nausea, hypoglycaemia, diarrhoea and liver failure [14], which necessitated this study.

The present study showed that the ethylacetate extract of *A. montanus* produced stronger inhibition of α-amylase than methanol extract. However, methanol extract will be more suitable to be used as anti-diabetic agent because of its mild inhibition of the enzymes, possessing higher IC_{50} than ethylacetate extract and acarbose. Previous studies have shown that any prospective anti-diabetic agent should be a mild inhibitor of α-amylase so as to prevent the drawback of synthetic drugs (like acarbose), which occur due to the excessive inhibition of the enzyme resulting in the abnormal bacterial fermentation of undigested carbohydrates in the colon [18,19]. Therefore, the Lineweaver-Burk plot of the inhibition depicted that methanol extract of *A. motanus* inhibited the enzyme in a non-competitive manner. This implies that the active components in the extract binds to a site other than the active site of the enzyme and combines with either free enzyme or the enzyme-substrate complex, possibly interfering with the action of both [20].

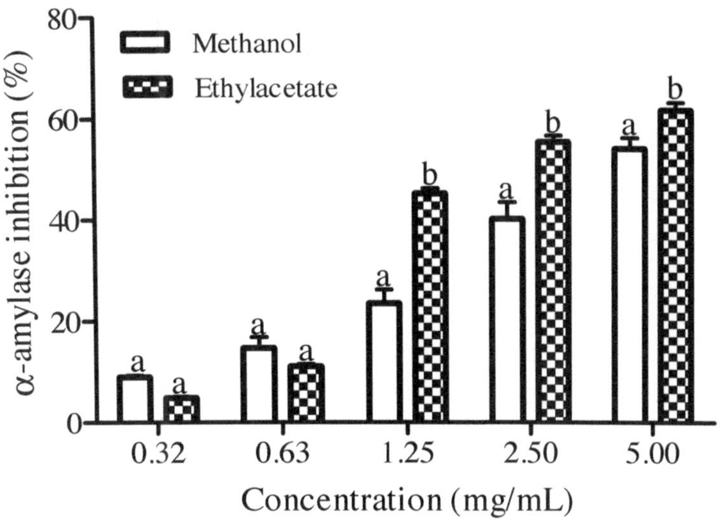

Fig. 1. Inhibitory potency of *A. montanus* leaf extracts against α-amylase activity. The values are expressed as means ± SEM of triplicate determinations. Means not sharing a common letter at the same concentration are significantly different (*P* = .05)

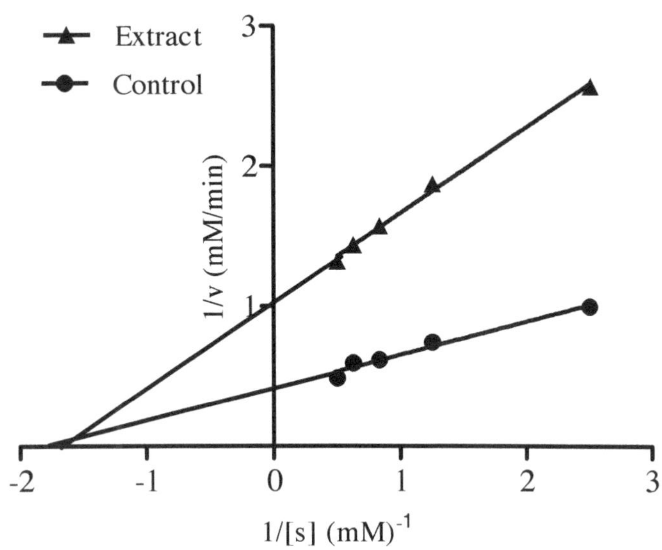

Fig. 2. Mode of inhibition of α-amylase by methanol extract of *A. montanus*

The stronger inhibition of α-glucosidase by the methanol extract of *A. montanus* at all concentrations tested compared to ethylacetate extract, culminated into having low IC_{50} which is also desirable of a good antidiabetic drug. The competitive inhibition of the enzyme by methanol extract of *A. montanus* suggest that the inhibitory component(s) in the plant binds reversibly to the active site of the enzyme and occupies it in a mutually exclusive manner with the substrate [21,22]. This may due to structural similarity between the inhibitor and the normal substrate (disaccharides), thereby slowing down the production of glucose and reducing hyperglycemia.

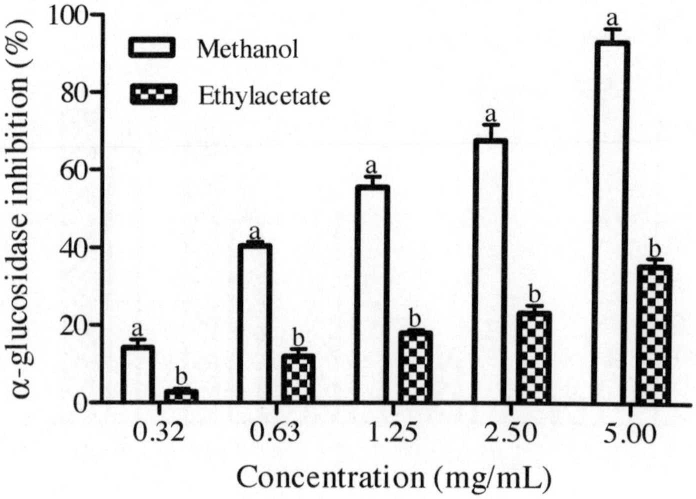

Fig. 3. Inhibitory potency of *A. montanus* leaf extracts against α-glucosidase activity. The values are expressed as means ± SEM of triplicate determinations. Means not sharing a common letter at the same concentrations are significantly different (*P* = .05)

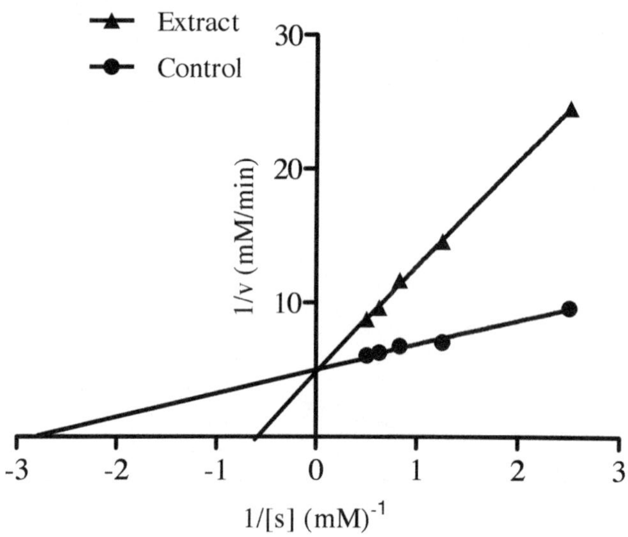

Fig. 4. Mode of inhibition of α-glucosidase by ethylacetate extract of *A. montanus*

Tannins are phenolic compounds which have been found to induce phosphorylation of insulin receptors and translocation of glucose transporter, thereby helping in the reduction of blood glucose level [23]. Studies have also shown the antioxidant and antidiabetic properties of saponins from different medicinal plants [24,25]. Therefore, it is probable that the inhibitory effect of *A. montanus* extracts on the activities of α-amylase and α-glucosidase may be due to the presence of these kinds of phytochemicals present in the extracts.

4. CONCLUSION

This study showed that methanol extract of *A. montanus* is a more potent inhibitor of α-amylase and α-glucosidase than ethylacetate extract. However, this methanol extract proved to be a non-competitive and competitive inhibitor of both α-amylase and α-glucosidase respectively. It can therefore be concluded that the hypoglycemic action of this plant may be due to the inhibition these diabetes-related enzymes studied.

CONSENT

It is not applicable.

ETHICAL APPROVAL

It is not applicable.

COMPETING INTERESTS

Authors have declared that no competing interests exist.

REFERENCES

1. Koyuturk M, Ozsoy-Sacan O, Bolkent S, Yanardag R. Effect of glurenorm on immunohistochemical changes in pancreatic β-cells of rats in experimental diabetes. Indian J Exp Biol. 2005;43(3): 268-7.
2. Nagappa AN, Thakurdesai PA, Rao NV, Singh J. Antidiabetic activity of *Terminalia catappa* Linn fruits. J Ethnopharm. 2003; 88(1):45-50.
3. International Diabetes Federation (IDF). Global diabetes scorecard-tracking progress for action. IDF, Brussels: Belgium. 2014;14.
4. Michael PK, Asim AB, Robert SB. The utility of oral diabetes medications in type 2 diabetes of the young. Current Diabetes Rev. 2005;1(1):83-92.
5. Okoli C, Akah P, Onuoha N, Okoye T, Nwoye A, Nworu C. *Acanthus montanus*: An experimental evaluation of the antimicrobial, anti-inflammatory and immunological properties of a traditional remedy for furuncles. BMC Complem Alter Med. 2008;1(8):27.
6. Songalem EA, Foyet HS, Ekobo S, Dimo T, Kamtchouing P. Antiinflammatory, lack of central analgesia and antipyretic properties of *Acanthus montanus* (Ness) T. Anderson. J. Ethnopharm. 2004;95(1): 63-8.
7. Ukwe CV, Ubaka CM. Hypoglycemic activity of leaves of *Acanthus montanus* T. Anderson (Acanthaceae) in rats. Int J Diab Dev Count. 2011;31(1):32-6.
8. Patrick-Iwuanyanwu KC, Weghu MO. Prevention of carbon-tetrachloride (CCl_4) induced liver damage in rats by *Acanthus montanus*. Asian J Biochem. 2008;3(4): 213-20.
9. Foyet HS, Asongalem EA, Nana P, Folefoc GN, Kamtchouing P. Tocolytic effect of *Acanthus montanus* in rat uterus. Pharmacologyonline. 2006;3:9-17.
10. Nana P, Asongalem EA, Foyet HS, Folefoc GN, Dimo T, Kamtchouing P. Maternal and developmental toxicity evaluation of *Acanthus montanus* leaves extract administered orally to Wistar pregnant rats during organogenesis. J Ethnopharm. 2008;116(2):228-33.
11. Djami TAT, Asongalem EA, Nana P, Choumessi A, Kamtchouing P, Asonganyi T. Subacute toxicity study of the aqueous extract from *Acanthus montanus*. Electronic J Biol. 2011;7(1):11-5.
12. Cheng AYY, Fantus IG. Oral antihyperglycemic therapy for type 2 diabetes Mellitus. Canadian Med Assoc J. 2005; 172(2):213-26.
13. Ogundajo AL, Kazeem MI, Evroh JE, Avoseh MM, Ogunwande IA. Comparative study on the phytochemical composition and hypoglycemic potentials of the leaves extracts of *Combretum paniculatum* and *Morinda morindoides*. Eur J Med Pl. 2015; 7(2):77-86.
14. Mccue PP, Shetty K. Inhibitory effects of rosmarinic acid extracts on porcine pancreatic α-amylase *in vitro*. Asia Pac J Cli Nutr. 2004;13(1):101-6.
15. Ali H, Houghton PJ, Soumyanath A. Alpha-amylase inhibitory activity of some Malaysian plants used to treat diabetes with particular reference to *Phyllanthus amarus*. J Ethnopharm. 2006;107(3): 449-55.
16. Kim YM, Jeong YK, Wang MH, Lee WY, Rhee HI. Inhibitory effects of pine bark extract on alpha-glucosidase activity and postprandial hyperglycemia. Nutr. 2005; 21(6):756-61.
17. Kazeem MI, Adamson JO, Ogunwande IA. Modes of inhibition of α- amylase and α-glucosidase by Aqueous extract of *Morinda lucida* Benth leaf. Biomed Res Int. 2013; 1-6.
18. Apostolidis E, Kwon Y-I, Shetty K. Inhibitory potential of herb, fruit, and fungal-enriched cheese against key enzymes linked to type 2 diabetes and hypertension. Innov Food Sci Emerg Tech. 2007;8(1):46-54.

19. Kwon Y-I, Apostolidis E, Shetty K. Inhibitory potential of wine and tea against α-amylase and α-glucosidase for management of hyperglycemia linked to type 2 diabetes. J Food Biochem. 2008; 32(1):15-31.
20. Mayur B, Sandesh S, Shruti S, Sung-Yum S. Antioxidant and α- glucosidase inhibitory properties of *Carpesium abrotanoides* L. J Med Pl Res. 2010;4(15):1547-53.
21. Matsuda H, Morikawa T, Yoshikawa M. Antidiabetogenic constituents from several natural medicines. Pure Appl Chem. 2002; 74(7):1301-8.
22. Kazeem MI, Ogungbe SM, Saibu GM, Aboyade OM. *In vitro* study on the hypoglycemic potential of *Nicotiana tabacum* leaf extracts. Bangladesh J Pharmacol. 2014;9(2):140-5.
23. Liu X, Kim JK, Li Y, Li J, Liu F, Chen X. Tannic acid stimulates glucose transport and inhibits adipocyte differentiation in 3T3-Li cells. J Nutr. 2005;135(2):165-71.
24. Yang C-Y, Wang J, Zhao Y, Shen L, Jiang X, Xie Z-G, et al. Anti-diabetic effects of *Panax notoginseng* saponins and its major anti-hyperglycemic components. J Ethnopharm. 2010;130(2): 231-6.
25. Zheng T, Shu G, Yang Z, Mo S, Zhao Y, Mei Z. Antidiabetic effect of total saponins from *Entada phaseoloides* (L.) Merr. in type 2 diabetic rats. J Ethnopharm. 2012; 139(3):814-21.

16

Pharmaceutical Quality Analysis of Ceftriaxone Sodium Brands Marketed in Southern Nigeria

Ogbonna Okorie[1], E. Omotoso Abayomi[2*] and Ebinyansi Onyinyechi[1]

[1]Department of Pharmaceutics and Pharmaceutical Technology, Faculty of Pharmaceutical Sciences, University of Port Harcourt, Rivers State, Nigeria.
[2]Department of Pharmaceutical and Medicinal Chemistry, Faculty of Pharmaceutical Sciences, University of Port Harcourt, Rivers State, Nigeria.

Authors' contributions

This work was carried out in collaboration between all authors. Author OO designed the study. Author EO wrote the protocol and author EOA wrote the first draft of the manuscript. Authors EOA and OO managed the literature searches and authors EOA and EO managed the experimental process and interpreted the data generated. All authors read and approved the final manuscript.

Article Information

Editor(s):
(1) Mohamed Fathy, Assiut University, Assiut, Egypt.
Reviewers:
(1) Ilham Zahir, University Sidi Mohamed Ben Abdellah, Morocco.
(2) Khasabuli Y. Osborn, The Kenya Medical Research Institute, Kenya.
(3) R. Revathi, The Erode College of Pharmacy, Tamil Nadu, India.
(4) Selçuk Yuksel, Pamukkale University, Turkey.

ABSTRACT

One of the paramount controversies between Physicians and Pharmacists is the issue of generic substitution. Prescribers are compelled to choose from such a large range of brands. The objective of this study was to compare the Pharmaceutical quality of innovator brand of injectable Ceftriaxone sodium with its generic brands that are marketed in Southern Nigeria. Seven brands of injectable Ceftriaxone sodium marketed in some pharmacies in Southern Nigeria were analysed. Standard physical and chemical tests for quality control of parenterals approved by the British Pharmacopoeia were performed on the branded sampled. The tested brands complied with the BP specifications for quality of Parenterals. Although one of the generic brands has content weight of Ceftriaxone greater than the upper limit specified (127.906%). The brands of Ceftriaxone sodium tested have been proven to be pharmaceutically and therapeutically equivalent. Though, there are variations among these brands due to the different manufacturing processes and formulation factors.

**Corresponding author: Email: abatoseb2001@yahoo.com, Abayomi.omotoso@uniport.edu.ng*

Keywords: Ceftriaxone sodium; pharmaceutical quality; quality control; generic substitution; pharmaceutical equivalence.

1. INTRODUCTION

Ceftriaxone sodium, chemically defined as, Disodium (6R,7R)-7-[[(2Z)-(2-aminothiazol-4-yl)(methoxyimino)acetyl]amino]-3-[[(2-methyl-6-oxido-5-oxo-2,5-dihydro-1,2,4-triazin-3-yl)sulphanyl]methyl]-8-oxo-5-thia-1-azabicyclo[4.2.0]oct-2-ene-2-carboxylate 3.5 hydrate; with the chemical formula, $C_{18}H_{16}N_8Na_2O_7S_3,3^1/_2H_2O$, and a calculated molecular weight of 661.59, is a third generation cephalosporin antibiotic. It has the following structural formula:

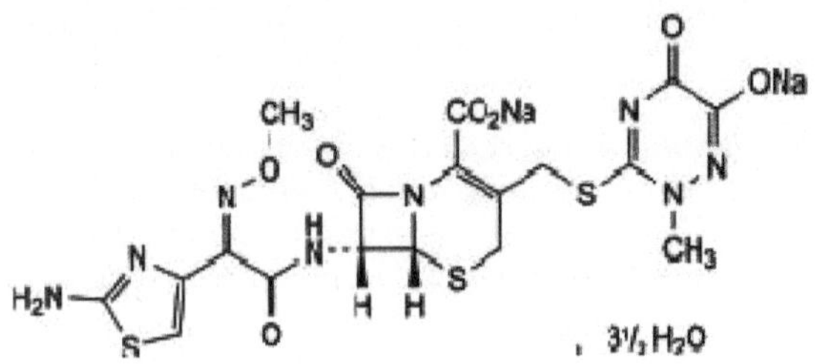

Fig. 1. Ceftriaxone sodium

Antibacterial action of Ceftriaxone sodium is produced through the inhibition of mucopeptide synthesis in the bacterial cell wall and by binding to one or more of the penicillin-binding proteins (PBPs) which in turn inhibits the final transpeptidation step of peptidoglycan synthesis in bacterial cell walls, thus hindering bacterial cell wall biosynthesis. This leads to subsequent cell death by lysis due to on-going activity of cell wall autolytic enzymes continues while cell-wall assembly is arrested [1,2]. Ceftriaxone sodium is well absorbed intramuscularly and possesses a complete bioavailability after intramuscular and intravenous administration. Urinary excretion is the major elimination pathway for Ceftriaxone sodium. As such, 33-67% of dose is excreted in urine as unchanged drug and the remaining fraction is eliminated in faeces through bile. Biliary elimination is significant for Ceftriaxone sodium [3,4].

A generic medicine is defined as an exact simulation of an established drug, not protected by a patent and promoted with the chemical name of the active ingredient. Generic drug formulation contains the same active pharmaceutical ingredient(s) in the same quantity as the reference listed drug (RLD) or innovator brand. There are legitimate concerns about the efficacy of generic formulations, and data show that cost-savings to the patient or the health care system may not be significant as expected [5].

The interchangeability of innovator brands with generic brands is dependent on the evidence of pharmaceutical equivalence, therapeutic equivalence and bioequivalence between the innovator and generic brands. Drug products are considered to be pharmaceutical equivalents if they contain the same active ingredients and are identical in strength or concentration, dosage form, and route of administration. Two pharmaceutically equivalent drug products are considered to be bioequivalent when the rates and extents of bioavailability of the active ingredient in the two products are not significantly different under suitable test conditions. Therapeutic equivalence in parenteral dosage forms is evaluated from pharmaceutical equivalence between the innovator brand and the generic brand, provided that the delivery of the active pharmaceutical ingredient(s) occurs directly in the systemic circulation (100% bioavailability) [6].

Generic brands must meet the official specifications for quality provided by different pharmacopoeias for a standard drug. Standards of a quality drug formulation including; safety, efficacy, purity, stability and potency; must be fully met by the generic formulation. Quality control requirements for parenteral dosage forms include; Visual inspection, clarity, color, and labelling; Uniformity of weight; Uniformity of content; Bacterial endotoxins-pyrogens; Sterility; and Particulate contamination: Visible and sub-visible particles [7].

Several investigations on the pharmaceutical quality of generic drug products have been carried out [8-11]. Previous studies mostly compared innovator brands and generic brands in terms of their physicochemical activities. The studies on Ceftriaxone sodium [12-14]. compared the quality of generic brands with Rocephin®. The limitations of the above studies include non-inclusion brands which are available in Nigeria and also no microbiological assay. Furthermore, as a result of usual controversies between Physicians and Pharmacists on the issue of generic substitution, this study provides evidence upon which such choices can be made in a more accurate, scientific and professional manner.

To the best of our knowledge, no such analysis for Ceftriaxone sodium generics available in Nigerian drug markets has been reported.

Therefore, the aim of this study was to compare the Pharmaceutical quality of innovator brand of Ceftriaxone sodium for injection with its generic brands that are marketed in Southern Nigeria in order to provide evidence of pharmaceutical and therapeutic equivalence that ensures interchangeability and generic substitution.

2. MATERIALS AND METHODS

2.1 Chemicals

The innovator brand (Rocephin®) and generic brands (Protedex® 'PC', Biocef® 'BC', Kincef® 'KC', Ebecef® 'EC', ZMC® 'ZC' and Xapo® 'XC') of Ceftriaxone sodium injection (1000mg) marketed in Nigeria were purchased from approved wholesale pharmacies in Southern Nigeria. These samples were stored at temperature <25℃ in a cool place, prevented from having direct access to light and thereafter tested within their expiration dates. The sampled generics represent the largest proportion of Ceftriaxone sodium for injection 1000 mg easily accessible in Nigeria. Table 1 provides the description of the Ceftriaxone brands sampled. Others include; Phosphate buffer solution pH 7.4, distilled water, ethanol, sterile water for injection, Sabouraund dextrose agar, Mueller-Hinton agar, plate count agar, GenScript ToxinSensor™ Chromogenic LAL Endotoxin Assay Kits (16 rxns) Cat. No. L00350C Lot No. C50181409 which contains Limulus Amoebocyte Lysate (LAL), LAL reagent water, *E. Coli* endotoxin standard, chromogenic substrate, buffer S for color-stabilizer #1, color-stabilizer #1, color-stabilizer #2 and color-stabilizer #3.

2.2 Physical Assessment and Physico-chemical Analysis

The primary and secondary packages of the brand samples were examined very carefully to check for required information such as manufacturers address, manufacturing dates, batch numbers, expiry date, and amount of active ingredients & National Agency for Food and Drug Administration and Control (NAFDAC) Registration number.

Melting point determination and pH value (acidity or alkalinity); were carried out on all brands sampled.

2.3 pH Determination

The pH value was determined using pH meter (PHS – 25 pH Meter, China). British Pharmacopoeia specification for pH of a solution containing the equivalent of 12.0% $^{w}/_{v}$ of Ceftriaxone sodium is 6.0 to 8.0.

2.4 Melting Point Determination

These tests were carried out on all brands sampled and the test were performed using procedures specified by the British Pharmacopoeia 2012, except where otherwise stated. The melting points of the brands were determined using melting point apparatus (Electrothermal, USA).

2.5 Pharmaceutical Quality Analysis

Color of vial content and reconstituted solution, clarity of solution, weight uniformity, content uniformity, sterility, bacterial endotoxin test, particulate matter determination: Visible matter; were carried out on all brand samples. These tests were performed according to British Pharmacopoeia 2012, except where otherwise stated.

2.6 Colour of Vial Content and of Reconstituted Solution

Color of vial content was assessed visually by examining a small quantity of powder placed on a flat white and then black background/surface. The color of the reconstituted solution was assessed by examining a 12% w/v aqueous solution in a clean colourless test tube placed against a white background. The British Pharmacopoeia 2012 specification for color of ceftriaxone sodium for injection is almost white or yellowish powder and the reconstituted solution should not be more coloured than reference solution.

2.7 Clarity of Solution

Samples were reconstituted as directed by the leaflet inserted in the drug package. Clarity of reconstituted solutions was observed against a visual inspection board with a black and white background under sufficient illumination. The presence of black particles was seen using white background whereas any white particles and fibres present were observed against black background. Rocephin® specification is

Table 1. Descriptions of the ceftriaxone sodium 1000 mg brands tested

Product	Manufacturer	Marketing company	Batch number	NAFDAC number	Manufacture date	Expiry date
ROCEPHIN®	Hoffmann-La Roche, Switzerland.	Swiss pharma, Nigeria.	B0112B03 F0527	04-7302	10/2013	10/2016
PROTEDEX®	GlaxoSmithKline, Italy.	GlaxoSmithKline, Nigeria.	T043	B4-0365	01/2014	01/2016
BIOCEF®	Shenzhen Pharmaceutical, China.	Biofem Pharmaceuticals Nigeria	20130802	A4-1459	08/2013	02/2016
KINCEF®	Yangzhou Pharmaceutical, China.	Kingzy Pharmaceuticals Nigeria	140572	A4-7429	05/2014	05/2017
EBECEF®	Swiss Parenterals PVT, India.	Elbe Pharma., Nigeria	XB-14007	04-8977	01/2014	12/2016
ZMC®	Shandong Pharmaceutical, China.	Demytex Pharma., Nigeria	140131	A4-8141	01/2014	01/2017
XAPO®	Swiss Parenterals, India.	Justeen Pharmaceuticals, Nigeria.	XB-13125	04-7267	09/2013	08/2016

(n = 10 per brand)

maximally six visible particles per container and maximum 20 per 10 containers, and maximum 600 sub-visible particles ≥25 mm per container. The British Pharmacopoeia specifies that a solution containing the equivalent of 1.20% w/v of ceftriaxone is clear.

2.8 Labelling Inspection

The label on the vials and the packs were inspected thoroughly and the written instructions were noted and compared with the British Pharmacopoeia specification for labelling of parenteral products and Ceftriaxone for injection.

2.9 Uniformity of Weight

The labels on ten containers of each brand were scraped off and their closures were also removed. Without labels and closures/caps these ten vials were weighed individually, then emptied, rinsed with water and ethanol, dried at 105^{0}C for 1 hour, cooled, and then weighed again. The weight of the vials with drug, and the weight of the empty vials were recorded. The weight difference was recorded as the weight of vial content. The percentage deviation of each vial-content from the average vial content was calculated and the results compared to the standards in the British Pharmacopoeia [7].

2.10 Uniformity of Content

The content of active substance of each brand sample was determined using ultraviolet (UV) spectrophotometry according to the method described by Bhaskar-Reddy and Subbareddy, 2013.

2.11 Sterility

The vial content was dissolved in the sterile water for injection (10 ml) provided with the preparation. The antimicrobial activity of the drug solution was neutralized by dilution in a sufficient quantity of sterile culture medium. As such, concentrated culture media (i.e. double strength) were used. Two culture media; double strength plate count agar and double strength sabouraund agar, were used for the test.

A 0.1 ml of drug solution was transferred into molten double strength plate count agar and another 0.1 ml was also transferred into molten double strength sabouraund dextrose agar. These were then transferred into sterile petri dishes, allowed to solidify, inverted and incubated; plate count agar at 35-37℃ and; sabouraund dextrose agar at 25℃. These were repeated for all brands.

Microbial growth on the incubated culture media was checked after 3, 7, and 14 days of incubation. Three vials per brand sample were tested.

2.12 Bacterial Endotoxins-pyrogens Test

Bacterial endotoxins were determined with GenScript ToxinSensor™ using the quantitative endpoint chromogenic method for the measurement of the endotoxin concentration. Three vials per product were tested. British Pharmacopoeia specification is an endotoxin limit concentration of 0.80 IU per mL.

2.13 Microbiological Assay

Antibiotic susceptibility assay was carried out using Muellar-Hinton agar; direct colony suspension, equivalent to a 0.5 McFarland standard for the clinical isolates of *Staphylococcus aureus;* and incubation conditions; 35± 2°C for 18 hours. The diameter of the zones of growth inhibition produced by the different brands was measured (CLSI, 2013).

2.14 Statistical Analysis

Data was entered in statistical software SPSS 14.0. ANOVA was performed to compare results of assay, Uniformity of weight, Bacterial endotoxin test, and Agar diffusion bioassay of different brands of Ceftriaxone sodium at a 0.05 level of significance.

3. RESULTS AND DISCUSSION

3.1 Physical Assessment: Physico-chemical Analysis

The physicochemical characters analyzed include pH, melting point, color of vial content and color of reconstituted solution and clarity of solution. The results obtained from these tests are expressed in Table 2.

pH is a critical variable and an important factor in the formulation of pharmaceutical products. It serves as a measure of the acidity/alkalinity of substances. The pH of a pharmaceutical product has a great influence on its solubility, stability, palatability and optimal microbial effectiveness (MIC_{max}) i.e. for antimicrobial agents. The product pH may reflect the intrinsic pH of the active pharmaceutical ingredient. All samples tested satisfied the British Pharmacopoeia [7] specification for the pH of ceftriaxone sodium for injection; 6.0 to 8.0.

Melting point is a physical property of drug substances and other chemicals. The melting point or range of a drug can be used as an indicator of purity of chemical substances. A pure substance is characterized by a very sharp melting point. Altered values of melting point temperature may indicate an admixed, impure substance or degradation product(s). Ceftriaxone sodium for injection, a formulation containing the active drug – Ceftriaxone and other excipients in the formulation, gave a melting point range that is lower than the melting point of pure Ceftriaxone. The degree to which the melting point is lowered is dependent on the excipients used in formulation. Hence, the generics of ceftriaxone sodium have different melting point ranges [15].

3.2 Pharmaceutical Quality Analysis

Parenteral drug products, especially those administered as liquid solutions should be free of particulate matter. For particulate matter determination: Sub-visible and visible particles, as a result of non-availability of the equipment for sub-visible matter determination, this study only looked at the visible matter content in the reconstituted solutions. On visual inspection of the reconstituted solutions of each brand sample, no visible particle was seen in samples KC, EC, ZC and RC. Though, visible particles were present in the reconstituted solutions of BC, PC & XC but their numbers were within the acceptable range (< 6 particles per vial or < 20 particles per 10 vials). The scope of this study does not include determination of exact identity of the observed particles. Some investigators suggest the presence of such particles in parenteral products may compromise tissue perfusion and impact the microcirculation, which may be clinically significant for the critically ill patients [16,17].

On inspection of the labels on the vials and the packs of different brands, all generics brands tested met the BP [7] specification for labelling of Ceftriaxone sodium for injection.

The average weight of all brand samples tested where within BP [7] specification for uniformity of weight of single dose preparations. They fall within 92.44-100.03% of the innovator product. This implies that there is an acceptable variation from the innovator brand. Although the intra-batch variation was high in two brands: Protedex® and Kincef®. The implication of this is that both brands may produce variable plasma concentration in the patient. The variations in the average weights of the different brands tested can be attributed to different formulation and manufacturing factors.

The content uniformity of the samples was assayed in phosphate buffer pH 7.4. Ceftriaxone showed maximum absorption at 320 nm. Linearity was observed in the concentration range 5-40 µg/ml and a calibration curve with correlation coefficient value 0.9961; slope 0.0033 and intercept 0.01 were obtained. The concentration of Ceftriaxone in the samples was obtained through extrapolation from the Beer-Lambert plot. These variations in content uniformity of the samples were attributed to formulation and manufacturing factors.

All the samples of Ceftriaxone sodium tested comply with the BP [7] specification for content uniformity of Ceftriaxone sodium for injection with exception of sample BC where the content was 127.91% against the standard value of 92-108%. The implication of the significant differences observed between other samples and BC may be due to non-adherence of manufacturer of sample BC to good manufacturing practices.

Sterility testing was carried out on the samples and no microbial growth was observed after 3, 7 & 14 days of incubation. The implication is that, neither bacteria nor fungi are present in the brand samples tested. Thus, the generic products tested comply with the BP 2012 specification of Sterility for parenteral products.

The standard specification of bacterial endotoxins for Ceftriaxone preparations is 0.8 IU/ml (BP). With exception of sample BC (0.8078 EU/ml) which technically (since it does not significantly differs from the upper limit) fails this test all other brands and the innovator product pass the test of content of bacteria endotoxin.

The samples of different brands of Ceftriaxone sodium tested produced distinct and clearly defined zones of growth inhibition on *Staphylococcus aureus* inoculated agar. The size of zones of inhibition produced with respect to the amount of drug used for the test indicates that the microorganism is susceptible to the antibacterial activities of the different brands of Ceftriaxone sodium tested. However, differences were observed in the magnitude of growth inhibition. ANOVA was adopted to compare the Zones of Inhibition produced by different brands of Ceftriaxone sodium. Results of ANOVA showed that there was significant influence of brand on the zones of growth inhibition of *Staphylococcus aureus* produced (p-value<0.05). This variation is attributed to formulation and manufacturing factors and thus account for why some of the brands are more efficacious than some other brands. The following order from maximum to minimum zone BC>KC>XC>EC>PC>RC>ZC was observed. The trend of zone of inhibition produced by various brands correlate with their content of ceftriaxone sodium. Therefore, sample BC with highest content produced the highest zone of inhibition. Thus, supporting the assertion of previous workers that there is a linear relationship between zone of microbial growth inhibition and the potency of antibiotics [18,19].

Table 2. Physical description and physicochemical characteristics of innovator and generic ceftriaxone sodium

Product	Physical description			Physicochemical characteristics	
	Color		Appearance	pH	Melting point (°C)
	Dry powder	Reconstituted solution			
Rocephin®	Off-white	Pale yellow	Fine powder	6.70	205-215
Protedex®	Off-white	Pale yellow	Fine powder	7.06	208-210
Biocef®	Off-white	Pale yellow	Fine powder	6.70	180-182
Kincef®	Off-white	Pale yellow	Fine powder	6.87	202-204
Ebecef®	Off-white	Pale yellow	Fine powder	6.66	210-216
ZMC®	Off-white	Pale yellow	Fine powder	6.87	180-185
Xapo®	Off-white	Pale yellow	Fine powder	6.88	220-222

Table 3. Pharmaceutical (chemical and microbiological) quality of innovator and generic brands of ceftriaxone sodium tested

Product	Visible particles	Average weight (mg) ± SEM	% content of ceftriaxone	Sterility	Endotoxin content (EU/mL)	Zones of inhibition (mm) ±SEM
Rocephin®	0	1190.5±5.31	100.00	No growth	0.4951	23.17±0.98
Protedex®	4	1190.8±15.67	105.72	No growth	0.6699	23.67±0.42
Biocef®	4	1178.2±5.98	127.91	No growth	0.8078	28.00±1.51
Kincef®	0	1100.5±10.19	97.87	No growth	0.7569	24.33±0.33
Ebecef®	0	1180.3±6.03	101.17	No growth	0.5861	23.83±0.65
ZMC®	0	1083.0±4.76	100.00	No growth	0.6061	21.33±0.21
Xapo®	2	1168.0±6.19	101.66	No growth	0.5067	24.33±0.21

4. CONCLUSION

The Pharmaceutical quality testing carried out on the innovator and six generics of ceftriaxone sodium for injection using standard quality control tests of Weight Uniformity, Uniformity of Content, Clarity, Sterility and Bacterial endotoxins-pyrogens with the aim of evaluating whether they are pharmaceutically equivalent and/or therapeutically equivalent, has been confirmed. The results obtained from this study match that of BP [7] standards and specifications, indicating that all brands tested can be pharmaceutically and therapeutically interchanged. Quality control tests are important and should be carried as one of the pharmacovigilance programs of drug regulatory agencies and by researchers in both developing and developed countries.

ETHICAL APPROVAL

It is not applicable.

ACKNOWLEDGEMENTS

We the author of this article wish to acknowledge tne contribution of Mrs Caleb of Pharmaceutical Microbiology Department, University of Port-Harcourt for her immense assistance in the microbiological aspect of this work,

COMPETING INTERESTS

Authors have declared that no competing interests exist.

REFERENCES

1. Frederick GH. Penicillin, cephalosporin, and other β– Lactam antibiotics. In: Brunton LL, Lazo JS, Parker KL (eds.) Goodman and Gillman's. The pharmacological basis of therapeutics. 11th ed. New York: McGraw Hills Medical Publishing Division; 2006.
2. Sweetman SC. (ed.) Martindale- the complete drug reference. London: Pharmaceutical Press; 2002.
3. Graumlich JF. β-Lactam antibiotics. In: Craig CR, Stitzel RE. Modern pharmacology with clinical applications. 6th edition. Philadelphia: Lippincott Williams & Wilkins; 2003.
4. Finkel R. (ed.) Lippincott's Illustrated reviews: Pharmacology. 4th edition. USA: Lippincott Williams & Wilkins; 2009.
5. Garattini L, Tediosi F. A comparative analysis of generics markets in Five European Countries. Health Policy. 2000; 51:149-162.
6. Snyman J. Editorial – bioequivalence: Should we trust generic antibiotics? South African Journal of Epidemiology of Infections. 2005;20(3):78-9.
7. British Pharmacopoeia. British Pharmacopoeia Commission. The Stationery Office, London. 2012;2.
8. Gasser UE, Fischer A, Timmermans JP, Arnet I. Pharmaceutical quality of seven generic Levodopa/ Benserazide Products compared with original Madopar®/ Prolopa®. BMC Pharmacology and Toxicology; 2013.
Available:http://www.biomedcentral.com/2050-6511/14/24
(Accessed 10 January 2015)
9. Betari N, Haidar S. Pharmaceutical quality of generic sitagliptin tablets compared with Januvia®. Journal of Applied Pharmacy. 2014;6(2):195-201.
10. Anjum F, Feroz M, Razvi N, Ghayas S, Ghazal L, Siddiqui SA. Assessment of pharmaceutical quality control and equivalence of various brands of

amlodipine besylate (5 mg) tablets available in the Pakistani market Under Bio-waiver Conditions. Int. J Pharm. and Pharm. Sci. 2014;6(2):909-913.

11. Rahim N, Naqvi SBS, Iqbal E, Nesar S, Khaliq UA, Hasan SK. Investigation on pharmaceutical quality of different brands of cefadroxil monohydrate available in Karachi, Pakistan. Indo- American J of Pharm Res. 2013;3(6):4577-4584.
12. Arnet I, Altermatt M, Roggo Y, Schnitzler G. Pharmaceutical quality of eight generics of ceftriaxone preparation for injection. Eastern Asia J of Chemotherapy. 2014;5(2):23-29.
13. Lambert PA, Conway BR. Pharmaceutical quality of ceftriaxone generic drug products compared with Rocephin®®. J Chemother. 2003;15(4):357–368.
14. Tange M, Yoshida M, Nakai Y, Uchida T. Comparison between original and generic versions of ceftriaxone sodium preparation for injection: Compatibility with calcium-containing product. Chem. Pharm Bull (Tokyo). 2012;60(4):29–34.
15. Allen LV, Popovich NG, Ansel HC. Dosage form design: Pharmaceutical and formulation considerations. In: Ansel's Pharmaceutical, Dosage Forms and Drug Delivery Systems. 9th Ed. Wolters Kluwer/Lippincott Williams & Wilkins; 2012.
16. Lehr HA, Brunner J, Rangoonwala R, Kirkpatrick CJ. Particulate matter contamination of intravenous antibiotics aggravates loss of functional capillary density in post-ischemic striated muscle. Am. J Resp. Crit Care Med. 2002: 165(4):514–20.
17. Kirkpatrick C, Ramzan R, Mykhaylo R, Mike B, Shahram G. Non-equivalence of antibiotic generic drugs and risk for intensive care patients. Pharm. Reg. Affairs. 2013;2(1):234-238
18. Salgado HRN, Alessio PV. Development and validation of a successful microbiological agar assay for determination of ceftriaxone sodium in powder for injectable solution. Pharmaceutics; 2012.
19. Manfio ML, Agarrayua DA, Machado JC, Schmidt CA. A fully validated microbiological assay to evaluate the potency of ceftriaxone sodium. Brazilian J of Pharm. Sci; 2013. Available:http://dx.doi.org/10.1590/S1984-82502013000400015 (Accessed on 10 January 2015)

17

Trend of HIV Seropositivity among Children at Teaching Tertiary Care Hospital in North India

Ritu Aggarwal[1*], Priyanka Yadav[1], Uma Chaudhary[1] and Vipul Kumar[2]

[1]Department of Microbiology, Pt. B.D. Sharma Institute of Medical Sciences, Rohtak, India.
[2]Department of Chest and TB, Pt. B.D. Sharma Institute of Medical Sciences, Rohtak, India.

Authors' contributions

This work was carried out in collaboration between all authors. Authors RA and PY designed the study. Author PY compiled the data retrospectively. Authors RA and PY wrote the protocol and the first draft of the manuscript. Authors RA, PY and VK managed the literature searches, discussion and revision of the manuscript. Author UC managed the investigational and administrative part of the manuscript part. All authors read and approved the final manuscript.

Article Information

Editor(s):
(1) Q. Ping Dou, Barbara Ann Karmanos Cancer Institute, Departments of Oncology, Pharmacology and Pathology, School of Medicine, Wayne State University, USA.
(2) Vasudevan Mani, Universiti Teknologi MARA (UiTM), Selangor, Malaysia.
Reviewers:
(1) Ketan Vagholkar, D.Y.Patil University School of Medicine, India.
(2) Rina G. Kaminsky, National Autonomous University of Honduras, Honduras.

ABSTRACT

Aim: The aim of this study is to ascertain the burden and trend of HIV sero-positivity among children attending ICTC in a teaching tertiary care hospital.
Study Design: Retrospective study.
Methodology: HIV seropositivity among children of age group 18 months- 14 years was determined by serological tests for HIV antibodies among children enrolled in ICTC of a teaching tertiary care hospital from Jan 2011 - Dec 2013 as per NACO guidelines.
Result: Of 2529 children tested for HIV infection, 10.4% were found to be seropositive. Statistically significant ($p < 0.05$) fall in the seropositivity was observed over the three years study period. In all the three years male children were more seropositive than female children (1.78:1). Most of the children were serodiagnosed late in our study, with mean age of 5.30 years / 63.64 months.
Conclusion: Our study reports a declining trend of sero-positivity (from 13.1% to 9.8%) among children attending ICTC. But the prevalence is still high (>9%) which calls for re-intensified efforts on health education and risk control programme.

**Corresponding author: Email: drritu252@yahoo.com*

Keywords: HIV; AIDS; NACO; children; paediatric; ICTC; sex ratio; seropositivity.

1. INTRODUCTION

Human Immunodeficiency Virus (HIV) continues to be a major global public health issue, having claimed more than 34 million lives so far. In 2014, 1.2 [1.0–1.5] million people died globally from HIV-related causes. There were approximately 36.9 [34.3–41.4] million people living with HIV at the end of 2014 with 2.0 [1.9–2.2] million people becoming newly infected with HIV in 2014 worldwide [1]. The HIV prevalence trend has witnessed significant decline among antenatal clinic attendees considered proxy for general population (0.49% in 2007 to 0.35% in 2012- 2013). Although the prevalence of HIV infection has declined in India but due to large population it stands third, in terms of absolute numbers of people living with HIV, next only to South Africa and Nigeria [2]. Heterosexual contact is the predominant mode of transmission among adults in India with an increasing number of women of childbearing age becoming infected with HIV. Consequently, children in India are increasingly getting infected, primarily from vertical transmission [3,4,5]. The vast majority of children born to HIV- infected mother acquire the infection in utero, at the time of delivery or postnatal through breast feeding [6]. Paediatric HIV is a major world health problem, which is progressing at an alarming rate. Data as per UNAIDS states that 2,40,000 new HIV infections occurred among children (0–14 years) in low- and middle-income countries in 2013 [7]. Children less than 15 years of age accounted for 7% (1.45 lakh) of all infections with an estimated to have around 14,500 new HIV infections among children in India in 2011 [2].

The knowledge of HIV infection among children is important as it will cause a parallel increase in heterosexual transmission and the number of infected women of a child bearing age. Although a lot of work has been done in different parts of world regarding extent and magnitude of paediatric HIV infection, there is a paucity of data on paediatric HIV infection in India. The HIV epidemic in India is heterogeneous in its distribution and disease burden is not same everywhere. This study is therefore an attempt to investigate the recent trend and magnitude of paediatric HIV infection in children attending Integrated Counselling and Testing Centre (ICTC).

2. MATERIALS AND METHODS

This is a retrospective analysis of the data from January 2011 to December 2013 done in ICTC, Department of Microbiology, Pt B.D. Sharma PGIMS Rohtak, a premier tertiary teaching hospital in North India and a referral hospital for Haryana and beyond. Case records of all the children in the age group of 18 months to 14 years, who were either walk-in clients or referred by clinicians, during the above mentioned study period were retrieved. Children <18 months of age were not included in the study as facility of DNA PCR for confirmation of reactive cases was not available. Written informed consent from parents or legal guardians was obtained before testing. Pre-test and post- test counselling was provided to all the parents or guardians accordingly and relevant demographic data was recorded. Blood sample was drawn by venepuncture and HIV testing was done as per National AIDS Control Organisation (NACO), India guidelines. Three HIV rapid test kits were used which were based either on different antigen or different principle. First test kit was of highest sensitivity. Samples with first test reactive were further confirmed with two other HIV tests with higher specificity. The HIV test kits utilized in the laboratory for the testing of these samples were provided by the NACO through Haryana State AIDS Control Society (HSACS). Details of the kits used in the study is mentioned in the Table 1. The sensitivity and specificity of different kits was provided by the manufacturer.

Table 1. Details of the test kits used in the study

Sr. no	Name	Manufacturer	Principle of test	Sensitivity	Specificity
1.	Comb-AIDS	J. Mitra & Co. Pvt. Ltd.	Dot immunoassay	100%	99.9%
2.	Pareekshak triline	Bhat bio-tech India Ltd.	Lateral flow immunochromatography	100%	99%
3.	Tridot	J. Mitra & Co. Pvt. Ltd.	Immunodiffusion	100%	100%

2.1 Statistical Analysis

Data analysis was done using Software Package for Social Sciences (SPSS) statistic version 19 for Windows. The chi square ($\chi 2$) test was used to evaluate the association between seropositivity rates and the age groups and p value of < 0.05 was considered statistically significant.

3. RESULTS

A total of 2529 children between 18months- 14 years comprising of 1545 male and 984 female children were screened during this study. The overall prevalence of HIV seropositivity in these three years was 10.4% with HIV-1 was the only viral serotype that was detected. Out of total 635, 857 and 1037 children tested, 83(13.1%), 79(9.21%) and 102(9.8%) were sero-positive for HIV in years 2011, 2012 and 2013 respectively as shown in Fig. 1. This trend of seropositivity over the three years was statistically significant with p value <0.05.

Fig. 2 shows gender wise distribution of HIV seropositive children. The HIV seropositivity was constantly high in male than female children in all three years but the difference was not statistically significant (p value >0.05).

Table 2 shows the age group wise distribution of seropositive children. The seropositivity rate was highest in the age group of >18 months- 05 years (22%), followed by age group >05-10 years and minimum in age group >10-14 years. However, this difference of seropositivity in various age groups was statistically insignificant (p value >0.05).

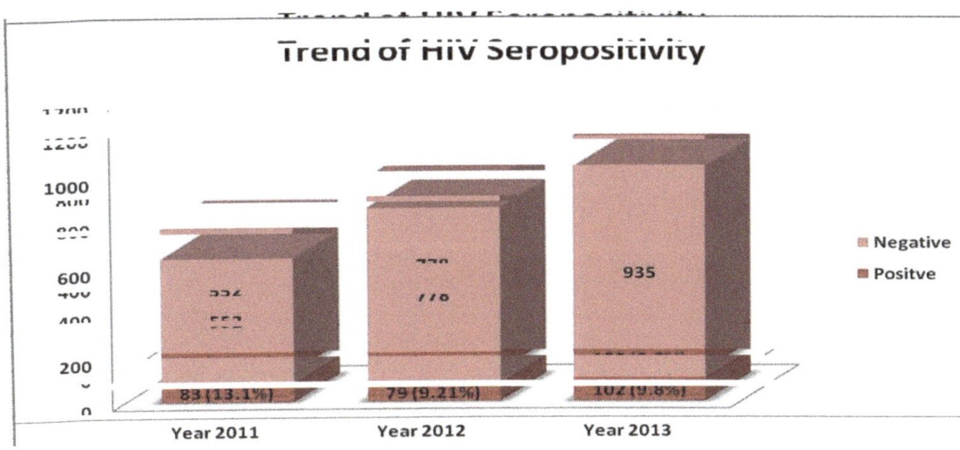

Fig. 1. Trend of HIV seropositivity
(Chi square -6.474, degree of freedom (dof) -2, p=0.039)

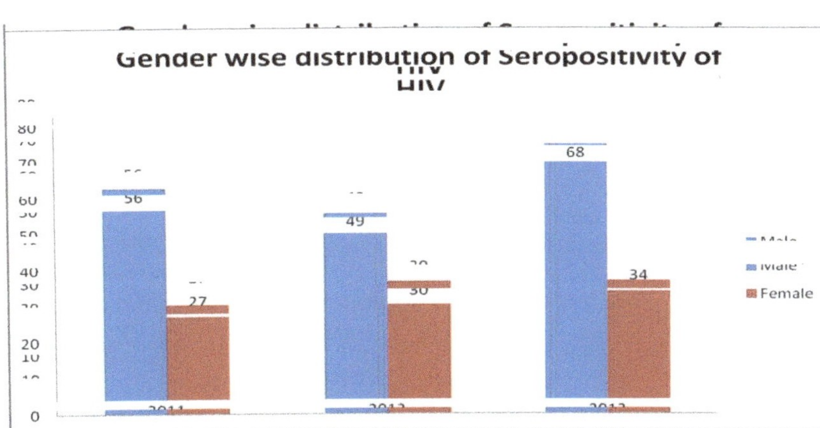

Fig. 2. Gender wise distribution of HIV seropositivity
Chi square -0.626, dof-2, p=0.7312

Table 2. Age group wise distribution of seropositivity of HIV

Age group	2011	2012	2013
18 m- 5 yrs	39	29	43
>5 - 10 yrs	27	22	32
>10 - 14 yrs	17	28	27

Chi square -4.694, dof-4, p=0.320

4. DISCUSSION

The overall seropositivity among paediatric age group observed in this study was 10.4%. Although actual prevalence of paediatric HIV infection in India is unknown, a wide range has been reported in literature. Quite higher rate of seropositivity of 20% has been reported by Bavdekar et al. [8]. Seropositivity of 11.2%, 8.9% and 8.18% was observed by Karande et al. [9], Parthasarathy et al. [10] and Agarwal et al. [11] respectively, is in accordance with the present study. Other workers have reported lower rates of seropositivity of 5.4% and 2.3% [12,13]. This difference in the prevalence may be due to different patient selection criteria followed by different authors. Moreover this difference in seropositivity of HIV among paediatric population reflects the seropositivity status in general population of that area.

In the present study, the number of attendees at ICTC has increased from 635 to 1037 but HIV seropositivity has declined from 13.1% to 9.8% in year 2011 and 2013 respectively. This fall in seroprevalence may be attributed to the effectiveness of the Prevention of Parent to Child Transmission (PPTCT) program by NACO, which was started in 2002. The different targeted interventions by National AIDS Control Programme along with increased involvement of Non- Government Organisations has increased awareness in general population and promoted safer sex practises, treatment of sexual and reproductive tract infections, safe blood transfusion services along with early diagnosis of HIV and early institution of anti retroviral therapy in pregnant females has ultimately lead to a parallel decrease in seropositivity in children.

In our study, attendance of male children ICTC exceeded that of female children by 561 (22%). This difference in sex ratio among attendees can be attributed to gender bias still prevailing in Indian society. In all three years, male children were more seropositive than female children. However this observation was insignificant statistically. Sex ratio for seropositive population was 1.78:1. Other studies conducted by Indian authors had also reported higher HIV seropositivity in male children [14,15,16]. However, studies conducted outside India had shown female predominance [17,18].

The children included in the study for HIV screening were of age 18 months to 14 years and majority of children were screened at more than five years of age. Mean age of diagnosis was 5.30 years / 63.64 months. Most of them were therefore diagnosed late. Late diagnosis has also been reported by various Indian studies as well as studies conducted outside India [15,19,20]. In contrast, a Nigerian teaching hospital has reported a lower mean age of diagnosis [21]. HIV seropositivity was highest in the age group of 18 months- 05 years. As majority of infection in children are acquired by vertical transmission.

5. CONCLUSION

Current HIV scenario in children is grim. Our study reports there is declining trend of sero-positivity (from 13.1% to 9.8%) among children attending ICTC. But the prevalence is still high (>9%) which calls for re-intensified effort on health education and risk control programme. Effective PPTCT programs, good diagnostic facilities and accessible and affordable ART are the need of the hour. To increase awareness among infected as well as general population so that they don't indulge in high risk behaviour and future transmission can be prevented.

ETHICAL APPROVAL

It is not applicable.

ACKNOWLEDGEMENT

We would like to acknowledge the Haryana AIDS Control Society for regular supply of HIV test kits and staff of Integrated Counselling and Testing Center at Microbiology Department, PGIMS Rohtak for their sincere technical support.

COMPETING INTERESTS

Authors have declared that no competing interests exist.

REFERENCES

1. WHO. Fact sheet: HIV/AIDS; 2014. Available:http://www.who.int/mediacentre/factsheets/fs360/en/ (Accessed 20 July 2015).

2. Department of AIDS Control Ministry of Health and Family Welfare Government of India. Annual Report, 2013-2014. Available:http://www.naco.gov.in/upload/Publication/Annual_Report/Annual_report_2012-13_English.pdf (Accessed 20 July 2015).
3. Madhivanan P, Mothi SN, Kumarasamy N, Yepthomi T, Venkatesan C, Lambert JS, et al. Clinical manifestations of HIV infected children. Indian J Pediatr. 2003; 70(8):615-20.
4. Merchant RH, Oswal JS, Bhagwat RV, Karkare J. Clinical profile of HIV infection. Indian Pediatr. 2001;38(3):239-46.
5. Pol RR, Shepur TA, Ratageri VH. Clinico-laboratory profile of pediatric HIV in Karnataka. Indian J Pediatr. 2007;74(12): 1071-5.
6. Alikor DE, Erhabor NO. Trend of HIV seropositivity among children in a tertiary health care institution in the Niger delta region of Nigeria. Afr J Health Sci. 2005; 12:108-13.
7. Statistical update children. Adolescents and AIDS digital release | 28 November; 2014.
8. Bavdekar SB, Agrawal R. Clinically directed selective screening for HIV infection in hospitalized children. Indian Pediatr. 2005;42:1191-7.
9. Karande S, Bhalke S, Kelkar A, Ahuja S, Kulkarni M, Mathur M. Utility of a clinically directed selective screening to diagnose HIV infection in hospitalized children in Bombay, India. J Trop Pediatr. 2002;48: 149–55.
10. Parthasarathy P, Mittal SK, Sharma VK. Prevalence of paediatric HIV in New Delhi. Indian J Pediatr. 2006;73:205–7.
11. Agrawal A, Thora S, Agrawal R. HIV seropositivity in hospitalized children on clinically directed selective screening: an experience from Central India. Pediatric Oncall [Serial online]; 2013. [Cited 2013 January 1]; 10. Art #4. Available:http://www.pediatriconcall.com/Journal/Article/FullText.aspx?artid=536&type=J&tid=&imgid=&reportid=60&tbltype=
12. Agarwal S, Sawant S, Shastri J. Pediatric HIV in Mumbai. Indian J Sex Transm Dis. 2011;32(1):57–8.
13. Shah I, Katira B. Seroprevalence of HIV infection in hospitalized paediatric patients at a tertiary care centre in Western India. HIV Medicine. 2007;8:265-6.
14. Lodha R, Upadhyay A, Kapoor V, Kabra SK. Clinical profile and natural history of children with HIV infection. Indian J Pediatr. 2006;73(3):201-4.
15. Shah I. Age- related clinical manifestations of HIV infection in Indian children. J Trop Pediatr. 2011;51(5):300-3.
16. Valsan PV, Cherian T, Anil J, Babu GP, Jacob JJ, Chellam K, et al. Clinical manifestations of HIV infection. Indian Pediatr. 2002;39:57-63.
17. Fru FS, Chiabi A, Nguefack S, Mah E, Takou V, Bonge JB, et al. Baseline demographic, clinical and immunological profiles of HIV-infected children at the Yaounde Gynaeco-Obstetric and Pediatric hospital, Cameroon. Pan Afr Med J. 2014; 17:1-6.
18. Fetuga MB, Ogunfowora OB, Oyegunle VN, Thanni LO. A ten-year review of paediatric HIV/AIDS among hospitalized children in a Nigerian Teaching Hospital. Nig J Paediatr. 2005;32(3):29-32.
19. Singh S, Jat KR, Minz RW, Arora S, Suri D, Sehgal S. Clinical profile of 516 children affected by HIV in a tertiary care centre in Northern India: 14 years of experience. Trans R Soc Trop Med Hyg. 2009;103(6): 627-33.
20. Diack MA, Signate SH, Diagne Gueye NR, Syllab A, Diouf A, Diagne I, et al. Epidemiological and clinical aspects of pediatric HIV infections in Albert-Royer Pediatric Hospital (Dakar, Senegal). Arch Pediatr. 2005;12(4):404-9.
21. Brown BJ, Oladokun RE, Odaibo GN, Olaleye DO, Osinusi K, Kanki P. Clinical and immunological profile of pediatric HIV infection in Ibadan, Nigeria. J Int Assoc Physicians AIDS Care (Chic). 2011;10(1): 49-53.

18

In vitro Antiplasmodial Activity and Phytochemical Screening of *Newbouldia laevis* Used in Treating Malaria-associated Symptoms

Enemakwu Thomas Andrew[1*], M. M. Adeyemi[1] and L. Salihu[1]

[1]*Department of Chemistry, Nigerian Defence Academy Kaduna, Nigeria.*

Authors' contributions

This work was carried out in collaboration between all authors. Author ETA designed the study, wrote the protocol and the first draft of the manuscript and conducted the research work. Author MMA supervised and guided the work. Author LS contributed in the interpretation and analysis of the results. All authors read and approved the final manuscript.

Article Information

Editor(s):
(1) Syed A. A. Rizvi, Department of Pharmaceutical Sciences, College of Pharmacy, Nova Southeastern University, USA.
Reviewers:
(1) Aina Oluwagbemiga Olanrewaju, Nigerian Institute of Medical Research, Nigeria.
(2) Abdullahi M. Nuhu, Kaduna Polytechnic, Nigeria.

ABSTRACT

This study investigated the *In vitro* antiplasmodial activity and phytochemical constituents of the leaves from *Newbouldia laevis* used in the local treatment of malaria. The crude ethanol extract from the medicinal plant (NL_{-01}) was fractionated into ethyl acetate (NL_{-01-01}), chloroform (NL_{-01-02}) and n-hexane (NL_{-01-03}) fractions. NL_{-01-03} has the highest weight of 1.7 g followed by NL_{-01-01} (0.9 g). SL_{-01-02} has the least weight of 0.7 g. *In vitro* antiplasmodial assays and phytochemical screening of ethyl acetate, chloroform and n-hexane fractions from the plant were further carried out. Alkaloids, saponins tannins, flavonoids, steroids and glycosides were detected in the extracts of the plant. Plant's leaves extracts and fractions were found to be active against *Plasmodium falciparum* with percentage elimination range of 43.18 to 79.54%. The results showed that percentage elimination increases as the concentrations of the extract and fractions increase. At 0.5 mg/cm^3, SL_{-01-01} has the highest activity of 54.54% while SL_{-01-02} has the least percentage elimination of 43.18%. At concentration of 5.0mg/cm^3, NL_{-01} has the highest activity of 79.54% while NL_{-01-02} has the least activity of 72.72%. The analysis of the results of the extract and that of the standard (positive

**Corresponding author: Email: enemakwuthomas@gmail.com*

control) using Mann-Whitny U test indicate that there is no significant difference between them at 95% confidence interval. Spearman rank correlation analysis of the plant samples with the positive control samples showed that there is correlation and the degree of relationship between the antiplasmodial activities of the plant samples and positive control samples is positively perfect ($\gamma_s = 1$).

TLC screening of the ethyl acetate fraction using ethyl acetate/n-hexane mixture in the ratio 1:4 revealed four spots on the plate.

Keywords: Newbouldia laevis; In-vitro antiplasmodia; phytochemical.

1. INTRODUCTION

Malaria is a vector borne disease, caused by protozoan parasites of the genus *Plasmodium* transmitted from the blood of an infected person and passed to a healthy human by a female anopheles mosquito bites. They are single celled organisms that cannot survive outside of their host(s) [1]. There are four main malaria causing parasites namely: *Plasmodium vivax, Plasmodium ovale, Plasmodium malariae* and *Plasmodium falciparum*. Additionally, in some parts of Southern Asia there are reports of *P. knowlesi* infecting human beings, [2] and [3]. The parasites multiply within red blood cells (RBC) causing symptoms that include anaemia as well as other general symptoms such as fever, chills, nausea and flu-like illness and in severe cases coma and death. Malaria is a worldwide public health concern. The World Health Organization (WHO) Malaria World Report, [4] reported an estimate of 207 million cases and 627, 000 deaths globally in 2012 alone. It has been reported that, over 70 countries are malaria endemic and globally, an estimated 3.4 billion people are at risk of malaria infection.

Despite the substantial progress made in the treatment of parasitic diseases, malaria remains a significant therapeutic challenge. Malaria treatment failures are due to *P. falciparum* developing reduced sensitivity to Artemisinin based Combination Therapy (ACTs), [5,6] and the parasites recrudescence after treatment with ACTs, [7]. It has been reported that ACT's reducing sensitivity has spread to Africa as well, [8].

Therefore, lack of new antimalarial drugs in the pipeline and reduced sensitivity, highlight the urgent need to search for new antimalarial drugs to replace the currently used or to expand the antimalarial drug arsenal. According to the WHO, [9] more than 80% of people living in developing countries still depend on herbal medicines to treat common diseases including malaria [10]. Evidently, more than 62% of new small chemical drugs approved in the United States of America between 1981 and 2007 were isolated from medicinal plants or synthesized from compounds isolated form plants.

2. EXPERIMENTAL SECTION

2.1 Sampling

The fresh leaves of the plant was collected from Eke-Avrugo Community in Igalamela-Odolu LGA of Kogi State, identified and authenticated by Prof. M.O Nwosu of Department of Plant Science and Biotechnology University of Nigeria Nsukka as *Newbouldia laevis* (UNH No_340b).

2.2 Preparation of the Plants Materials

The leaves of the plant, *Newbouldia laevis* were collected, washed and air-dried for two weeks after which they were grinded, subsequently sieved into powder form and stored in air tight containers for further use.

2.3 Maceration

A weight of 200 g of the powdered plant sample was macerated in 95% ethanol (1 litre) at room temperature for 2 weeks. This was then filtered using a no.1 whatmans filter paper. The solvent was evaporated using a rotary evaporator (R110) at 40℃. The *Newbouldia laevis* ethanol extracts was weighted (22.739g) and labeled as NL_{-01}, [11].

2.4 Merceration of the Crude Extracts (NL_{-01})

The ethanol extract (NL_{-01}) was extracted successively with chloroform, n-hexane and ethyl acetate according to the protocols described by Fatope et al. [12].

2.5 Phytochemical Screening

A weight of 10 g of the pulverized plant sample (*Newbouldia laevis*) was macerated in 50 cm^3 each of the following solvents: Ethyl acetate, Chloroform, n-hexane and Ethanol for one (1) week. The filtrates obtained from the solvent fractions were subjected to phytochemical screening. The phytochemicals screened include alkaloids, saponins tannins, flavonoids, steroids and glycosides [13-15].

2.5.1 Test for tannins

1 cm^3 each of the fractions was separately added to 1 cm^3 of distilled water in test tubes. A few drops of 10% ferric chloride was added and observed for brownish green or a blue-black colouration.

2.5.2 Test for saponin

1 cm^3 each of the fractions were separately mixed with 4 cm^3 of distilled water and shaken vigorously for a stable persistent froth.

2.5.3 Test for flavonoid

1 cm^3 of 10% NaOH was mixed with 1 cm^3 each of the fractions, shaken vigorously and observed for the development of a yellow colouration.

2.5.4 Test for cardiac glycosides

1 cm^3 of concentrated sulphuric acid was gently poured on the walls of an inclined test tube containing 1 cm^3 each of the fractions separately. 10% Ferric chloride solution was added in drop wise and a brown ring was observed.

2.5.5 Test for steroids

To test the presence of steroid phytochemicals, 1 cm^3 each of the fractions were separately dissolved in 10 cm^3 chloroform and equal volume of concentrated sulphuric acid (H_2SO_4) added by sides of test tube. The upper layer turned red and sulphuric acid layer turned yellow with green fluorescence. This indicated the presence of steroids.

2.5.6 Test for alkaloids

2.5.6.1 Preparation of wagner's reagent

This was prepared by dissolving 1.0 g of I_2 crystals and 3.0 g of KI in distilled water and making up to the mark in 50cm^3 volumetric flask.

2.5.6.2 Test

4 cm^3 of 1% hydrochloric acid was added to 1 cm^3 each of the fractions in separate test tubes, mixed and the solutions warmed in a warm bath. The presence of turbidity or precipitate after the addition of 1 ml of Wagner's reagent confirmed the presence of alkaloid.

2.6 Malaria Parasite Assay

2.6.1 Preparation of test solution

A stock solution of 10 mg/cm^3 of the extract and fractions were prepared by dissolving 0.02 g of the dried extract and fractions separately in 2 cm^3 of 1% Dimethyl sulphoxide (DMSO). The following concentrations 0.5 mg/cm^3, 1.0 mg/cm^3, 2.0 mg/cm^3 and 5.0 mg/cm^3 were prepared from the stock solutions of each of the extract and fractions by serial dilution using:

$$C_1V_1 = C_2V_2$$

C_1 = concentration of the stock solution, C_2 = final or expected concentration
V_1 = volume of stock solution, V_2 = final volume (that is V_1 + volume of solvent).

0.5 mg/cm^3 was prepared by diluting 0.05 cm^3 of the stock solution with 0.95 cm^3 of DMSO. 1.0 mg/cm^3 was prepared by diluting 0.1 cm^3 of the stock solution with 0.9 cm^3 of DMSO. 2.0 mg/cm^3 was prepared by diluting 0.2 cm^3 of the stock solution with 0.8 cm^3 of DMSO. 5.0 mg/cm^3 was prepared by diluting 0.5cm^3 of the stock solution with 0.5 cm^3 of DMSO.

Artemetther lumefantrine anti-malaria drug was used as Positive control prepared in the same way as test solutios. RPMI 1640 and 1% DMSO don't affect the development of P. *falciparum* in the culture medium, [16].

2.6.2 Sourcing of malaria parasites for the assay

Malaria parasites infected blood sample of patients were collected from Hematology Department Bayero University Hospital, Kano. The samples were immediately transferred into K3-EDTA disposable plastic sample bottles corked, mixed thoroughly and then transported to the Microbiology laboratory at Bayero University in a thermo flask containing water maintained at 4℃ as demonstrated by [17].

2.6.3 Determination of *Plasmodium falciparum* (positive blood samples) using the thin smear method

The method described by Dacei and Lewis was adopted. Using a clean capillary tube, a small drop of the blood sample was placed at the centre of a clean glass slide at least 2 mm from one end. A cover slip was placed at angle 45° in front of each drop and drawn backward to make a contact with each drop. The drop was run along the full length of the edge of the cover slip. Smears were formed by moving the cover slip forward on each glass slide. The thin smears were dried and immersed in methanol for few seconds. Geimsa's stain was dropped on each smear, and allowed to stay for about 10 minutes. Excess stain was washed with clean tap water. The smears were dried in air by hanging the glass slides inverted in a rack. Each dried smear was microscopically observed under a high power objectives (x100) using oil immersion. An average parasitaemia was determined using the reading of 3 microscopic fields.

2.6.4 Separation of the erythrocytes (0.5% *Parasitaemia*) from the serum of the blood samples

50% dextrose solution (0.5 cm^3) was added to each of the blood samples (5 cm^3) defibrinated, and then centrifuged at 2500 rpm for 15 minutes in a spectra merlin centrifugation machine. Supernatant layers were separated from the sediments. The latter was diluted with normal saline [17] and centrifuged at 2500 rpm for 10 minutes. The resulting supernatants were discarded. Samples with higher parasitaemia (above 0.5%) were diluted with fresh malaria parasite negative erythrocytes [18].

2.6.5 Determination of *Plasmodium falciparum* initial count

The method described by Dacei and Lewis was adopted. Using a clean dropper pipette, a small drop of the defibrinated erythrocyte blood sample above was smeared on microscopic slide and stained by Giemsa's staining techniques. The mean number of erythrocytes appearing as blue discoid cells containing life rings of the parasite (that appeared red pink) was estimated as the initial count of the parasite before incubation.

2.6.6 Preparation of *Plasmodium falciparum* culture medium

Venous blood (2 cm^3) from the main vein of white healthy rabbits pinnae was withdrawn using a disposable 5 cm^3 syringe (BD 205 WG) into EDTA bottles. This was defibrinated by allowing it to settle for at least one hour [17]. The defibrinated blood was centrifuged at 1500 rpm using spectre merlin centrifuge for 10 minutes and the supernatant layer was collected in a sterilized tube. The sediment was further centrifuged at 1500 rpm for five minutes, and the supernatant layer was added to the first test tube. The sediments were discarded and the serum collected was supplemented with the salt of RPMI 1600 medium (KCl 5.37 mM, NaCl 10.27 mM, $MgSO_4$ 0.4 mM, $NaHPO_4$ 17.73 mM, $Ca(NO_3)_2$ 0.42 mM, $NaHCO_3$ 2.5 mM, and glucose 11.0 mM. (BDH Ltd, UK). The medium was sterilized with 40 µg/cm^3 gentamicin sulphate [19].

2.6.7 *In-Vitro* assay of the activity of the extracts and fractions on *plasmodium falciparum* culture

A 0.1 cm^3 of test solution and 0.2 cm^3 of the culture medium were added into EDTA bottle containing 0.1 ml of 0.5% parasitaemia erythrocytes and mixed thoroughly. The sensitivity of the parasites to the samples was determined microscopically after incubation for 48 hours at 37°C. The incubation was undertaken in glass bell jar containing a lighted candle to ensure the supply of required quantity of CO_2 about 5% O_2 gas, 2% and nitrogen gas 93% as demonstrated by Muktar [20].

2.6.8 Determination of the activity

At the end of the incubation period of 48 hours, the sample was centrifuged to remove the culture media and a drop of the sample (red blood cell only) was smeared on microscopic slide and stained by Giemsa's staining techniques. The mean number of erythrocytes appearing as blue discoid cells containing life rings of the parasite (that appeared red pink) was estimated and the average percentage elimination by the samples was determined. The activity of the test samples was calculated as the percentage elimination of the parasites after incubation period of 48 hours, using the formula below;

$$\% = \frac{N}{Nx} \times 100$$

Where,

% = Percentage activity of the test sample
N = Total number of parasites eliminated by the sample,
Nx = Total number of parasitized RBC.
Note: RBC = Red Blood Cells [20]

2.7 Thin Layer Chromatography (TLC)

TLC was conducted on the ethyl acetate fractions of the medicinal plant. This was carried out using aluminium plate silica gel (20x20). Ethyl acetate and chloroform solvent mixture was used in the following ratio 1:1, 1:4, 1:9, 0.5:9.5, 2:3; and ethyl acetate and n-hexane solvent mixture in the following ratio, 1:1, 1:4, 1:9, 4:1, 2:3.

3. RESULTS

The results of all the experiment conducted are presented as given below:

Table 1. Results of ethanol extracts of leaves

Plants	Colour of solution	Weight of extracts (g)	Percentage yield (%)
NL-01	Deep green	22.739	11.37

NL-01 = Ethanol extract of Newbouldia leavis

Table 2. Results of macerated fractions from crude ethanol extract of the plant

Fractions	Colour of the solution	Weight of extracts (g)	Percentage yield (%)
NL_{-01-01}	Deep green	0.9	7.92
NL_{-01-02}	Dark green	0.7	6.17
NL_{-01-03}	Greenish yellow	1.7	14.95

NL_{-01-01} = Ethyl acetate fraction of Newbouldia laevis from crude ethanol extract; NL_{-01-02} = Chloroform fraction of Newbouldia laevis from crude ethanol extract; NL_{-01-03} = n-hexane fraction of Newbouldia laevis from crude ethanol extract

Table 3. Results of phytochemical screening of the various fractions of plants

Phytochemicals	NL_A	NL_C	NL_E	NL_H
Tannins	-ve	-ve	+ve	-ve
Saponins	-ve	NI	-ve	+ve
Flavonoid	+ve	+ve	+ve	+ve
Steriods	+ve	+ve	+ve	+ve
Alkaloids	+ve	NI	+ve	-ve
Cardiac glycoside	+ve	+ve	+ve	+ve

+ve = present, –ve = absent; NI = not intense; NL_A = Newbouldia laevis ethyl acetate fraction; NL_C = Newbouldia laevis chloroform fraction; NL_E = Newbouldia laevis ethanol fraction; NL_H = Newbouldia laevis n-hexane fraction

Table 4. Results of Antimalarial activity of fractions from the leaves of *Newbouldia laevis*

Fraction	Concentration (mg/cm^3)	Average no. of parasite before incubation	Average N number of parasite after 48 hrs	Percentage elimination at the end of incubation. (%)
NL_{-01}	0.5	44	21	52.27
	1.0	44	15	65.91
	2.0	44	12	72.72
	5.0	44	9	79.54
NL_{-01-01}	0.5	44	20	54.54
	1.0	44	18	59.9
	2.0	44	15	65.91
	5.0	44	11	75.00
NL_{-01-02}	0.5	44	25	43.18
	1.0	44	19	56.81
	2.0	44	16	63.63
	5.0	44	12	72.72
NL_{-01-03}	0.5	44	22	52.00
	1.0	44	18	59.90
	2.0	44	13	70.45
	5.0	44	10	77.27

Table 5. Results of antimalarial activity of positive control

Control	Concentration (mg/cm^3)	Average No. of parasite before incubation	Average Nnumber of parasite after 48hrs	Percentage elimination at the end of incubation. (%)
Positive	0.5	44	11	75
	1.0	44	6	86.36
	2.0	44	4	90.90
	5.0	44	3	93.18

Table 6. Results of TLC of ethyl acetate fractions of the leaves of the plants Ethyl acetate/hexane solvent mixture

Plants	Ethyl acetate/hexane ratio	Number of spots	Retention factor (R_f)
NL	1:4	4	0.09, 0.36, 0.53, 0.98

NL= Newbouldia laevis

4. ANALYSIS OF RESULTS

Mann-Whitney U Test and Spearman' Rank Correlation where adopted for the analysis of the results.

Mann-Whitney U Test Analysis of antiplasmodial results of *Newbouldia laevis* Mann-Whitney U Test is used to determine whether there is a difference at 0.05 significance level between the results of the positive control and the test samples.

5. DISCUSSION

Ethanol extract of the *Newbouldia laevis* medicinal plant yielded 22.739 g as shown in above Table 1. Table 2 shows the weights of ethyl acetate, chloroform and n-hexane fractions from crude ethanol extract of the plant. It also shows the colour of the solutions of the fractions. NL_{-01-03} has the highest weight of 1.7 g followed by NL_{-01-01} (0.9 g). NL_{-01-02} has the least weight of 0.7 g.

Table 3 shows the result of phytochemical screening of the various fractions of the medicinal plant. Six phytochemicals (alkaloids, saponins tannins, flavonoids, steroids and glycosides) with promising antiplasmodial activity were screened for. From the results, it showed that the leaves of the plant sample contained the phytochemicals screened for in one or more of the solvent fractions. Tannins were absent in less polar solvent such as n-hexane, chloroform and ethyl acetate fractions except in ethanol fraction. Saponins were found to be present mainly in the less polar solvent fractions such as NL_C and NL_H although not intense in NL_C. Alkaloids were found to be present in more polar fractions such as ethanol and ethyl acetate; and absent in n-hexane fraction. Flavonoids, steroids and cardiac glycoside were found to be present in all the fractions.

Table 4 above show the antiplasmodial (antimalarial) activities of fractions from the leaves of *Newbouldia laevis*. Their percentage activities were investigated at various concentrations of 0.5 mg/cm^3, 1.0 mg/cm^3, 2.0 mg/cm^3 and 5.0 mg/cm^3. It was found that all fractions were active against the *plasmodium* parasite. The results showed that percentage elimination increases as the concentrations of the extract and fractions increase. At 0.5 mg/cm^3, NL_{-01-01} has the highest activity of 54.54% followed by NL_{-01} (52.27%) while NL_{-01-02} has the least percentage elimination of 43.18%. At concentration of 5.0 mg/cm^3, NL_{-01} has the highest activity of 79.54% followed by NL_{-01-03} (77.27%) while NL_{-01-02} has the least activity of 72.72%.

Table 5 above shows the results of antimalarial activity of the positive control. At 5.0 mg/cm^3, the percentage elimination activity is 93.18% and at 0.5 mg/cm^3, the percentage activity is 75%. Table 6 above shows the result of thin layer chromatography of large scale ethyl acetate extracts of the leaves of the medicinal plant. Also, TLC screening of the ethyl acetate fraction using ethyl acetate/n-hexane in the ratio 1:4 revealed four spots on the plate. The results of antiplasmodial activities of the positive control were compared with that of the results of the antiplasmodial activities of the plant test samples. Random sampling technique was used to resize the results of the antiplasmodial activities of the plants to the corresponding number of results in the positive control as shown in Table 7.

Table 7. Results of antiplasmodial activity of positive control and resized results of antiplasmodial activity of the plant samples

Concentration mg/cm^3	0.5	1.0	2.0	5.0
SL Test sample	52.27	61.36	75.00	84.10
Positive Control	75	86.36	90.90	93.18

The analysis of the results of the extract and that of the standard (positive control) using Mann-Whitny U test indicated that there is no significant difference between them at 95% confidence interval. Spearman rank correlation analysis of the plant samples with the positive control samples showed that there is correlation and the degree of relationship between the antiplasmodial activities of the plant samples and positive control samples is positively perfect ($\gamma_s = 1$).

Table 6 shows the result of thin layer chromatography of ethyl acetate extract of the leaves of the medicinal plant. The result reveals ethyl acetate/n-hexane solvent mixture 1:4 has the highest number of spots and better retention factor compared to the rest hence will be used for further chromatographic work in order to isolate the most active antimalarial compound(s) and subject them to structural elucidation.

6. CONCLUSION

This study as a contribution to the evaluation of ethnomedicinal plants for search of new chemical constituents with known antiplasmodial properties has proven that the medicinal plant used for this study is active against *Plasmodium falciparum* parasite. Tannins, Saponins, Flavonoid, Steriods, Alkaloids and Cardiac glycoside were found to be present in the medicinal plant screened.

The phytochemical screening and *in vitro* antiplasmodial activity of the ethanol extracts as well the fractions from the plant supported the use of this plant to treat malaria associated symptoms in traditional settings. Data analysis of the results of the plant's samples and that of the standard (positive control) using Mann-Whitny U test indicate that there is no significant difference between them. Spearman rank correlation analysis of the plant samples with the positive control samples showed that there is correlation and the degree of relationship is positively perfect ($\gamma_s = 1$).

The identification and isolation of the bioactive components of this plant will serve as a basis for in-depth pharmacological evaluation of these bioactive phytochemicals for antimalarial drugs development. Additionally, this can also assist in herbal drug formulations of the selected plants.

Further works will include actual identification of single chemical entity responsible for antiplasmodial activity from the leaves of the medicinal plant, *Newbouldia laevis,* using ethyl acetate fraction.

CONSENT

It is not applicable.

ETHICAL APPROVAL

It is not applicable.

COMPETING INTERESTS

Authors have declared that no competing interests exist.

REFERENCES

1. Snow RW, Guerra CA, Noor Am, Mijint HY, HAY SI. The global distribution of clinical episodes of *Plasmodium falciparum* Malaria. Nature. 2005;434(7030):214-7.
2. White Nicholas J, Pukrittayakamee, Sasithon, Hien Tran Tinh, Faiz, Olugbenga M Abul, Mokuolu A, Dondorp Arjen M. Malaria; 2013.

   DOI:org/10.1016/S0140-6736 (13) 60024-0
3. Kantele A, Jokiranta TS. Review of cases with the emerging fifth human malaria parasite, *Plasmodium knowlesi.* Clinical Infectious Diseases. 2011;52(11):1356-1362.
4. WHO. World malaria report. Geneva Switzerland; 2013.
5. Whegang SY, Tahar R, Foumane VN, Soula G, Gwét H, Thalabard JC, Basco LK. Efficacy of non-artemisinin and artemisinin-based combination therapies

for uncomplicated *falciparum* malaria in Cameroon. Malaria Journal. 2010;9:56.

6. Lin JT, Juliano JJ, Wongsrichanalai C. Drug-resistant malaria: The era of ACT. Current Infectious Disease Reports. 2010; 12(3):165-173.
7. Dondorp AM, Yeung S, White L, Nguon C, Day NP, Socheat D, von Seidlein L. Artemisinin resistance: Current status and scenarios for containment. Nature Reviews Microbiology. 2010;8(4):272-280.
8. Mita T, Tanabe K, Kita K. Spread and evolution of *Plasmodium falciparum* drug resistance. Parasitology International. 2009;58(3):201-209.
9. World Health Organization fact sheet no. 134: Traditional medicine. World Health Organization; 2008.
10. Ginsburg H, Deharo E. A call for using natural compounds in the development of new antimalarial treatments – An introduction. Malar J. 2011;10(Suppl 1):S1.
11. Sylvia Ndeshihafela Nafuka. *In vitro* antiplasmodial activity and phytochemicals screening of ethnomedicinal plants used to treat malaria associated symptoms. International Science and Technology Journal of Namibia. 2014;2(1):78-93.
12. Fatope MO, Ibrahim H, Takeda Y. Screening higher plants reputed as pesticides using the brine shrimp lethality assay. Inter. J. of Pharmacognosy. 1993; 31(4):250-256.
13. Harbone JB (ed.) Methods of plants analysis. Phytochemical Methods Chapman and Hall London; 1973.
14. Sofowora AE, Medicinal and traditional medicine in Africa. Vol. 2 Spectrum Books Ltd. 1993;142-146.
15. Trease GE, Evans WC. Pharmacognosy (11th edition). Braille TRida Canada Macmillan Publishers, Canada. 1989;257.
16. Josué WP, Nadia NAC, Claire KM, Jeannette Y, Mbida M. *In Vitro* sensitivity of *Plasmodium falciparum* field isolates to methanolic and aqueous extracts *of Cassia alata* (Fabaceae). Altern Integ Med. 2014; 3:159.
DOI: 10.4172/2327-5162.1000159
17. Dacie JV, Lewis SM. Practical Haematology fourth edition Black well Publishers, USA. 1968;65-66.
18. Hanne IZ, Dan S, Jette C, Lars H, Henri Jerzy WJ. *In-vitro P. falciparum* sensitivity assay. Antimicrobial Agents and Chemotherapy. 2002;42(6):1441-1446.
19. Trager W. Cultivation of malaria parasites. British Mee Bull. 1982;38(2):129-31.
20. Mukhtar MD, Bashir M, Arzai AH. Comparative *in vitro* studies on antiplasmodial acticvity of some Nigerian and foreign brands of chloriquine oral formulation marketed in Kano. African Journal of Biotechnology. 2006;5(24): 2464-2468.

19

Preparation and Characterization of sPLGA Complex Microspheres as a Promising Carrier for Cucurbitacin B

Yi Zhang[1,2], Yue Liu[1], Hewei Shao[1] and Xiaoyan Han[1*]

[1]Tianjin Key Laboratory of Chemistry and Analysis of Chinese Materia Medica, College of Chinese Materia Medica, Tianjin University of Traditional Chinese Medicine, Tianjin 300193, China.
[2]Department of Experimental Teaching, Tianjin University of Traditional Chinese Medicine, Tianjin 300193, China.

Authors' contributions

This work was carried out in collaboration between all authors. Authors YZ and XH designed the study, wrote the protocol and wrote the first draft of the manuscript. Author HS managed the literature searches, analyses of the study performed the spectroscopy analysis and author YL managed the experimental process. All authors read and approved the final manuscript.

Article Information

Editor(s):
(1) Mohamed Fathy, Assiut University, Assiut, Egypt.
Reviewers:
(1) Megha Shah, Gujarat University, India.
(2) Syed Umer Jan, University of Balochistan, Quetta, Pakistan.

ABSTRACT

The purpose of this research was to develop a new kind of GA-CS/sPLGA complexed Microspheres delivery system for CuB. In this work, star-shaped poly(lactic-co-glycolic acid) (sPLGA-COOH) and chitosan modified with glycyrrhetic acid (GA-CS) were successfully synthesized. The GA-CS/sPLGA complexed Microspheres for CuB was prepared by emulsion evaporation method. Futhermore, CuB-loaded Microspheres formulations were optimized. The release behaviour of CuB-loaded Microspheres in vitro were also examined. It was showed that CuB-loaded amount of Microspheres could reach 58.78%±1.288 by adding GA-CS into the external water phase. The size of corresponding CuB-loaded Microspheres was 370±16.14 nm in diameter, and zeta potential was negative 10.86±0.4790 mV measured by laser light particle size/zeta potential analysis. The results indicated that the complexed GA-CS/sPLGA Microspheres

**Corresponding author: Email: 15022611743@163.com*

raised the entrapment efficiency for CuB. *In vitro* drug release demonstrated that complexed GA-CS/sPLGA Microspheres had many advantages such as sustained release and low initial drug burst.

Keywords: Cucurbitacin B; star poly(lactic-co-glycolic acid); complexed microspheres; chitosan modified by glycyrrhetic acid.

ABBREVIATIONS

CuB: Cucurbitacin B; PLGA: Poly(lactide-co-glycolide); CS: Chitosan; PTOL: Pentaerythritol, PVA: Polyvinyl Alcohol; star-PLGA-OH: Star poly(lactic-co-glycolic acid) terminated with hydroxyl groups; star-PLGA-COOH (or star-PLGA): Star poly(lactic-co-glycolic acid) terminated with carboxyl group; GA-CS: Chitosan modified with glycyrrhetic acid; $Sn(Oct)_2$: Stannous octoate; DCC: Dicyclohexylcarbodiimide; NHS: N-hydroxysuccinimide; SDS: Sodium dodecyl sulfate; PBS: Phosphate buffered saline.

1. INTRODUCTION

CuB belongs to the family of tetracyclic triterpenes, which can be extracted from the calyx melo of Cucumis melo L., a Chinese medicinal plant [1]. Cucurbitacin used clinically contain mostly CuB and CuE, which are effective against chronic hepatitis and primary liver carcinoma. However, their nonspecific cytotoxicity and insolubility in water had hindered their clinical applications [2,3]. To overcome such limitations, nanometer scale devices were used for CuB entrapment [4-6], such as liposomes and solid lipid nanoparticles.

The most commonly used polymer in controlled release dosage forms were poly lactic acid (PLA), PLGA, poly (lactic-co-glycolic acid), poly caprolactone (PCL) and Chitosan (CS) etc. Polylactic-co-glycolic acid (PLGA) is FDA-approved biodegradable polymer. Owing to its excellent biocompatibility, PLGA is often used for drug delivery [7]. It was reported that both drug entrapment and release performances can be improved by using star PLGA polymer as drug carrier [3,8]. Chitosan (CS) is a kind of amino polysaccharide with high affinity for cell membrane and is widely used as drug carriers [9,10]. In addition, chitosan has many reactive groups on the surface, such as amino groups, which can be used for grafting appropriate ligand to obtain the active targetability.

In this article, four-arm star poly(lactic-co-glycolic acid) and chitosan modified with glycyrrhetic acid (a targeting ligand) were synthesized. The Chinese Traditional Medicine (Cucurbitacin B, CuB) was used as a model drug and the drug-loaded GA-CS/sPLGA Microspheress were constructed by electrostatic interaction of positive GA-CS and negative sPLGA. It is expected that the complexed Microspheres will have great potential to both raise the drug-loaded amounts and improve the drug release behavior [11,12].

2. EXPERIMENTS

2.1 Materials

Glycolide and D,L-lactide were purchased from Beijing Yuan-Sheng Rong Technology Co., Ltd. (China). PTOL (AR) and PVA (molecular weight, 30,000-70,000) were purchased from Beijing J&K Scientific Ltd. (China). Chitosan (low molecular weight, 85% deacetylation degree) was purchased from Jinan Haidebei Marine Bioengineering Ltd. Co. (China). Succinic anhydride (AR) was purchased from TCI Development Ltd. Co. (China). $Sn(Oct)_2$ was purchased from Sigma Company. Glycyrrhetic acid (purity 99%) was purchased from Fujie Pharmaceutical Co. Ltd. (China). Cucurbitacin B (purity 95.5%) was purchased from Tianjin Institute of Pharmaceutical Research Ltd. Co. (China). All other chemicals were of analytical grade and all materials were used without further purification.

2.2 Instruments

^{1}H-NMR spectra were performed on a Varian UNITY-plus 400 spectrometer. Tetramethylsilane was used as an internal standard. Both GA-CS and sPLGA were dissolved in $CDCl_3$ solvent.

UV-vis absorption spectra of the samples were recorded at room temperature using a UV-2401 UV-vis spectrophotometer (SHIMADZU).

The mean size and zeta potential of drug-loaded Microspheres were determined by a 3000HS

Malvern instrument (Worcestershire, UK). All the measurements were repeated three times.

The amount of CuB contained in the samples were determined by SofTA, CoMetro-6000 HPLC equipped with a Hypersil ODS C_{18} column (200 mm×4.6 mm, 5 μm). All the measurements were repeated three times.

2.3 Synthesis and Characterization of star-PLGA-COOH

Lactide and glycolide (monomer), PTOL (initiator) and $Sn(Oct)_2$ (catalyst)) were added in dichloromethane to meltingly polymerize in a sealed tube [3,13]. The stoichiometric ratios were monomer:initiator:catalyst=10000:100:1 mol/mol). Before heating, the tube was repeatedly passing nitrogen gas to remove trace air. The reaction was conducted for eight hours at 160℃ in oil bath. After the reaction finished, the reaction mixture was dissolved in dichloromethane, and pure star-PLGA-OH was obtained by precipitation twice with anhydrous methanol, and vacuum dried overnight.

The detailed synthetic procedure of star-PLGA-COOH was as follows. Two times amount of succinic anhydride reacted with star-PLGA-OH for 24 h at room temperature under continuous stirring. The solvent (1,4-dioxane) was removed after the reaction finished. Then the concentrated solution was dissolved in hot water and extracted three times with dichloromethane. Finally, star-PLGA-COOH was obtained by methanol recrystallizing and vacuum dried, whose structure was further characterized by ^{1}H-NMR.

2.4 Preparation and Characterization of Chitosan modified with Glycyrrhetic Acid

According to the reference [14,15], carboxyl group of glycyrrhetic acid was activated with DCC/NHS, then a condensation reaction was conducted between chitosan and the activated ester of glycyrrhetic acid. The structure of product was characterized by H^1-NMR.

2.5 Preparation of Drug-loaded Complexed sPLGA Microspheress

Briefly, 160 mg sPLGA-COOH and 40 mg CuB were dissolved in 2 mL dichloromethane as the oil phase, and an apropriate amount of GA-CS (or CS) was dissolved in 20 mL 2% PVA solution as the water phase. Under ultrasound action the oil phase was slowly dropped into water phase to form a stable emulsified solution in an ice bath (0℃). The obtained solution was then poured into a large amount of 2% PVA solution, and the mixed solution was continually stirred for 6 h to volatilize dichloromethane completely. Pure CuB-loaded Microspheres were obtained by centrifugation at 3,500 rpm for 30 min, followed by washing with 2% aqueous solution of ethanol (3×10 mL) and vacuum drying for 48 hours.

Drug entrapment efficiency, drug-loaded amount, particle size and zeta patential were chosen as indexes, and the preparation formulation of drug-loaded Microspheres was optimized by changing the amount and types of chitosan added in the external water phase.

2.6 Determination of the Content and Entrapment Efficiency of CuB

5 mg CuB-loaded Microspheres were put into a 10 mL volumetric flask. Then 2 mL of dichloromethane was added to dissolve the Microspheres completely under ultrasound action. Finally, 8 mL of methanol was added and the solution was filtered through 0.22 μm microporous membrane. After abandoning primary filtrate, subsequent filtrate was collected. CuB concentration in the filtrate was determined by HPLC under the following chromatographic conditions [Chromatographic column: Shim-pack VP-ODS C_{18} (200 mm×4.6 mm, 5 μm), mobile phase of methanol: water (70:30), flow rate: 1 mL·min^{-1}, column temperature: 30℃, detection wavelength: 228 nm, injection volume: 20 μL]. Based on the standard curve of CuB and the following formulas, the drug-loaded amount and entrapment efficiency were calculated.

The amount of drug-loaded Microspheress = The drug weight contained in the Microspheres/The total weight of Microspheres×100%;

The entrapment efficiency = The drug weight contained in the Microspheres/The total weight of the drug×100%.

2.7 *In vitro* Release Investigation of Drug-loaded Microspheres

10 mg of drug-loaded Microspheres were dispersed in 10 mL PBS solutions. The solution was then placed in the dialysis bags. The release medium was PBS solution (containing 0.5% SDS) at pH 7.4 in 37℃ water bath oscillator. Samples were withdrawn at appropriate time

intervals and we added an amount of PBS solution equal to that withdrawn. CuB concentration of the supernatant was determined by HPLC after centrifuging. The cumulative release curves were drawn by calculating cumulative release amount at each time interval.

2.8 Statistical Analyses

All experiments were repeated at least three times. Results are expressed as means ± standard deviation. A difference between means was considered significant if the p value was less than or equal to 0.05.

3. RESULTS AND DISCUSSTION

3.1 Characterization of sPLGA and Chitosan Modified with Glycyrrhetic Acid

The structure of star-PLGA-OH and star-PLGA-COOH was confirmed by ^{1}H-NMR. The ^{1}H-NMR spectrum of star-PLGA-OH was shown in Fig. 1. The chemical shifts of δ=1.27 and 3.7 corresponded to CH_3 and CH of the initiator PTOL respectively. The chemical shift of δ=1.58 and 5.17 corresponded to CH_3 and CH of lactide respectively. The chemical shift 4.82 corresponded to CH_2 of the glycolide. The rest peaks were impurities peaks. The results showed that the glycolide/lactide copolymer had been synthesized successfully. After the reaction of star-PLGA-OH with succinic anhydride, the peak of δ=2.72 appeared in the spectrum of Fig. 1b, which corresponded to CH_2 chemical shift of succinic anhydride (δ=2.62) and indicated successful synthesis of star-PLGA-COOH.

New peaks at 2.5~2.7 ppm was shown in spectrum C compared with spectrum D in Fig. 1. These new peaks corresponded to the methyl, GA methyl and methylene protons respectively, so it was inferred that GA-CS polymer had been successfully synthesized.

The UV-vis spectra of GA, CS and GA-CS in solution were examined. The methanol solution of GA had a characteristic absorption peak at 248 nm, while the GA-CS in methanol solution had a characteristic absorption peak at 258 nm, which was characteristic absorption of GA. However CS solution had no obvious absorption in the 200~400 nm, which furtherly support that coupling reaction of GA and CS was successful.

3.2 GA-CS/sPLGA Complexed Micro-spheress´ Preparation and the Effect of GA-CS Concentration on the Microspheress´ Properties

Microspheres drug delivery systems are of considerable therapeutic interest. Currently, this field is dominated by the use of poly(lactide-co-glycolide) type Microspheress. Copolymer poly(lactic-co-glycolic acid) (PLGA) nano-technology has been approved by the US FDA for the use of drug delivery, diagnostics and other applications of clinical and basic science research, including cardiovascular disease, cancer, vaccine and tissue engineering. However, because of the deficiency of suitable functional groups on their surface, conventional PLGA Microspheres lack the possibility of surface modifications for specialized targeting or other purposes. Such modifications are thought to greatly improve the effectiveness of Microspheres delivery systems.

To solve this problem, sPLGA and chitosan modified with glycyrrhetic acid were synthesized and sPLGA complexed Microspheres was constructed by means of chitosan and modified chitosan with glycyrrhetic acid. The decision to choose glycyrrhetic acid as a targeting ligand was that glycyrrhetic acid accumulated in rat hepatocytes by a ligand-receptor interaction and had good hepatoma cellular targeted efficiency [14-17].

The effect curves of varied GA-CS amounts added in the external water phase on the properties of CuB-loaded complexed Microspheres was shown in Fig. 2. The zeta potential of Microspheres increased as the amount of the GA-CS with positive potential was added gradually in negative sPLGA system. Meanwhile the size of the PLGA Microspheres increased as GA-CS concentration increased in the external water phase. Most importantly, the adding of GA-CS improved the amount CuB-loaded of Microspheres. It was shown that the amount of drug loaded was 58.78%±1.288 when 80% GA-CS was added. However continuously increasing of GA-CS concentration led to highly viscous solutions and broad size distribution of Microspheres. Statistical evaluation proved that no significant difference was observed for zeta potential and the size of CuB-loaded microspheres by adding GA-CS in the Fig. 2 ($p<0.05$). Similarly, no significant difference bserved for drug-loaded amount and drug entrapment efficiency in the Fig. 2 ($p<0.05$).

So the Microspheres were employed for the subsequent experiment, which were prepared by adding 80% GA-CS in the external water phase. It was shown that GA-CS had the stabilizing and auxiliary emulsifying effect during Microspheres formation.

3.3 The Effect of CS/GA-CS Type Added on Complexed Microspheress´ Properties

Two types of complexed Microspheres´ properties were also examined and compared with the uncomplexed mirospheres. The value of particle size and zeta potential for the Microspheres under the conditions that two types of CS was added (both 80 % added) was shown in Table 1. Zeta potential Microspheres differed significantly between uncomplexed sPLGA and complexed sPLGA Microspheres. It was shown in Table 1 that complexed sPLGA shifted the negative zeta potential of uncomplexed sPLGA Microspheres to positive values. As can be seen from the Table 1, the size of the Microspheres increased as CS or GA-CS was added. The size distribution of sPLGA Microspheres were narrow.

In addition, entrapment efficiency is an important index to evaluate drug-loaded Microspheres. Drug entrapment efficiency was improved by adding either CS or GA-CS into the external water phase. The results of the experiment indicated that adding PVA and GA-CS into the external water phase might have a better synergistic effect on the improvement of drug entrapment efficiency than adding PVA or CS (GA-CS) alone. It was shown that the maximum amount of CuB loaded Microspheres prepared by

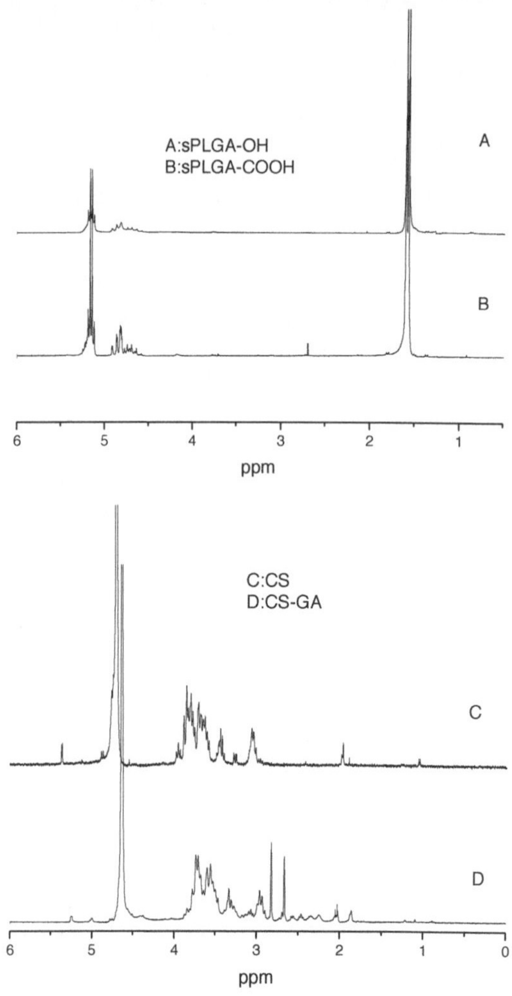

Fig. 1. H[1]-NMR spectrum of star-PLGA-OH (A), star-PLGA-COOH (B), CS (C) and GA-CS (D)

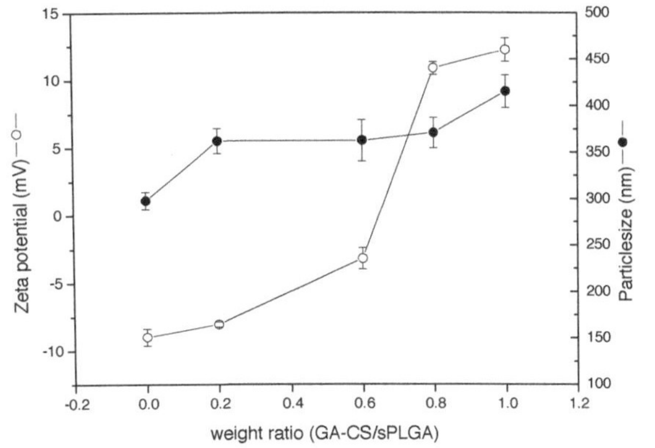

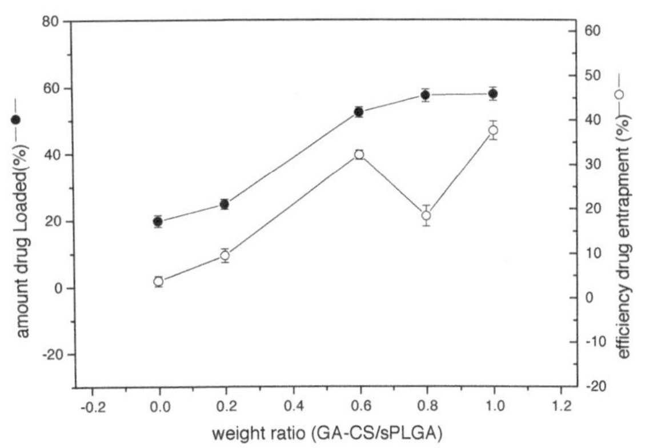

Fig. 2. Influence of different amount of GA-CS added in GA-CS/sPLGA microspheres on (A) Particle size, zeta potential, (B) Drug-loaded amount and drug entrapment efficiency

Table 1. Properties of produced Microspheres under different conditions: sPLGA/CS[2] (CS-GA[3] or none added[1])

Formulation code	mass ratio	Size (nm)	PDI[a]	Zeta potential (mv)	Drug loaded (%)	Drug entrapment (%)
sPLGA/CS-GA[3]	1:0.8	370±16.14	0.032±0.0041	10.86±0.4790	58.78±1.288	18.0±0.7079
sPLGA/CS[2]	1:0.8	459±21.57	0.025±0.0064	12.03±0.6541	49.20±0.6378	17.25±0.7405
sPLGA[1]	1:0	295±12.48	0.016±0.0049	-8.92±0.2576	19.56±0.8029	3.67±0.0941

a: PDI was the polydispersity index.

adding 80% GA-CS into the external water phase was 58.78%±1.288, the size of corresponding Microspheres was 370±16.14 nm in diameter, and zeta potential was 10.86±0.4790 mV. Optimized test CuB-loaded sPLGA/CS-GA complexed microspheres exhibited good propertities than other formulations [18,19].

3.4 *In vitro* Release Study of CuB-loaded Microspheres

In vitro drug release profile reveals fundamental information on the Microspheres´ composition and structure. The release curves of two kinds of CuB-loaded Microspheres *in vitro* was shown in Fig. 3. The cumulative release amount of drug-loaded Microspheres decreased when GA-CS added in the external water phase. The burst release reduced and the release rate had the tendency of slowing down. When the release time was close to 300 h, the cumulative releasing amount hadn't reached 70% yet. This was because the complexing of GA-CS with sPLGA Microspheres restricted the drug's diffusion through the Microspheres. The propertities *in vivo* of CuB-loaded microspheres, such as pharmacokinetic parameters or adverse effects will be further studied in subsequent work.

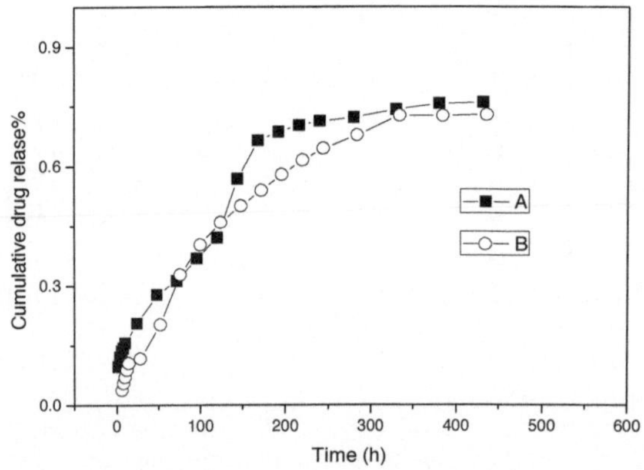

Fig. 3. ***In vitro*** **release profiles of the CuB-loaded Microspheres: sPLGA(A), sPLGA/GA-CS (B)**

4. CONCLUSIONS

In this work, we developed a new kind of drug-loaded complexed Microspheres from sPLGA-COOH and GA-CS by electrostatic interaction. The ligand GA was introduced to the Microspheres by adding GA-CS in the external water phase. We have shown that GA-CS could be used as a stabilizer and a auxiliary emusifier to prepare sPLGA complexed Microspheres by emulsion evaporation method. The results showed that the complexed Microspheres had higher CuB entrapment efficiency, smaller drug burst release and a slower sustained release than the uncomplexed ones. In summary, sPLGA/GA-CS complexed mirospheres are suitable drug carrier for CuB and these results are helpful in subsequently drug targeting experiment.

CONSENT

It is not applicable.

ETHICAL APPROVAL

It is not applicable.

ACKNOWLEDGEMENTS

This work was financially supported by National Natural Science Foundation of China (81202921) National Training Programs of Innovation and Entrepreneurship for Undergraduates (201310063012).

COMPETING INTERESTS

Authors have declared that no competing interests exist.

REFERENCES

1. Ren FB, Hong B. Advances in the pharmacological and clinical study of the Cucurbitacin treating for hepatitis and primary carcinoma of the liver. Chin J Inte Trad West Med. 1986;6:633-635.
2. Jayaprakasam B, Seeram NP, Nair MG. Anticancer and antiinflammatory activities of Cucurbitacins from *Cucurbita andreana*. Cancer Letters. 2003;189:11-16.
3. Zhang Y, Shao HW, Liu Y, Han XY. Study on preparation of star PLGA Cucurbitacin - loaded microspheress and its propertities. Advanced Materials Research. 2014;884: 630-634
4. Sarthak KP, Afsaneh L, Phillip C. Roles of nonpolar and polar inter-molecular Interactions in the improvement of the drug loading capacity of PEO-b-PCL with Increasing PCL content for two hydrophobic cucurbitacin drugs. Biomacromolecules. 2009;10:2584-2591
5. Wang WY, Zhao XL, Hu HY. Galactosylated solid lipid nanoparticles with cucurbitacin B improves the liver targetability. Drug Deliv. 2007;17:114-122.
6. Wang JW, Zhou XM, Cao YL. The antitumor activities of Cucurbitacin liposome for injection both *in vitro* and *in vivo*. Asian J Tradit Med. 2007;2:97-103.
7. Jan S, Khan GM, Muhammad S, Khan H, Khan KA, Shah K. Formulation, evaluation and effect of 3 new polymers and co-excipients on *in-vitro* controlled release patterns of flurbiprofen matrix tablets Lat. Am. J. Pharm. 2013;32(9):1335-1341.
8. Liang XF, Wang HJ, Luo H. Preparation and characterization of novel

biodegradable multifunctional microspheres. Acta Chim Sinica. 2008;66:2178-2183.

9. Ouyang CP, Liu Q, Zhao SX. Synthesis and characterization of star-shaped poly(lactide-co-glycolide) and its drug-loaded microspheress. Polym Bull. 2012; 68:27-36

10. Ta HT, Dass CR, Larson I, Choong PFM, Dunstan DE. A chitosan-dipotassium orthophosphate hydrogel for the delivery of Doxorubicin in the treatment of osteosarcoma. Biomaterials. 2009;30: 3605-3613.

11. Majeti NV, Ravi K. A review of chitin and chitosan applications. React Funct Polym. 2000;46:1-27.

12. Mao SJ, Bi YQ, Jin H. Preparation, characterization and uptake by primary cultured rat hepatocytes of liposomes surface-modified with glycyrrhetinic acid. Pharmazie. 2007;62:614-619.

13. Zhang CN, Wang W, Liu T. Doxorubicin-loaded glycyrrhetinic acid-modified alginate nanoparticles for liver tumor chemotherapy. Biomaterials. 2012;7: 2187-2196.

14. Ma GL, Zhao SX, Jin X. Folate conjugated micelles based on star shaped PLGA-PEG-NH2 copolymers as novel tumo-targeted nanocarriers. Chem J Chinese U. 2012;33:1854-1859.

15. Tian Q, Wang XH, Wang W. Self-assembly and liver targeting of sulfated chitosan nanoparticles functionalized with glycyrrhetinic acid. Nanomed Nanotechnol Biol Med. 2012;8(6):870-879.

16. Han XY, Zhang Y, Zhao PL. Synthesis of glycyrrhetinic acid-modified chitosan cligosaccharide-stearic acid drug carrier and its micellar properties. Chin Tradit Herbal Drugs. 2011;3:505-509.

17. Manca ML, Antimisiaris S. PLGA, chitosan or chitosan-coated PLGA microparticles for alveolar delivery? A comparative study of particle stability during nebulization. Colloids and Surfaces B: Biointerfaces. 2008;62(2):220-231.

18. Chung YI, Kim JC, Kim YH. The effect of surface functionalization of PLGA nanoparticles by heparin or chitosan-conjugated pluronic on tumor targeting. J. Control. Release. 2010;143(3):374-382.

19. LI Y, Han CY, Li JM, Qin L, Tang SJ. Optimization of preparation of nanostructured lipid carriers loaded with cucurbitacin B by central composite design and response surface methodology. Chinese Journal of Pharmaceuticals. 2014; 45(11):1042-1045.

20

Molecular Mechanisms of the Modulatory Effect of Vitamin E on Tacrolimus (FK506)-Induced Renal Injury in Rats

Hassan Afify[1], Abdel-Aziz H. Abdel-Aziz[2], Mahmoud Nour El-Din[1], Amany Balah[2] and El-Sayed Akool[1,2*]

[1]Department of Pharmacology and Toxicology, Faculty of Pharmacy, Egyptian-Russian University, Cairo, Egypt.
[2]Department of Pharmacology and Toxicology, Faculty of Pharmacy, Al-Azhar University, Cairo, Egypt.

Authors' contributions

This work was carried out in collaboration between all authors. Authors ESA, AAHAA and AB designed the study. Author HA performed the experiments. Authors HA and MNED carried out the statistical analysis. Authors ESA and AB wrote the first draft of the manuscript. All authors read and approved the final manuscript.

Article Information

Editor(s):
(1) Rafik Karaman, Bioorganic Chemistry, College of Pharmacy, Al-Quds University, USA.
Reviewers:
(1) Weiting Wang, Tianjin Institute of Pharmaceutical Research, China.
(2) Pratibha Ravindra Kamble, Ohio State University Medical centre, USA.
(3) Hayrettin Ozturk, Abant Izzet Baysal University, Turkey.

ABSTRACT

Aim: This study was designed to evaluate the possible modulatory effect of vitamine E on tacrolimus (FK506)-induced renal injury in rats.
Methods: Twenty-four male Wistar rats (6 animals in each group) were used in this study. The first group (Control) received normal saline intraperitoneal (i.p.) daily for 21 days. The second group received FK506 (1 mg/kg/day i.p.) daily for 21 days. The third group was administered Vitamin E (250 mg/kg/day by oral gavage) 5 days before and concurrently during FK506 administration daily for 21 days. The fourth group received Vitamin E alone (as previously described in the third group).
Results: Administration of FK506 significantly increased blood urea nitrogen and serum creatinine

**Corresponding author: Email: elsayed.akool@yahoo.com*

levels. In addition, FK506 has also reduced the renal content of reduced glutathione, as well as the enzymatic activities of superoxide dismutase and catalase. Furthermore, these effects were associated with an increase in lipid peroxidation, inducible NO-synthase (iNOS), and NF-κB expression. Moreover, histopathological examinations showed severe damage of the renal tissues in animals treated with FK506. Interestingly, it was found that concomitant administration of vitamin E along with FK506 ameliorated all these parameters and improved renal function. Furthermore, the immunosuppressive effect of FK506 was not affected by vitamin E.

Conclusion: The findings of the present study suggest that concomitant use of vitamin E might be useful in reducing nephrotoxicity induced by FK506.

Keywords: Tacrolimus; Vitamin E; Nephrtoxicity; ROS; iNOS; NF-κB.

1. INTRODUCTION

Solid organ transplantation has become one of the most important fields in modern medicine due to its contribution in decreasing the mortality rate of patients with organs failure. However, the risk of transplant rejection threatens the success of the transplantation procedure. Transplant rejection can be prevented by the use of an immunosuppressive agent to suppress the reaction of the immune system to the transplanted tissue. Tacrolimus (FK506) is one of the calcineurin inhibitors that suppress T-cell activation by inhibiting the cellular phosphatase calcineurin [1,2]. The mechanism involves binding of FK506 to the FK binding protein 12 (FKBP12). The tacrolimus-FKBP12 complex then binds to calcineurin and mediates inhibition of phosphatase activity of calcineurin. This inhibition prevents the dephosphorylation and nuclear translocation of the nuclear factor of activated T cells (NFAT) and subsequent transcription of IL-2 and other cytokines. Calcineurin inhibitors (CNI) are among the most efficient immunosuppressive agents and therefore are widely used in organ transplantation and for the treatment of many inflammatory diseases. However, the clinical use of the calcineurin inhibitor FK506 is strongly limited by acute and chronic nephrotoxicity which remains a major clinical problem [2-4]. The mechanisms of FK506-induced renal injury are not fully elucidated. However, one of the possible mechanisms of FK506-induced nephrotoxicity is thought to be over production of reactive oxygen species (ROS) and a consequent imbalance between oxidants and endogenously produced antioxidants [4,5]. The harmful effects of ROS induced by FK506 can be antagonized by using a powerful antioxidant agent [4,5]. One of the most important natural antioxidants is vitamin E (Vit E) [6,7]. Vit E has eight naturally occurring components including α, β, γ, and δ derivatives of tocopherol and tocotrienol. In 1989, it has been reported that α-tocopherol has high activity as a chain-breaking antioxidant [8]. Furthermore, α-tocopherol has been demonstrated to be the most abundant lipid-soluble antioxidant in humans and it has been detected in cellular and sub-cellular membranes [9]. Thus it was interesting to investigate the potential protective role of Vit E against FK506-induced nephrotoxicity in rats.

2. MATERIALS AND METHODS

2.1 Animals

Male Wistar albino rats weighing 200-230 g were housed in a 12 h dark/light cycle animal facility with controlled humidity and constant temperature. The animals were fed a standard diet and water was supplied *ad libitum*. The animals were kept under observation for one week before the treatments for adaptation. The experimental protocol used in this study was approved by the Institutional Animal Ethics Committee.

2.2 Drugs and Chemicals

FK506 was purchased from Astellas Pharma Inc., Japan. Vit E was purchased from Pharco Pharmaceuticals, Alexandria, Egypt. Nuclear factor kappa-B (NF-κB), inducible NO-synthase (iNOS) and catalase (CAT) ELISA kits were purchased from ElAab Science Co., Ltd., China. Superoxide dismutase (SOD), reduced glutathione (GSH), and thiobarbituric acid reactive substances (TBARS) assay kits were purchased from Trevigen (USA), Oxford biomedical research (Oxford MI, USA), and Cell Biolabs (USA) respectively. Interleukin-2 (IL-2) ELISA kit was purchased from Uscn Life Science Inc, Wuhan, China. Creatinine and blood urea nitrogen (BUN) assay kits were purchased from Bioassay system (USA).

2.3 Experimental Design

Twenty-four male Wistar albino rats were used in this study. The animals were randomly divided into four groups, 6 animals in each. The first group (Control) received normal saline intraperitoneal (i.p.) daily for 21 days. The second group received FK506 (1 mg/kg/day i.p.) [10] daily for 21 days. The third group was administered Vit E (250 mg/kg/day by oral gavage) [11] 5 days before and concurrently during FK506 administration daily for 21 days. The fourth group received Vit E alone (as previously described in the third group). 24 h after the last treatment, blood samples were collected for the determination of serum levels of creatinine, BUN as well as IL-2. After terminal bleeding, animals were sacrificed by cervical dislocation. The left kidney was dissected immediately after death, washed with ice cold phosphate buffered saline (PBS) and kept at -20°C till used. The right kidney was fixed in 10% neutral-buffered formal saline for histopathological investigation.

2.4 Assessment of BUN and Serum Creatinine

The serum levels of BUN and creatinine were determined by commercial kits according to the manufacturer's instructions (Bioassay system, USA).

2.5 Assessment of Serum Cytokine

The serum level of IL-2 was determined by enzyme-linked immunosorbent assay (ELISA) according to the manufacturer's instructions (Uscn Life Science Inc, Wuhan, China).

2.6 Determination of Oxidative Damage Markers

2.6.1 Determination of lipid peroxides

The by-product of lipid peroxidation malondialdehyde (MDA) in renal tissues was measured using a TBARS assay kit according to the manufacturer's instructions (Cell Biolabs, Inc., USA). Briefly, Tissue samples were homogenized in ice-cold PBS containing 1X BHT (Butylated hydroxytoluene) and centrifugated at 10,000 g for 5 min at 4°C to collect the supernatant. The unknown MDA containing samples or MDA standards were first reacted with thiobarbituric acid (TBA) at 95°C. After a brief incubation, the samples and standards can be read spectrophotometrically. The MDA content in unknown samples was determined by comparison with the predetermined MDA standard curve.

2.6.2 Determination of iNOS expression

The protein level of iNOS in renal tissues was determined by enzyme-linked immunosorbent assay (ELISA) according to the manufacturer's instructions (ElAab Science Co., Ltd., China).

2.6.3 Determination of NF-κB expression

Total NF−κB level in renal tissues was determined by enzyme-linked immunosorbent assay (ELISA) according to the manufacturer's instructions (ElAab Science Co., Ltd., China).

2.7 Determination of Endogenous Antioxidants

2.7.1 Determination of GSH content

Renal content of GSH was determined by colorimetric assay according to the manufacturer's instructions (Oxford biomedical research, Oxford MI, USA). Briefly, the method is based on the reaction of GSH with Ellman's reagent [5, 5'-dithiobis-2-nitrobenzoic acid (DTNB)] which gives rise to a product that can be quantified spectrophotometrically at 412 nm.

2.7.2 Determination of SOD activity

Renal SOD activity was determined by assay kit according to the manufacturer's instructions (Trevigen, USA). In Trevigen's superoxide dismutase assay, superoxide radicals generated from the conversion of xanthine to uric acid and hydrogen peroxide by xanthine oxidase, converts nitroblue tetrazolium (NBT) to NBT-diformazan. NBT-diformazan absorbs light at 550 nm. SODs reduce superoxide radical concentrations and thereby lower the rate of NBT-diformazan formation. The extent of reduction in the appearance of NBT-diformazan is a measure of SOD activity.

2.7.3 Determination of CAT activity

Renal CAT activity was determined by enzyme-linked immunosorbent assay (ELISA) according to the manufacturer's instructions (ElAab Science Co., Ltd., China).

2.8 Histopathological Examination

Kidney specimens from all animals were immediately dissected and fixed in 10% neutral-buffered formal saline for at least 72 hours. All the specimens were washed in tap water for half an hour and then dehydrated in ascending grades of alcohol, cleared in xylene and embedded in paraffin. Serial sections of 6μm thick were cut and stained with Haematoxylin and eosin [12] for histopathological investigation.

2.9 Statistical Analysis

Results are expressed as means ± SD. Statistical analysis was performed using one way ANOVA followed by Turkey-Kramer as a post-hoc test. *P*-values below 0.05 were considered as indication for statistically significant differences between conditions compared.

3. RESULTS

3.1 Effects of FK506 and/or Vit E on Serum Creatinine and BUN Levels

Treatment of rats with FK506 produced a significant increase in BUN (Fig. 1A) and serum creatinine levels (Fig. 1B). However, concomitant administration of Vit E along with FK506 significantly reduced the levels of BUN (Fig. 1A) and serum creatinine (Fig. 1B) as compared to FK506 alone treated animals. No significant changes were observed in rats treated with Vit E alone.

3.2 Effects of FK506 and/or Vit E on Oxidative Damage Markers

3.2.1 Effects of FK506 and/or Vit E on lipid peroxides

Administration of FK506 significantly induced lipid peroxidation as indicated by an increase in the by-product of lipid peroxidation MDA. On the other hand, lipid peroxidation is significantly attenuated in animals treated with FK506 in combination with Vit E as compared to FK506 alone treated animals (Fig. 2A). No significant changes were observed in animals treated with Vit E alone.

3.2.2 Effects of FK506 and/or Vit E on iNOS expression

As demonstrated in Fig. 2B, administration of FK506 significantly induced iNOS expression. However, concomitant administration of Vit E along with FK506 significantly reduced iNOS expression as compared to FK506 alone treated animals. The basic level of iNOS expression was not changed in rats treated with Vit E alone.

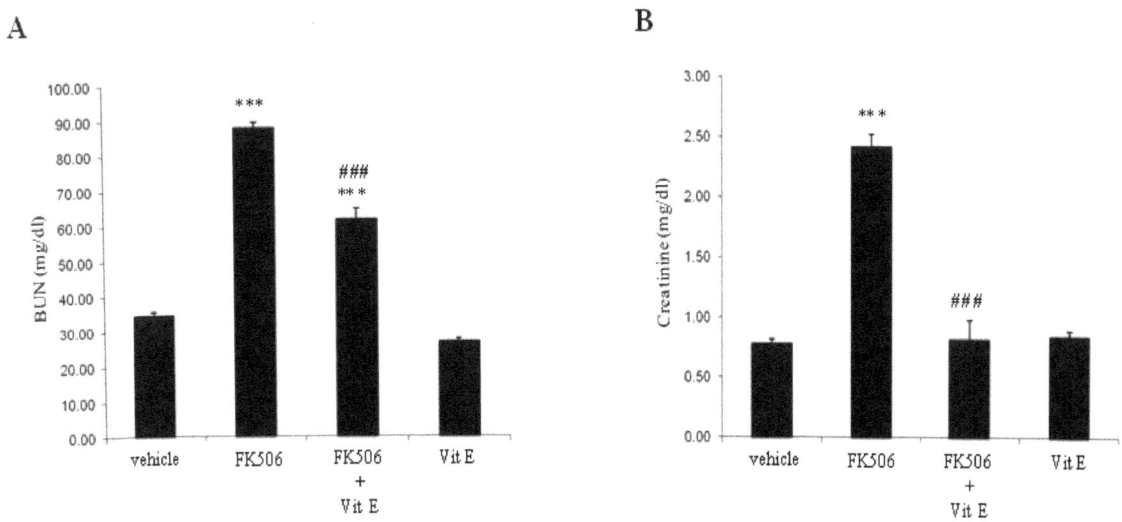

Fig. 1. Effects of FK506 and/or Vit E on BUN (A) and serum creatinine (B) in male Wistar albino rats

*Data represent means ± S.D. (n=6), *** p < 0.001 versus control, ### p < 0.001 versus FK506 alone-treated animals*

3.2.3 Effects of FK506 and/or Vit E on NF-κB Expression

NF-κB expression was highly induced in animals treated with FK506 alone. On the other hand, concomitant administration of Vit E along with FK506 significantly reduced the expression of NF-κB as compared to FK506 alone treated animals (Fig. 2C). NF-κB expression was not altered in animals treated with Vit E alone.

3.3 Effects of FK506 and/or Vit E on Endogenous Antioxidants

3.3.1 Effects of FK506 and/or Vit E on GSH Content

As shown in Fig. 3A, treatment of animals with FK506 significantly reduced the renal content of GSH. However, GSH level in animals treated with FK506 in combination with Vit E was highly increased compared to FK506 alone treated animals. Renal GSH content in rats treated with Vit E alone significantly increased compared with control group.

3.3.2. Effects of FK506 and/or Vit E on SOD Activity

Administration of FK506 produced a significant reduction in SOD activity. On the other hand, concomitant administration of Vit E along with FK506 significantly increased SOD activity as compared to FK506 alone treated group (Fig. 3B). SOD activity in rats treated with Vit E alone significantly increased compared to control group.

3.3.3 Effects of FK506 and/or Vit E on CAT activity

Treatment of animals with FK506 significantly reduced CAT activity. However, CAT activity in rats treated with FK506 in combination with Vit E was significantly increased as compared to FK506 alone treated animals (Fig 3C). No significant changes were observed in animals treated with Vit E alone.

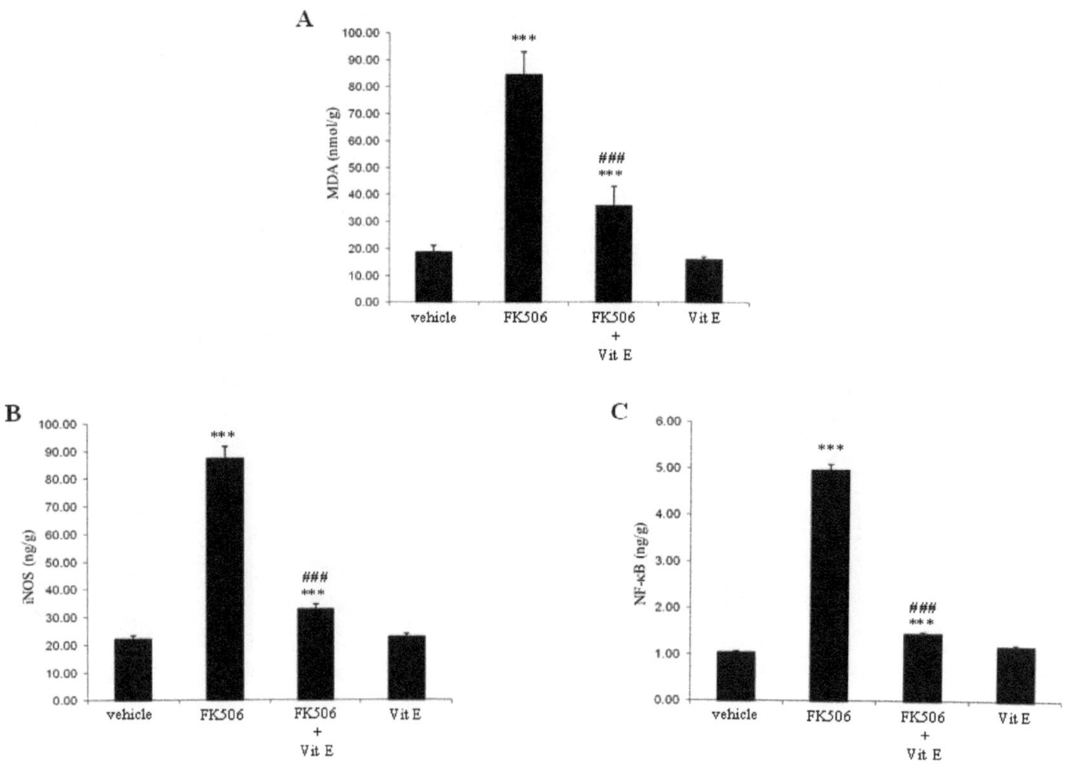

Fig. 2. Effects of FK506 and/or Vit E on renal content of MDA (A) as well as iNOS (B) and NF-κB Expression (C) in male Wistar albino rats

*Data represent means ± S.D. (n=6), *** $p < 0.001$ versus control, ### $p < 0.001$ versus FK506 alone-treated animals*

3.4 Histopathological Examination

As shown in Fig. 4, histopathological examinations showed sever damage of the renal tissue in FK506 alone-treated rats as indicated by necrotic damaged tubule & glomerular tufts segmentation (Fig. 4B). However, concomitant administration of Vit E along with FK506 improved the histopathological changes to a great extent as indicated by improvement in the tubular damage (Fig. 4C).

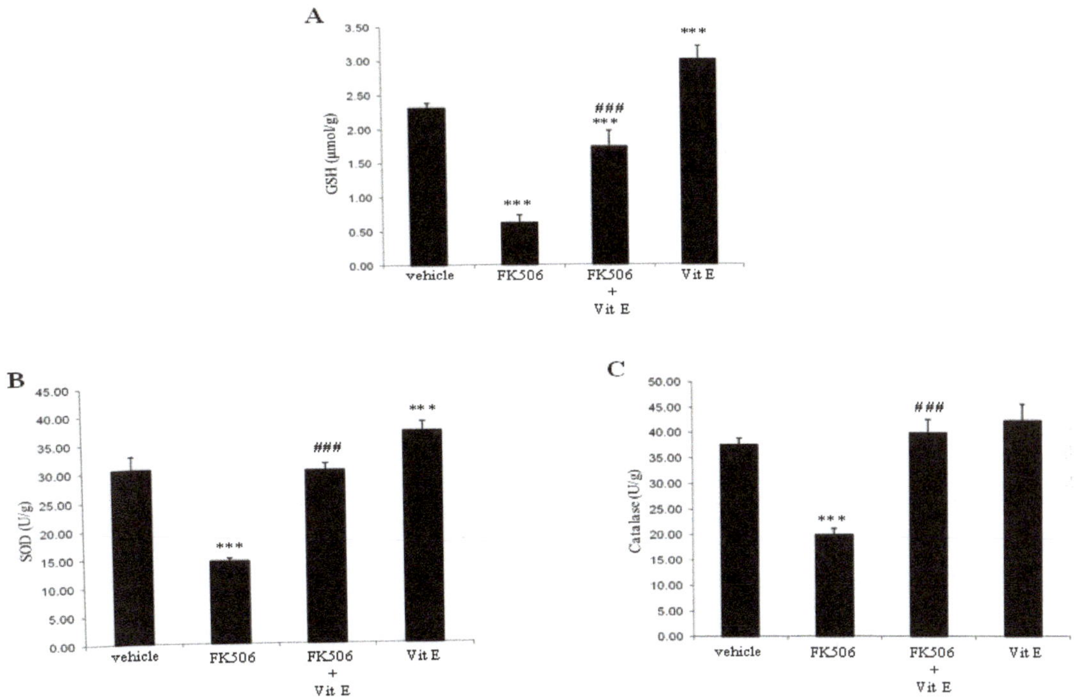

Fig. 3. Effects of FK506 and/or Vit E on renal content of GSH (A) as well as renal enzymatic activities of SOD (B) and CAT (C) in male Wistar albino rats

*Data represent means ± S.D. (n=6), *** p < 0.001 versus control, ### p < 0.001 versus FK506 alone-treated animals*

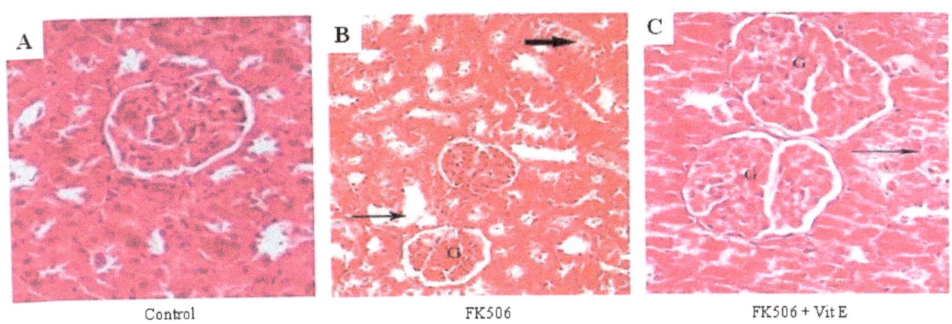

Fig. 4. A. A photomicrograph of a section of the kidney of a control rat showing the normal structure of the tissue (H&E 200). B. A photomicrograph of a section of the kidney of FK506 alone-treated rats showing sever damage of tubules, where some tubules show only dilatation of lumen (thin arrow), others show necrotic material in their lumen with degeneration of lining cells (thick arrow). The glomeruli show segmentation of their tuft of capillaries (G) (H&E 200). C. A photomicrograph of a section of the kidney of rats received FK506 + Vit E showing many tubules with vacuolated epithelium lining (thin arrow). The glomeruli show segmentation of their tuft of capillaries (G). In comparison to FK506 alone-treated group the necrotic tubules show improvement (H&E 200)

3.5 Effects of FK506 and/or Vit E on Serum Level of IL-2

To test whether the immunosuppressive effect of FK506 would also be affected in the presence of Vit E, serum IL-2 level was measured as a marker of the immunosuppressive efficiency of FK506 [13]. As shown in Fig. 5, treatment of animals with FK506 produced a significant reduction in the serum IL-2 level as expected. On the other hand, no significant changes were observed in rats treated with FK506 in combination with Vit E as compared to FK506 alone treated animals.

4. DISCUSSION

FK506 is one of the most efficient immunosuppressive agents that are commonly used in organ transplantation. However, the clinical use of FK506 is strongly limited by acute and chronic nephrotoxicity which remains a major clinical problem. Recently, it has been reported that over production of ROS and consequently oxidative stress plays a major role in FK506 (parent drug)-induced renal toxicity [4,5,14]. In 2012, Akool et al. [15] demonstrated that mitochondrial enzymes may represent the main sources of ROS induced by FK506 in the kidney. In addition, it was found that the antioxidant melatonin has the ability to protect against FK506-induced renal oxidative stress in rats [5]. In the present work, it was found that treatment of rats with FK506 resulted in a decline in renal function as indicated by significant increase in BUN and serum creatinine levels as well as histopathological changes. These data are in agreement with previous findings by several researchers who reported significant alteration in BUN and serum creatinine levels as well as histopathological changes following FK506 administration [16,17]. Interestingly, concomitant administration of Vit E along with FK506 improved the renal function as indicated by significant reduction in BUN and serum creatinine levels compared with FK506 alone-treated rats. Furthermore, administration of Vit E along with FK506 improved the histopathological changes to a great extent as indicated by improvement in the tubular damage. Previously, it has been demonstrated that FK506 generates ROS in renal cells [4,14]. Furthermore, alterations in renal function and structural damage have been shown to be associated with lipid peroxidation induced by FK506 [16,17]. In the present study, Vit E was found to attenuate lipid peroxidation induced by FK506 indicating that Vit E has the ability to exert cells protection against oxidative damage induced by FK506. The highly reactive peroxynitrite ($ONOO^-$) that is usually produced by the reaction between nitric oxide (NO) and superoxide (O_2^-) has been demonstrated to be involved in renal cellular damage [18]. Moreover, it has been reported that renal injury induced by FK506 is associated with the production of NO [5]. In the present work, it was observed that Vit E has the ability to inhibit the expression of iNOS (that catalyze the production of NO) induced by FK506 in renal tissues indicating that Vit E has the ability to exert cells protection against oxidative damage induced by FK506 via inhibition of iNOS expression and consequently NO level.

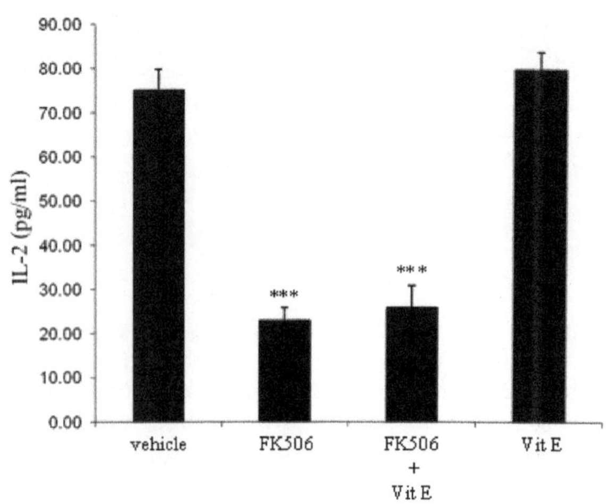

Fig. 5. Effects of FK506 and/or Vit E on serum level of IL-2 in male Wistar albino rats
*Data represent means ± S.D. (n=6), *** p < 0.001 versus control*

Furthermore, it was found that Vit E has the ability to inhibit FK506-induced NF-κB expression that plays an important role in the transcription of the inflammatory enzyme iNOS and other inflammatory genes in response to oxidative stress [19-21]. An efficient endogenous antioxidant defense system operates to scavenge the reactive oxygen species. The most important endogenous antioxidants are GSH, SOD and CAT [22-25]. In agreement with previous study [17], it was found that treatment of rats with FK506 produced a significant reduction in the endogenous antioxidants GSH, SOD and CAT. This reduction in oxygen radical scavenger system due to the toxic effects of FK506 leads to oxidative stress and renal injury. Interestingly, concomitant administration of Vit E along with FK506 significantly increased the renal level of GSH as well as SOD and CAT activities which play a major role in cells protection against oxidative damage. Moreover, the present work demonstrates that the immunosuppressive effect of FK506 was not affected in the presence of Vit E. In the present work, Vit E was found to protect against oxidative damage induced by FK506 as indicated by improvement not only in histopathological changes but also in renal function. These positive effects of Vit E were associated with an increase in oxygen radical scavenger system (endogenously produced) and decrease in the oxidative damage markers.

5. CONCLUSION

The findings of present work demonstrate that Vit E has the ability to protect against FK506-induced nephrotoxicity due to its ability to restore the balance between oxygen radical formation and the endogenous oxygen radical scavenger system which was disturbed by FK506 in renal tissue. These findings suggest that concomitant use of Vit E might be useful in reducing renal toxicity induced by FK506 via inhibition of ROS, iNOS, and NF-κB expression.

CONSENT

It is not applicable.

ETHICAL APPROVAL

All procedures performed in this study were approved by the Institutional Animal Ethics Committee.

COMPETING INTERESTS

Authors have declared that no competing interests exist.

REFERENCES

1. Schreiber SL, Crabtree GR. The mechanism of action of cyclosporine A and FK506. Immunol Today. 1992;13:136-142.
2. Naesens M, Kuypers DRJ, Sarwal M. Calcineurin inhibitor nephrotoxicity. Clin J Am Soc Nephrol. 2009;4:481-508.
3. Hisamura F, Kojima-Yuasa A, Kennedy DO, Matsui-Yuasa I. Protective effect of green tea extract and tea polyphenols against FK506-Induced cytotoxicity in renal cells. Basic Clin Pharmacol Toxicol. 2006;98:192-196.
4. Akool El-S, Doller A, Babelova A, Tsalastra W, Moret K, Schaefer L, Pfeilschifter J, Eberhardt W. Molecular mechanisms of TGF beta receptor-triggered signaling cascades rapidly induced by the calcineurin inhibitors cyclosporin A and FK506. J Immunol. 2008;181:2831-2845.
5. Ara C, Dirican A, Unal B, Bay Karabulut A, Piskin T. The effect of melatonin against FK506-induced renal oxidative stress in rats. Surg Innov. 2011;18:34-38.
6. Wolf R, Wolf D, Ruocco V. Vitamin E: the radical protector. J Eur Acad Dermatol Venereol. 1998;10:103-117.
7. Ohkatsu Y, Kajiyama T, Arai Y. Antioxidant activities of tocopherols. Polymer degradation and stability. 2001;72:303-311.
8. Burton GW, Ingold KU. Vitamin E as an in vitro and in vivo antioxidant. Ann N Y Acad Sci. 1989;570:7-22.
9. Cordero Z, Drogan D, Weikert C, Boeing H. Vitamin E and risk of cardiovascular diseases: A review of epidemiologic and clinical trial studies. Crit Rev Food Sci Nutr. 2010;50:420-440.
10. Mitamura T, Yamada A, Ishida H, Fujihira S, Ohara K, Noguchi H, Mine Y. Tacrolimus (FK506)-induced nephrotoxicity in spontaneous hypertensive rats. J Toxicol Sci. 1994;19:219-26.
11. Kongkham S, Sriwong S, Tasanarong A. Protective effect of alpha tocopherol on contrast-induced nephropathy in rats. Nefrologia. 2013;33:116-123
12. Drury RVA, Walligton EA. Carltons Histological techniques, 5th ed, Oxford University Press, New York, Pronto; 1980.
13. Tocci MJ1, Matkovich DA, Collier KA, Kwok P, Dumont F, Lin S, Degudicibus S,

Siekierka JJ, Chin J, Hutchinson NI. The immunosuppressant FK506 selectively inhibits expression of early T cell activation genes. J Immunol. 1989;143:718-726.

14. Jeon SH, Park HM, Kim SJ, Lee MY, Kim GB, Rahman MM, Woo JN, Kim IS, Kim JS, Kang HS. Taurine reduces FK506-induced generation of ROS and activation of JNK and Bax in Madin Darby canine kidney cells. Hum Exp Toxicol. 2010;29:627-633.
15. Akool ES, Gauer S, Osman B, Doller A, Schulz S, Geiger H, Pfeilschifter J, Eberhardt W. Cyclosporin A and tacrolimus induce renal Erk1/2 pathway via ROS-induced and metalloproteinase-dependent EGF-receptor signaling. Biochem Pharmacol. 2012;83:286-295.
16. Silva WT, dos Santos JG, Watanabe M, Vattimo MFF. Renoprotective effects of wine flavonoids in nephrotoxicity of the immunosuppressant Tacrolimus. Acta Paul Enferm. 2011;24:388-392.
17. Al-Harbi NO, Imam F, Al-Harbi MM, Iqbal M, Nadeem A, Al-Shahrah OA, Korashy MH, Al-Hosaini AK, Ahmed M, Bahashwar S. Treatment with aliskiren ameliorates tacrolimus-induced nephrotoxicity in rats. J Renin Angiotensin Aldosterone Syst; 2014 [Epub ahead of print].
18. Josephine A, Amudha G, Veena CK, Preetha SP, Varalakshmi P. Oxidative and nitrosative stress mediated renal cellular damage induced by cyclosporine A: Role of sulphated polysaccharides. Biol Pharm Bull. 2007;30:1254-1259.
19. Nanxin LI, Karin M. Is NF-kB the sensor of oxidative stress? FASEB J. 1999;13:1137-1143.
20. Tak PP, Firestein GS. NF-κB: A key role in inflammatory diseases. J Clin Invest. 2001;107:7-11.
21. Aktan F. iNOS-mediated nitric oxide production and its regulation. Life Sciences 2004;75: 639-653.
22. Meister A, Anderson ME. Glutathione. Ann Rev Biochem. 1983;52:711-760.
23. Inselmann G, Lawerenz HU, Nellessen U, Heidemann HAT. Enhancement of cyclosporin a induced hepato- and nephrotoxicity by glutathione depletion. Eur J Clin Invest. 1994;24:355-359.
24. Deisseroth A, Dounce AL. Catalase: Physical and chemical properties, mechanism of catalysis and physiological role. Physiol Rev. 1970;50:319-375.
25. McCord JM, Keele BB Jr, Fridovich I. An enzyme-based theory of obligate anaerobiosis: The physiological function of superoxide dismutase. Proc Natl Acad Sci USA. 1971;68:1024-1027.

Effectiveness of Systemic Administration of Amoxycillin and Metronidazole versus Azithromycin in Generalized Aggressive Periodontitis – A Randomized Controlled Clinical Trial

Archana Mootha[1*], Sankari Malaiappan[1], Sheeja S. Varghese[1] and N. D. Jayakumar[1]

[1] *Department of Periodontics, Saveetha Dental College and Hospitals, Velappanchavadi, Chennai – 600077, India.*

Authors' contributions

This work was carried out in collaboration between all authors. All authors read and approved the final manuscript.

Article Information

Editor(s):
(1) Salvatore Chirumbolo, Clinical Biochemist, Department of Medicine, University of Verona, Italy.
Reviewers:
(1) Arda Isik, Erzincan University, Turkey.
(2) Ilham Zahir, University Sidi Mohamed Ben Abdellah, Morocco.

ABSTRACT

Aim: To evaluate the effect of systemic Amoxycillin and Metronidazole against Azithromycin as an adjunct to non-surgical therapy and correlate the clinical periodontal parameters at baseline, 10 days and 30 days in subjects with generalized aggressive periodontitis (GAP).
Study Design: Randomized controlled clinical trial.
Place and Duration of the Study: The study was conducted in Saveetha Dental College and Hospitals from February 2015 to August 2015.
Methods: Subjects were recruited from the outpatient department of Periodontics and were categorized as GAP according to AAP criteria. A total of 16 patients with GAP were included in the study. Clinical periodontal parameters like sulcus bleeding index [SBI], gingival index [GI], Probing depth [PD] and clinical attachment loss [CAL] were recorded at baseline. The subjects were then randomly allotted into Group 1 [Amoxycillin+Metronidazole] and Group II [Azithromycin]. After

*Corresponding author: Email: archanamootha@gmail.com

evaluation of clinical parameters at baseline, scaling and root planning [SRP] was done in both the Groups and systemic antibiotics, namely combination of Amoxycillin and Metronidazole in Group I and Azithromycin in Group II were administered. Subjects were recalled at day 10 and 30 for re-evaluation of clinical parameters. Within Group comparison was made using paired "t test" and inter Group comparison was made using Un-paired "t test".

Results: Intra-Group comparisons of clinical parameters between baseline and 30 days, in both the Groups were statistically significant ($P<0.05$). The difference from baseline to 30 days follow up in sulcus bleeding index (8.7±0.59 versus 4.1±0.38 mm) and clinical attachment loss (8.8±0.48 versus 4.6±0.39 mm) was statistically significant between the Groups ($P<0.05$). Whereas no statistical significance was found with gingival index and probing depth between the Groups ($P>0.05$).

Conclusion: Systemic administration of Azithromycin as an adjunct to SRP in subjects with GAP resulted in better improvement of clinical periodontal parameters compared to a combination of Amoxycillin and Metronidazole.

Keywords: Azithromycin; generalized aggressive periodontitis; SRP; non-surgical therapy; adjunctive systemic antibiotics.

1. INTRODUCTION

Periodontitis is an infectious polymicrobial disease affecting the attachment apparatus of the teeth [1,2]. It is categorized as aggressive periodontitis and chronic periodontitis, each of which can be sub classified as localized or generalized type [3]. Chronic periodontitis can be managed adequately by disruption of local factors whereas mechanical therapy alone is inadequate in aggressive periodontitis as it is a disease entity with microbial invasion deep into epithelium and connective tissue [4]. Generalized aggressive periodontitis (GAP) is an inflammatory disease of the periodontal tissues caused by infection with highly virulent periodontal pathogens in susceptible individuals [5]. Clinically, it is characterized by rapid interproximal attachment loss with radiographic evidence of bone loss affecting at least three permanent teeth other than the first molars and incisors, eventually leading to loss of teeth [6,7]. Various drugs like Amoxycillin, Metronidazole, Tetracyclines, Ciprofloxacin, Azithromycin have been used as an adjunctive measure for its management [8,9]. These antibiotics are chosen because of various reasons like activity against anaerobic flora, higher concentrations in gingival crevicular fluid [10], sustained for longer duration in the tissues, and anticollagenolytic properties [11-13]. Azithromycin is recently administered in periodontitis [14]. Previously studies have compared the effectiveness of Azithromycin in comparison to Metronidazole in chronic periodontitis [15] but no study has compared the effects of Amoxicillin and Metronidazole versus Azithromycin in aggressive periodontitis. Thus the aim of this study is to evaluate the effectiveness of systemic Amoxycillin and Metronidazole against Azithromycin as an adjunct to non-surgical therapy and correlate the clinical periodontal parameters at baseline, 10 days and 30 days in subjects with GAP.

2. MATERIALS AND METHODS

The study population comprised of native residents of South India who were recruited from the Department of Periodontics, Saveetha Dental College and Hospitals, Chennai. The patients were categorized as GAP patients according to the 1999 American academy of Periodontology (AAP) criteria. Sixteen subjects were included in the study and randomly allocated to Group I or Group II. The study was verbally explained to each patient and a signed informed consent was obtained from all the participants. Ethical approval was obtained from the institutional Scientific Review Board committee (SRB) and patients were informed prior to commencement of the study (SRB reference number: SRB/SDMDS12ORT17). The power of the study was set to 90%.

2.1 Inclusion and Exclusion Criteria

Systemically healthy subjects who were between the age of 16 and 30 when first diagnosed with GAP and had a minimum of 20 teeth present, who did not receive any antibiotics or underwent periodontal treatment during the last 6 months were included in the study. Pregnant or lactating women, subjects with systemic disease, history of drug allergies, long term antibiotic/ antiinflammatory therapy and those not willing to give consent for the study were excluded.

A detailed medical and dental history was taken following which clinical and radiographic examination was done for all the study subjects by a single examiner. Orthopantomogram (OPG) was taken for all the sixteen subjects (Fig. 1). Baseline full-mouth clinical parameters, i.e; Sulcus bleeding index (SBI), gingival index (GI), probing depth (PD), and clinical attachment loss (CAL) were recorded. The probing depth was measured on all the six sites from the crest of the gingival margin to the base of the pocket using a graduated manual probe (University of North Carolina (UNC) 15-mm probe; Hu-Friedy) as shown in Fig. 2. CAL was recorded from the cemento-enamel junction (CEJ) to the base of the pocket using the same probe. Microbial analysis was not performed in this study.

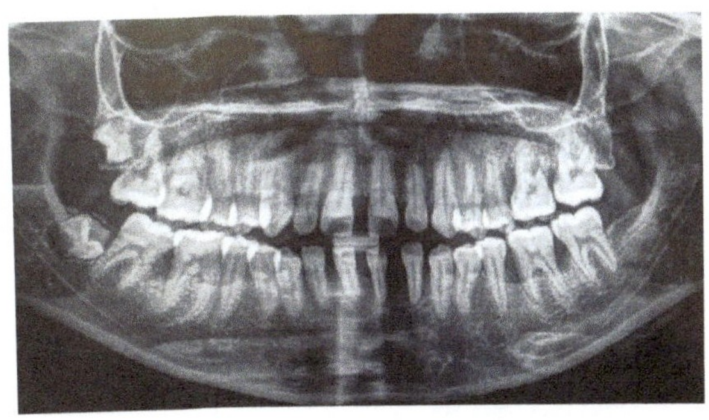

Fig. 1. OPG showing angular defect in relation to permanent first molars

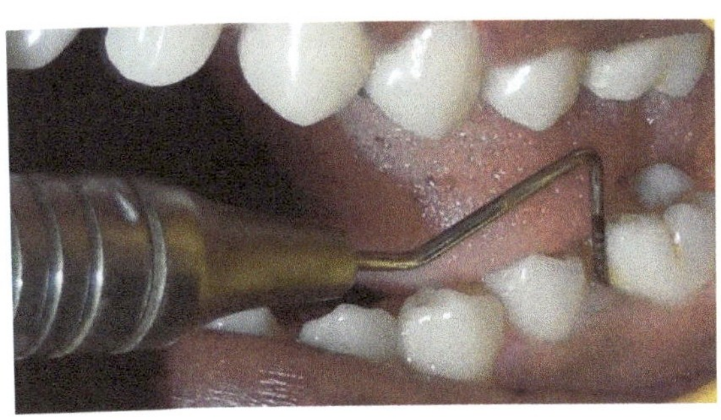

Fig. 2. Deep pocket present in relation to permanent first lower molar

The subjects were randomly divided into two Groups (Group I and Group II) using lottery method based on the antibiotic regimen. During this visit, subjects underwent full-mouth scaling and root planning under LA, following which, systemic antibiotics were prescribed. Patients assigned to Group I (n = 8) were given a combination of Amoxycillin 500mg plus Metronidazole 400mg, three times a day for 8 days (12). Patients assigned to Group II (n = 8) were given Azithromycin 500mg once a day for 5 days (14). Subjects were recalled after 10 and 30 days for re-evaluation and recording of clinical parameters.

The mean values of bleeding on probing (SBI), gingival index (GI), probing depth (PD), and clinical attachment loss (CAL) within the Groups were compared using the 'Student paired "*t*" Test'. Inter-group comparisons were made by 'un-paired t test'. *P* value of <0.05 was considered as statistically '*significant*' and *P* value < 0.001 was considered as statistically '*highly significant*'.

3. RESULTS

Tables 1-4 describe the comparison of mean values and the statistical significance in clinical parameters between Groups.

Table 1. Comparison of SBI values between Group I and Group II

	Baseline	30 days	*P* value
Group I (n=8)	8.4±0.37	4.7±0.5	0.0001*
Group II (n=8)	8.7±0.59	4.1±0.38	0.0001*
Inter Group comparison – SBI (t test)	0.023		

Sulcus bleeding index (SBI), Group I- Amoxycillin+Metronidazole, Group II- Azithromycin

Tables 1 and 2 show *high statistical significant* intra-group difference in SBI and GI between baseline and 30 day follow up in both the Groups. Tables 3 and 4 shows high *statistically significant* intra-group difference with relation to PD and CAL in Group II; and *significant* intra-group difference with relation to PD and CAL in Group I.

Table 2. Comparison of GI values between Group I and Group II

	Baseline	30 days	*P* value
Group I (n=8)	4.8±0.13	0.4±0.15	0.0001*
Group II (n=8)	4.5±0.43	0.6±0.16	0.0001*
Inter Group comparison – GI (t test)	0.211		

Gingival index (GI), Group I- Amoxycillin+Metronidazole, Group II- Azithromycin

The inter-group comparisons of SBI (P = 0.023) and CAL (P = 0.059) were statistically significant at 30 days follow up, whereas no significant inter-group difference was found with relation to GI (P = 0.211) and PD (P = 0.063).

Table 3. Comparison of PD values between Group I and Group II

	Baseline	30 days	*P* value
Group I (n=8)	8.0±0.58	4.82±0.40	0.018
Group II (n=8)	8.1±0.46	4.63±0.46	0.001*
Inter Group comparison – PPD(t test)	0.063		

Probing depth (PD), Group I-Amoxycillin+Metronidazole, Group II- Azithromycin

Table 4. Comparison of CAL values between Group I and Group II

	Baseline	30 days	*P* value
Group I (n=8)	8.8±0.44	5.53±0.28	0.02
Group II (n=8)	8.8±0.48	4.6±0.39	0.001*
Inter Group comparison – CAL(t test)	0.059		

Clinical attachment loss (CAL), Group I-Amoxycillin+Metronidazole, Group II- Azithromycin

4. DISCUSSION

GAP is a polymicrobial infectious disease with microbial invasion into epithelium and connective tissues [6]. Pathogenic bacteria may persist on the various tooth surfaces even after periodontal surgical procedures. Reservoirs of pathogenic microflora include the furcation area of roots [16], dentinal tubules [17], lateral canals, areas inaccessible to instrumentation, deep anatomical defects, including the soft tissue wall of the pocket, where bacteria are present in deeper layers of connective tissue and bone [18,19]. Current literature suggests that the clinical results of mechanical debridement can be improved by the adjunctive use of systemic antibiotics in the management of aggressive and refractory periodontitis [20]. Sites that are refractory to treatment can be managed with local drug delivery. Since there is generalized involvement in GAP, a systemic regimen of antibiotics is required.

It is known that microbes like *Actinobacillus actinomycetemcomitans (Aa), Porphyromonas gingivalis (Pg), Tanerella forsythia (Tf), Treponema denticola (Td)* play an etiological role in the pathogenesis of aggressive periodontitis. Studies with microbial studies have concluded that treatment of GAP was not complete without the elimination of these microorganisms and that the efficacy of mechanical treatment was limited. Thus, use of different antibiotics either single or a combination of drugs as an adjunct to SRP have been recommended to successfully eliminate these periodontal pathogens [21]. Similar results have been reported by Kapoor and Prakasam et al. [22,23] where patients with LAP positive for Aa, Pg, and Tf, were given Doxycycline or Amoxycillin plus Metronidazole combination before SRP. Baltacioglu et al. [24] reported that treatment of aggressive periodontitis with SRP plus systemic antibiotics provided clinical benefits over treatment with SRP alone, which reduced the need for periodontal surgery.

The use of Amoxicillin/Metronidazole as an adjunct to non-surgical therapy was supported by a systematic review by Sqolastra et al. [25]. Azithromycin has been recently administered in AgP as an adjunct to non-surgical therapy [26]. In addition Azithromycin had been proven to concentrate locally in saliva, healthy and pathological gingival tissue, reach concentrations greater than the minimum inhibitory concentrations of microbes associated with pathophysiology of periodontal disease and has been reported to have high penetrability in fibroblasts [27].

5. CONCLUSION

Due of the relative absence of RCT's in GAP, no definitive guidelines exist regarding the most effective antibiotic regime, dosage and time of administration of drug. Therefore, this study was undertaken in order to evaluate the effects of a combination of systemic Amoxycillin and Metronidazole versus Azithromycin as an adjunct to nonsurgical therapy among subjects with GAP and compare their effects on clinical parameters at 30 day recall.

On clinical examination, a statistically significant decrease in SBI, GI, PD and CAL was noted between the baseline and 30 days in both the Groups. Patients treated with Azithromycin showed a greater decrease in SBI and CAL scores between the Groups compared to the Amoxycillin+Metronidazole Group. These results are in accordance with the results of studies by Ercan et al. [28] where Amoxycillin and Metronidazole were administered to patients as an adjunct to mechanical therapy. The findings of this study indicate that when patients with GAP were given Azithromycin as an adjunct to non-surgical therapy demonstrated a significant improvement in SBI and CAL compared to those with Amoxycillin+Metronidazole during 30 days.

As CAL is the most ideal indicator of periodontal tissue destruction, the significant decrease in its values between the Groups should be noted. Short duration of follow up and small sample size are drawbacks of this study. Further studies with a larger sample size and longer evaluation period are essential to evaluate the long term disease activity.

Within the limitations of the study, the results indicate that systemic administration of Azithromycin as an adjunct to non-surgical therapy resulted in improvement of clinical periodontal parameters compared to a combination of Amoxycillin+Metronidazole. Since this is a study with a small sample size, further RCT's with a larger sample size and longer follow up with microbial analysis are required for proving the consistency and clinical applicability of the results.

COMPETING INTERESTS

Authors have declared that no competing interests exist.

REFERENCES

1. Hajishengallis G, Lamont RJ. Beyond the red complex and into more complexity: The polymicrobial synergy and dysbiosis (PSD) model of periodontal disease etiology. Mol Oral Microbiol. 2012;27(6):409-419.
2. Md A Nahid, Mercedes Rivera, Alexandra Lucas, Edward KL Chan, Kesavalu L. Polymicrobial infection with periodontal pathogens specifically enhances MicroRNA miR-146a in ApoE$^{-/-}$ Mice during experimental periodontal disease. Infect Immun. 2011;79:1597-1605.
3. highfield J. Diagnosis and classification of periodontal disease. Aust Dent J. 2009; 53(1):11-26.
4. Standards for reporting chronic periodontitis prevalence and severity in epidemiologic studies. Birte Holtfreter, Jasim M Albandar, Thomas Dietrich, Bruce A Dye, Kenneth A Eaton, Paul I Eke, et al. J Clin Periodontol. 2015;43(5):407-412.
5. Jasim M Albandar. Aggressive periodontitis: Case definition and diagnostic criteria. Periodontol 2000. 2014;65(1):13-26.
6. Wim Teughels, Rutger Dhondt, Christel Dekeyser, Marc Quirynen. Treatment of aggressive periodontitis. Periodontol 2000. 2014;66(1):107-133.
7. Roshna T, Nandakumar K. Generalized aggressive periodontitis and its treatment options. Case Rep Med. 2011;2012:1-17.
8. Keestra JAJ, Grosjean W Coucke, Quirynen M, Teughels W. Non-surgical periodontal therapy with systemic antibiotics in patients with untreated chronic periodontitis: A systematic review and meta-analysis. J Periodont Res. 2014; 50(3):294-314.
9. Vishakha Patil, Rohono Mali, Amita Mali. Systemic anti-microbial agents used in periodontal therapy. J Indian Soc Periodontol. 2013;17:162-68.
10. Nidhi Jain, Pin-Chuang Lai, John D Walters. Effect of gingivitis on azithromycin concentrations in gingival crevicular fluid. J Perioodntol. 2012;83:1122-28.
11. Reza Amid, Mohammad Bagher Tabeie, Mahdi Kadkhodazadeh, Amir Reza Mehdizadeh, Navid Youssefi. Local concentration of systemic amoxicillin and metronidazole in healthy and inflamed gingiva: A comparative *in vivo* study. Drug Metabol Personal Ther. 2012;27(2):113-118.
12. Lai PC, Ho W, Jain N, Walters JD. Azithromycin concentrations in blood and gingival crevicular fluid after systemic administration. J Periodontol. 2011;82(11): 1582-6.
13. Bangalore Varadhan Karthikeyan, Devireddy Venkata Tejaswi, Munivenkatappa Lakshmaiah Venkatesh Prabhuji. Non-Antibacterial implications of tetracyclines in the management of periodontitis: An Update. J Immunodefic Disor. 2013;2:1-7.
14. Francisco Walker, Mustafa Gomes, Muniz N Camila, Carvalhode Oliveira, Rosimary de Sousa, Carvalho, et al. Azithromycin: A new concept in adjuvant treatment of periodontitis. Eur J Pharmacol. 2013;705: 135–39.
15. Jawna Mammdoh K. Efficacy of azithromycin in comparison to metronidazole in the treatment of chronic periodontitis. Al-Rafidain Dent J. 2011;11: 323-30.
16. Abdullah Seckin Ertugrul, Hacer Sahin. Relationship between furcation defects and periodontal disease. Univ Res J Med Dent. 2012;1(9):108-114.

17. Silvio Taschieri, Massimo Del Fabbro, Lakshman Samaranayake, Jeffrey WW Chang, Stefano Corbella. Microbial invasion of dentinal tubules: A literature review and a new perspective. J Investig Clin Dent. 2014;5(3):163-170.
18. Joseph M DiRienzo. Breaking the gingival epithelial barrier: Role of the aggregatibacter actinomycetemcomitans cytolethal distending toxin in oral infectious disease. Cells. 2014;3(2):476-499.
19. Annapurna Ahuja, Baiju CS, Vipin Ahuja. Role of antibiotics in generalized aggressive periodontitis: A review of clinical trials in humans. J Indian Soc Periodontol. 2012;16(3):317-323.
20. Cleverton Correa Rabelo, Magda Feres, Cristiane Gonçalves, Luciene C Figueiredo, Marcelo Faveri, Yu-Kang Tu, et al. Systemic antibiotics in the treatment of aggressive periodontitis. A systematic review and a Bayesian Network meta-analysis. J Clin Periodontol. 2015;42(7): 647-57.
21. Fabrizio Sgolastra, Ambra Petrucci, Roberto Gatto, Annalisa Monaco. Effectiveness of systemic amoxicillin/ metronidazole as an adjunctive therapy to full-mouth scaling and root planing in the treatment of aggressive periodontitis: A systematic review and meta-analysis. J Periodontol. 2012;83(6):731-743.
22. Kapoor A, Malhotra R, Grover V, Grover D. Systemic antibiotic therapy in periodontics. Dent Res J. 2012;9:505-15.
23. Prakasam A, Elavarasu SS, Natarajan RK. Antibiotics in the management of aggressive periodontitis. J Pharm Bioallied Sci. 2012;2:252-55.
24. Baltacioglu E, Aslan M, Sarac O, Saybak A, Yuva P. Analysis of clinical results of systemic antimicrobials combined with nonsurgical periodontal treatment for generalized aggressive periodontitis: A pilot study. J Can Dent Assoc. 2011;77:97.
25. Sgolastra F, Petrucci A, Gatto R, Monaco A. Effectiveness of systemic amoxicillin/ metronidazole as an adjunctive therapy to full-mouth scaling and root planing in the treatment of aggressive periodontitis: A systematic review and meta-analysis. J Periodontol. 2012;83(6):731-43.
26. Emingil G1, Han B, Ozdemir G, Tervahartiala T, Vural C, Atilla G, Baylas H, Sorsa T. Effect of azithromycin, as an adjunct to nonsurgical periodontal treatment, on microbiological parameters and gingival crevicular fluid biomarkers in generalized aggressive periodontitis. J Periodontal Res. 2012;47(6):729-39.
27. Chirayu Shah, Monali Shah, Deepak Dave, Prasad Nadig, Amit Shah. Azithromycin I Perioodntics. Adv Hum Biol. 2012;2(3):1-5.
28. Ercan E, Uzun BC, Ustaoglu G. Effects of azithromycin versus metronidazole-amoxicillin combination as an adjunct to nonsurgical periodontal therapy of generalized aggressive periodontitis. Niger J Clin Pract. 2015;18:506-10.

22

Preliminary Shelf Life Studies of *In-vitro* Antioxidant Potential of Gamma Irradiated Dried Mushrooms (*Pleurotus ostreatus* Ex. Fries) Kummer in Ghana

N. K. Kortei[1*], G. T. Odamtten[1,2], V. Appiah[1], M. Obodai[3], D. L. Narh Mensah[3], P. T. Akonor[3], M. Wiafe- Kwagyan[2], M. Ayim- Akonor[4] and R. M. Adaboro[5]

[1]*Department of Nuclear Agriculture and Radiation Processing, Graduate School of Nuclear and Allied Sciences, P.O.Box LG 80, Legon, Ghana.*
[2]*Department of Botany, University of Ghana, P.O.Box LG 55, Legon, Ghana.*
[3]*Food Research Institute- Council for Scientific and Industrial Research, P.O.Box M20, Accra, Ghana.*
[4]*Animal Research Institute- Council for Scientific and Industrial Research, P.O.Box AH20, Achimota, Ghana.*
[5]*Ghana Atomic Energy Commission, Applied Radiation Biology Centre, P.O.Box AE 1, Atomic, Ghana.*

Authors' contributions

This work was carried out in collaboration between all authors. Authors NKK, GTO and VA designed the study, wrote the protocol and wrote the first draft of the manuscript. Authors MO, VA and DLNM managed the literature searches, analyses of the study performed the spectroscopy analysis. Authors RMA, PTA and MWK managed the experimental process and authors MO and GTO identified the species of mushrooms. All authors read and approved the final manuscript.

Article Information

Editor(s):
(1) Vasudevan Mani, Universiti Teknologi MARA (UiTM), Selangor, Malaysia.
Reviewers:
(1) Mutemi Muthangya, South Eastern Kenya University, Kenya.
(2) Ali Mohamed Elshafei, National Research Centre, Egypt.

ABSTRACT

Aim: Antioxidant potential of dried and gamma irradiated mushrooms (*Pleurotus ostreatus*) were assessed over a 12 months storage period.
Place and Duration of Study: Laboratory work was carried out at the Applied Radiation and Biological Centre, Radiological and Medical Research Institute, Ghana Atomic Energy

**Corresponding author: Email: nii_korley_1@yahoo.com*

Commission, Accra. From 25th June 2013 to 25th June 2014.
Methodology: Mushrooms were stored in polythene and polypropylene packs and were irradiated with ionizing radiation from a cobalt-60 source at doses of 0.5, 1, 1.5, 2 kGy at a dose rate of 1.7 kGy/hr at room temperature of 28-30℃. The control was not irradiated. Total phenolic contents, flavonoids and free radical scavenging activity DPPH (2, 2'-diphenyl-1-picrylhydrazyl) were examined at 0, 3, 6 and 12 months of storage using aqueous, ethanol and methanol extracts by Folin-Ciocalteu's method.
Results: Total phenolic content ranged from 0.50±0.01- 10.96±1.7 mg/GAE, flavonoids ranged from 1.64±0.05- 8.90±0.6 mg/QE, DPPH radical scavenging activity also ranged from 6.85±0.10-13.03±0.04% and IC_{50} values also ranged from 0.069 - 1.071 mg/ml. Both extracts and the treatment doses of mushrooms stored in polythene and polypropylene packs differed significantly ($P<0.05$). Good linear correlation was confirmed between the values for the total phenolic content and antioxidant activity of mushroom extracts.
Conclusion: *Pleurotus ostreatus* could be regarded as a promising candidate for natural mushroom sources of antioxidants with high value due to the presence of high phenolic compounds which contribute to high antioxidant activity. Employing low dose gamma radiation by the local food industry could enhance the hygienic quality, extend shelf-life, and preserve nutrients and anti-nutrients.

Keywords: Antioxidant; gamma radiation; Pleurotus ostreatus; total phenolic content; flavonoids; IC_{50}.

1. INTRODUCTION

Mushrooms have been used for many years as nutritional food and food flavouring materials as well as medicines [1-3]. Because of their flavour and aroma, mushrooms are greatly appreciated in many countries. In Ghana, several mushroom species are collected from the wild in forest zones during rainy seasons [4,5] and used for diverse purposes for thousands of years [6] an activity which dates back the emergence of ethnomycology as a discipline in many parts of the world. The use of familiar mushroom species such as *Termitomyces robusta, Termitomyces globulus, Coprinus disseminatus, Volvariella volvacea* (Domo in Akan language) and *Pleurotus* spp. as blood tonic, treatment for blood pressure in hypertensives, etc are well documented by some researchers [7-9]. Nonetheless, the consumption of some species of mushrooms not properly identified and documented, causes minimal exploitation of their full potential and results in the mushrooms remaining mysterious. A lot of mushrooms have had their potency either exaggerated or underutilized. Some special mushrooms species according to oral folklore [10] has had attention to date due to speculative peculiar attributes such as natural sex enhancing boosters for men, rheumatism treatment, purgative drugs and hallucinative effects etc. when consumed while others unfortunately, have become extinct as a result of human activities during farming (weedicide, fungicides, fertilizer etc. application), urbanization and annual wild fire outbreak.

The poor identification and documentation as outlined by [11] of edible and medicinal species of mushrooms in many developing nations including Ghana over the years have created some degrees of inconsistencies in their usages relative to folk medicine practice, food and mythological beliefs. Their relevance in modern day pharmaceutics and nutraceuticals is a product of human experimentation over time. Factors that may be anthropogenic, ethnographic, ethnoecological/ environmental have been implicated in mushrooms underutilization and under-exploration of mushrooms in West Africa.

These observations still form the basis of modern scientific studies of fungal medicinal activities, especially in the field of cancer development. It is therefore essential and noteworthy how reliable these facts collected by traditional West African medicine are in the study of medicinal mushrooms [12-14].

Polyphenols are secondary metabolites distributed moderately in fungi which have important primary roles as defense against plant and mushroom pathogens and fungivore aggression or mycophagy and as response to various strenuous abiotic conditions, such as drought and ultraviolet or gamma radiation [15]. According to Lima et al. [16], some synthetic phenolic antioxidants such as Butylatedhy-droxyanisol (BHA), Tert-butylhydroquinone (TBHQ), Butylatedhydroxytoluene (BHT), 2-Tert-butyl-4-methylphenol (TBMP) and gallic acid esters are currently used in food industry and are considered harmful to human health. Studies by some researchers [17,18] have shown that high doses of TBHQ exert negative health effects on laboratory animals, such as DNA damage, which may lead to stomach tumors. BHA has also been reported to have the same genotoxic and carcinogenic effects in some animal tissues [19]. The current concern about adverse effects of synthetic antioxidants should be reiterated. Mushrooms as nutraceuticals may represent an alternative source of accessible natural antioxidants and a possible food supplement or exploited for other pharmaceutical applications. Explaining the mechanisms of polyphenols metabolism, it is an essential step in appreciating their health effects *in vivo*. Gut absorption and metabolism of these compounds depend on their connection with microbes of the intestines [20].

A debate has been raised about the role of fungi derived mycochemicals on the gut microflora since food is the main source of intake of natural polyphenols. The gut microbes may be altered in composition, biological activity and the mychochemicals could be converted by the colonic microbiota to bioactive compounds like steroids, terpenoids, β-glucans etc. that can affect host health [21,22]. Polyphenols are widely known to possess certain antimicrobial properties which suggest a development into new food preservatives [23] owing to the increasing consumer demands on the food industry to avoid synthetic preservatives, or to develop innovative therapies for the treatment of various microbial infections [24,25] considering the increase in microbial resistance against predictable antibiotic therapy [26].

Sequences of chemical reactions results in an imbalance between oxidant and antioxidant reactions and is typically referred to as oxidative stress [27,28]. Both classes of substances (oxidants and antioxidants) are generated in an oxidation- reduction (redox) set-up, where oxidations involve electron loss and reduction, electron gain [29,30] and has been implicated as causes of a lot of degenerative diseases such as atherosclerosis, cancer, and tissue damage in rheumatoid arthritis [31,32]. Reactive species are commonly identified as substances leading to the oxidation of lipids (lipoxidation), glucose (glycation) and proteins (carbonylation). The reaction products generated in lipoxidation are represented by malondialdehyde, glyoxal, acrolein, 4-hydroxy-nonenal (HNE). Those generated by glycation are methylglyoxal and glyoxal. These compounds react with proteins and amino acids resulting in amino-glycated end products (AGEs) [33]. Brownlee [34] outlined that AGEs are involved in regular events, which may trigger obesity and insulin resistance, diabetes mellitus II and inflammation, and could correspond to important activators of inflammation in various tissues. These outcomes appear quite encouraging but, on the other hand, most of them resulted from fresh and non pretreated sample materials.

Radiation treatments of biological systems have been employed for various processes: reduction of microbial contamination of food, sterilization of materials and increasing the safety and shelf life of foods [35]. The major constraint when using a gamma irradiated phenolic derivative that proves to possess elevated antioxidant and antimicrobial efficacy concerns its stability when stored for a long period of time. There are several reports on effect of irradiation processing on phenolic and flavonoid content as well as antioxidant activity from several plant and food products. Although, some studies report that, gamma irradiation does maintain or enhance the anti-oxidant properties; there are a few examples wherein the antioxidant properties of the food material were decreased [35].

This paper evaluates the stability of total phenolic content, total flavonoid content and antioxidants in dried mushrooms stored for 12 months period following gamma irradiation.

2. MATERIALS AND METHODS

Analytical ethanol, methanol and sodium hydrogen carbonate NAHCO3 were purchased from Sigma-Aldrich, USA. Standards of phenolic acids (gallic acid [3, 4, 5-Trihydroxybenzoic acid]) and of flavonoids, Potasium Acetate, Quercetin [3, 3',4', 5, 7-Pentahydroxyflavone], and 2,2-dyphenyl-1-picrylhydrazyl (DPPH) were obtained from Sigma Chemicals Co., St Louis, MO, USA. The Folin-Ciocalteu's phenol reagent, and Aluminium chloride (AlCl3) were from FlukaChemie AG, Buchs, Switzerland.

Micropipette 100-1000 µl (Iso lab, Germany), sensitive balance (Sartorius, Germany), ultra sonic bath, electric shaker (Vortex Genie 2, USA), Waring blender, moisture analyzer balance (Precisa, Switzerland), centrifuge (Shanghai surgical instruments factory, China), pH-meter (TOA HM-60S, Japan), spectrophotometer (Jasco V-530, USA) were used for sample preparation and antioxidant activity determination.

Pleurotus ostreatus originally from Mauritius, was cultivated on *Triplochiton scleroxylon* sawdust composted for 28 days, supplemented with 1% $CaCO_3$ and 10% wheat bran [36] at the Mushroom Unit of Food Research Institute-C.S.I.R, Accra, Ghana. Cultivation and harvesting was from the period between September and December, 2012. Mushroom fruit bodies were solar-dried at temperature range of 20- 40 πC to a moisture content of about 12%. Dried mushroom parts were cut up to average size of 2 cm x 3 cm, stored in tight-sealed polythene and polypropylene containers at room temperature. Samples for analysis were ground to powder and stored until needed.

2.1 Irradiation of Mushroom Materials

Forty (40) grams of dried mushrooms were packed into the various containers and irradiated at doses of 0, 0.5, 1, 1.5 and 2 kGy at a dose rate of 1.7 kGyhr -1 from a cobalt 60 source (SLL- 515, Hungary) with an average dose distribution ratio of0.69 in air at the Radiation Technology Centre (R.T.C) of the Ghana Atomic Energy Commission (G.A.E.C). The absorbed dose was determined by using Lithium fluoride photo-fluorescent film dosimeter (SUNNA Dosimeter System, UK).

2.2 Preparation of Mushroom Extracts

Methanolic, de-ionised water (aqueous) and ethanolic extracts of mushrooms were prepared by mixing 10% powder in solvent by constant agitation on a shaker (150 rpm, 30℃, 24 h) [37,38]. Extracts were filtered through Whatman filter paper (No. 1) and the filtrate was centrifuged (10000 rpm, 10℃, 10 min) to obtain a clear supernatant. Its yield was determined and 10 mg/ml stock solution prepared, which was stored in amber coloured bottles at 4℃ till further studies.

2.3 Determination of Total Phenolic Contents in the Mushroom Extracts

The concentration of phenolics in mushroom extracts was determined using spectrophotometric method [39]. Methanolic solution of the extract in the concentration of 1 mg/ml was used in the analysis. The reaction mixture was prepared by mixing 50 ml of methanolic solution of extracts, 2.5 ml of 10% Folin-Ciocalteu's reagent (v/v) dissolved in water and 2.5 ml 7.5% $NaHCO_3$. Blank was concomitantly prepared, containing 50 ml methanol, 2.5 ml 10% Folin-Ciocalteu's reagent dissolved in water and 2.5 ml of 7.5% of $NaHCO_3$. The samples were thereafter incubated in a thermostat at 45 πC for 45 min. The absorbance was determined using spectrophotometer at λmax = 760 nm. The samples were prepared in triplicate for each analysis and the mean value of absorbance was obtained. The same procedure was repeated for the standard solution of gallic acid and the calibration line was constructed. Based on the measured absorbance, the concentration of phenolics was read (mg ml^{-1}) from the calibration line; then the content of phenolics in extracts was expressed in terms of mg of gallic acid equivalent per gram of extract (mg of GAE/g of extract).

Concentration (mg/GAE) = Concentration x Volume /Weight of sample (1)

2.4 Determination of Flavonoid Concentrations in the Mushroom Extracts

The content of flavonoids in the examined mushroom extracts was determined using a modified spectrophotometric method [40]. The sample contained 500 ml of ethanol solution of the extract in the concentration of 1 mg/ml and 100 ml of 10% $AlCl_3$ solution dissolved in 1500 ml ethanol. The samples were incubated for an hour at room temperature. The absorbance was determined using spectrophotometer at λmax = 415 nm. The samples were prepared in triplicate for each analysis and the mean value of absorbance was obtained. The same procedure was repeated for the standard solution of 500 ml of Quercetin, 100 ml of Potassium acetate (10%) and the calibration line was constructed. Based on the measured absorbance, the concentration of flavonoids was read (mg/ml) on the calibration line; then, the content of flavonoids in extracts was expressed in terms of Quercetin equivalent (mg of QE/g of extract).

2.5 Evaluation of Antioxidant Activity and Ic_{50}

The ability of the mushroom extract to scavenge DPPH free radicals was assessed by the standard method [41], adopted with suitable modifications [42]. The stock solutions of extracts were prepared in methanol to achieve the concentration of 1 mg ml^{-1}. Dilutions were made to obtain concentrations of 0.01, 0.05, 0.1, 0.15

and 0.2 mg ml^{-1}. Diluted solutions of sample (200 ml each) were mixed with 3800 ml of methanolic solution of DPPH. After 30 min incubation in darkness at room temperature (23πC), the absorbance was recorded at 517 nm. Control sample contained all the reagents except the extract. Percentage inhibition was calculated using equation (2). The data were presented as mean values ± standard deviation (n =2).

$$\% \text{ inhibition} = (A_C - A_S)/A_C \times 100 \qquad (2)$$

A_c and A_s are absorbance readings for the control and test sample respectively.

IC_{50} value is the concentration of sample required to scavenge 50% of DPPH free radical and was calculated by plotting a graph of concentration and % inhibition. A linear regression was estimated to plot x-y and fit data with a straight line. From linear equation y= mx+ c.

Where y= 50 and x calculated.

2.6 Statistical Analysis

Duplicate experimental measurements were carried out and expressed as average of two analyses ± standard deviation. The degree of correlation between variables was done using a SPSS (Chicago, IL) statistical software package (SPSS for Windows, version XIV, 2004). Significances of differences were conducted with a Duncan's Multiple Range Test (DMRT). Linear regression analysis was used to determine total phenolics, total flavonoid contents and antioxidant activity using using Excel for Microsoft Windows 2003.

3. RESULTS AND DISCUSSION

The total phenolic content of the various extracts was compiled in Table 1. For 0- 3 months of storage, aqueous ranged 1.96±0.05 - 10.96±1.7 mgGAE/g. Methanol and ethanol extracts ranged from 0.56± 0.01- 4.81±0.4 mgGAE/g and 1.32 ± 0.02- 2.36±0.2 mgGAE/g respectively.

Generally, fairly superior values of antioxidant activity were recorded. However, there was a general decrease in total phenolic contents in all the extracts which caused some significant ($P<0.05$) differences. Periods of 6-12 months resulted in ranges of 1.90±0.05- 10.60±1.65 mgGAE/g, 1.20-2.38 mgGAE/g and 0.50- 4.81 mgGAE/g for aqueous, ethanol and methanol respectively. There was an apparent effect of 1 kGy irradiation dose generating greater quantity of TPC of 10.60- 10.96 mgGAE/g (Table 1). Irradiation dose of 0.5 kGy produced the most amounts of phenols for all the extracts while 2 kGy recorded least for the extracts.

The increase in phenolic compounds by gamma radiation could be attributed to their release from glycosidic components and the degradation of larger phenolic compounds into smaller ones or significant activation of phenol producing enzymes by gamma irradiation [43]. Conversely, an increase in the radiation dose 1 to 2 kGy did not result in a corresponding increase in the phenolic compounds but rather a decrease in the phenolic compound (Table 1). These results may indicate degradation or insolubilization of phenolic compounds when they are exposed to gamma irradiation [44]. However, studies need to be conducted with more samples to confirm the results.

Comparatively among the extracts, aqueous samples yielded the most of phenols of a range of 1.96-10.96 mgGAE/g (Table 1). Kumari et al. [45] also showed similar results with Triphala, where they reported a significant increase in gallic acid concentration and total phenolics in the water extract due to irradiation that leads to increase in antioxidant property. The phenolic compounds are usually hydrophilic and therefore would be extracted more in aqueous solvents than in methanol. Phenolic compounds such as *p*-Hydroxybenzoic acid, *p*- Coumaric acid and Cinnamic acid have been reported for *P.ostreatus* strain EM 1 [46]. Unekwu et al. [47] recorded significantly ($P<0.05$) higher values of a range of 97.16- 248.80 mgGAE/g for mushrooms species including *P. ostreatus, P. pulmonarius, Auricularia auricula, Hericium erinaceus, Lactarius deliciousus, Cantarellus cibarius, Termitomyces robustus* and *T. manniformis*. In contrast, studies by some researchers [48-50] reported lower values of 0.55 mgGAE/g (*Lentinula edodes*), 8.72 mgGAE/g (*A. fuscosuccinea*), 4.61 mgGAE/g (*A. mesenterica*), 1.04 mgGAE/g (*Tremella fuciformis*) which were within the range of results obtained in this work.
Also, results obtained compares well with common fruits and vegetables noted for their relatively high phenolic constituents such as apple (29.63±0.64 mg/g), banana (9.04±0.32 mg/g), lemon (8.19±0.35 mg/g), orange (8.12±0.11 mg/g), pineapple (9.43±0.15 mg/g), strawberry (16.00±0.12 mg/g), pear (7.06±0.16 mg/g), and grape (4.96±0.26 mg/g) [51,52].

Studies by some researchers [53,54] show that phenolic compounds have inhibitory effects on mutagenesis and carcinogenesis in humans, when up to 1.0 g ingested daily from a diet rich in mushrooms, fruits and/or vegetables. With regards to packaging material appropriateness, there was no significant (P>0.05) difference between polythene and polypropylene.

The total flavonoid content of the various extracts was compiled in Table 2. Flavonoid contents of doses and solvent extracts differed significantly ($p < 0.05$). Post irradiation storage studies of 0-3 months recorded a range of 3.09±0.2-8.92±0.6, 1.64±0.05- 7.86±0.4 and 2.10±0.1-5.37±0.5 mgQE/g for aqueous, ethanol and methanol respectively. 6-12 months also recorded ranged

Table 1. Effect of irradiation on total phenolic content of dried mushrooms stored in packaging materials for 12 months period

Time (month)	Package	Dose applied (kGy)	Extracts		
			Aqueous (mgGAE/g)	Ethanol (mgGAE/g)	Methanol (mgGAE/g)
0	Polythene	0	3.84±0.4 c	2.00±0.1 b	2.40±0.1 c
		0.5	5.00±0.3 d	2.36±0.2 bc	2.36±0.2 c
		1	4.63±0.3 c	1.54±0.18 b	4.81±0.4 d
		1.5	2.78±0.1 b	1.32 ± 0.02 a	2.83±0.1 c
		2	1.96±0.05 a	1.32±0.02 a	1.96±0.05 b
	Polypropylene	0	2.54±0.1 b	1.32±0.02 a	1.96±0.05 b
		0.5	4.46±0.3 c	1.96±0.05 bc	1.93±0.02 b
		1	10.96±1.7 e	1.53±0.04 b	1.35±0.03 a
		1.5	4.46±0.8 c	1.89±0.07 b	0.56±0.01 a
		2	2.50±0.2 b	1.76±0.05 b	1.40±0.03 a
3	Polythene	0	3.74±0.3c	1.70±0.05a	2.38±0.1c
		0.5	5.11±0.3d	2.31±0.2c	2.36±0.3c
		1	4.60±0.3c	1.50±0.14a	4.80±0.3d
		1.5	2.75±0.1b	1.31±0.02a	2.83±0.2c
		2	1.94±0.05a	1.30±0.01a	1.92±0.05b
	Polypropylene	0	2.54±0.1b	1.32±0.01a	1.91±0.02b
		0.5	4.42±0.3c	1.93±0.05c	1.93±0.03b
		1	10.90±1.7e	1.50±0.03a	1.32±0.02a
		1.5	4.40±0.6c	1.84±0.05b	0.51±0.02a
		2	2.48±0.2b	1.73±0.03b	1.43±0.03b
6	Polythene	0	3.70±0.30c	1.20±0.01a	2.26±0.2c
		0.5	5.03±0.3cd	2.36±0.3c	2.27±0.2c
		1	4.59±0.40c	1.54±0.13b	4.79±0.3d
		1.5	2.70±0.20b	1.27±0.02a	2.83±0.2c
		2	1.90±0.05a	1.30± 0.01a	1.91±0.05b
	Polypropylene	0	2.57±0.10b	1.32±0.01a	1.96±0.02b
		0.5	4.41±0.30c	1.96±0.05b	1.92±0.02b
		1	9.87±1.60e	1.53±0.03b	1.35±0.02a
		1.5	4.42±0.60c	1.89±0.05bc	0.50±0.01a
		2	2.50±0.20b	1.70 ±0.02bc	1.26±0.02a
12	Polythene	0	3.84±0.40c	2.00±0.30b	2.41±0.1c
		0.5	4.81±0.20cd	2.38±0.4c	2.36±0.4c
		1	4.63±0.30c	1.54±0.03b	4.81±0.3d
		1.5	2.73±0.20b	1.32±0.02a	2.83±0.2c
		2	1.94±0.06a	1.30±0.02a	1.92±0.04b
	Polypropylene	0	2.54±0.20b	1.32±0.01a	1.96±0.05b
		0.5	4.42±0.30c	1.96±0.05b	1.93±0.04b
		1	10.60±1.65e	1.51±0.03b	1.30±0.02a
		1.5	4.46±0.70c	1.81±0.05b	0.46±0.01a
		2	2.44±0.30b	1.73±0.02b	1.22±0.03a

Means with same letters in a column are not significantly (P>0.05) different

3.09-8.75, 1.64-7.86 and 2.00-5.37 mgQE/g for aqueous, ethanol and methanol respectively. There were marginal decrements in flavonoid contents over storage period which caused significant ($p<0.05$) changes in aqueous and ethanolic extracts but caused no significant ($P>0.05$) change in methanolic extracts. The decrease might be attributed to some changes in the molecular conformation as a result of low moisture levels which might have solidified or aggregated to immobilize the flavonoids.

There is reduction of the radical scavenger after exposure to high doses of gamma radiation due to displacement from the B-ring to the 2.3-double bond, pointing to a relatively small reactivity (because of the absence of high density spin on a given site) for these intermediate species [55,56]. The survival of such intermediate species after irradiation apparently does not abolish the antioxidant properties and can maintain the radioprotective effects of flavonoids - A feature already noticed in gamma-irradiated strawberry [35,57]. Our results are in harmony with the presence of stabilized quinones, which have been observed after H-abstraction from the B-ring of flavonoids in radiolytic solutions [58]. Irradiation can cause oxidative damage and impair flavor in food. However, the action of effective and radiostable natural antioxidants may prevent chemical oxidation of biomolecules in irradiated foods. Irradiation dose of 0.5 kGy recorded greatest amounts of flavonoids in general for all the extracts. In terms of packaging material suitability, there was no significant ($P>0.05$) difference between polythene and polypropylene. Mujic et al. [53] reported values ranging from 1.61- 5.04 mgCE/g for *L. edodes, Agrocybe aegerita* and *Hericium erinaceus* which were in agreement with our results. Also, Lin et al. [59] reported comparatively low flavonoid values of 2.18 mg QE/g for white variety of *A. fuscosuccinea*, 0.78 mgQE/g for *Tremella fuciformis* and 0.49 mg QE/g for *A. polytricha*. However, values recorded from this work, were higher than works of Obodai et al. [60] and Iwalokun et al. [61] who reported values ranging between 0.2- 2.03μg of RE/g of dry weight and absence of flavonoid extracts in *Pleurotus* sp. The antioxidant concentration in a food material according to Lele et al. [62] depends upon the time of evaluation, like analyzing immediately after the irradiation treatment or after certain period of time duration.

Table 3. shows the percentage inhibition of each extract (aqueous, ethanolic and methanolic) against their DPPH radical scavenger for dried and gamma irradiated mushrooms which were calculated from calibration curves. The analysis of variance (ANOVA) showed that concentration significantly ($P<0.05$) affected percent inhibition. Dried and gamma irradiated *P.ostreatus* stored at 0-3 months, ranged 7.02±0.10- 12.71±0.02, 7.44±0.16- 11.22±0.15 and 8.79±0.06- 13.03±0.04% mgGAE/g for the respective extracts. Storage months 6 to 12 also recorded ranges 7.02±0.10- 12.71±0.02, 7.44±0.16 – 10.81±0.15 and 8.79±0.06- 13.03±0.04% mgGAE/g. Interaction of gamma radiation and storage period resulted in a general significant ($P<0.05$) decrease in percentage inhibition. The process of reduction of free radicals through the system of hydrogen donation from antioxidant compounds. Free radicals used are synthetic DPPH reacts with an antioxidant compound through the donation of electrons from an antioxidant compound to get a pair of electrons. DPPH radical compound deep purple would fade to yellow if it is reduced by antioxidants into non radical DPPH. When the free electron of DPPH radical has been paired with electrons from traps compounds (antioxidants) it would reduce DPPH to radical (DPPH-H), and form stable compounds are DPP Hydrazine [61]. There were significant ($P<0.05$) differences recorded between the aqueous and ethanol extracts. Methanol extracts however, recorded no significant differences with increasing radiation dose. Packaging did not influence results significantly. Present data cannot adequately elucidate the influence of type of extract on yield and activity of DPPH in *P. ostreatus*. Future studies are required to answer this question.

3.1 Half Maximal Inhibitory Concentration (Ic_{50})

This quantitative measure indicates how much of a particular drug or other substance (inhibitor) is needed to inhibit a given biological process (or component of a process, i.e. an enzyme, cell, cell receptor or microorganism) by half [62]. It is commonly used as a measure of antagonist drug potency in pharmacological research. According to [62], IC_{50} represents the concentration of a drug that is required for 50% inhibition in vitro.

The antioxidant activity with $IC_{50}< 0.01$ mg ml^{-1} value corresponds to good antioxidant activity and are included in the category of powerful antioxidants class [63,64].

Table 4. illustrates the amount of each extract needed for 50% inhibition (IC_{50}). IC_{50} mg ml^{-1} of the extracts were in the order aqueous < methanol <ethanol and corresponded to a range of 0.069- 0.073, 0.22- 0.27 and 1.020- 1.071 mg ml^{-1} respectively over the 12 month storage period. IC_{50} of the standard compound quercetin was 0.00287mg ml^{-1}.

The highest radical scavenging activity was shown by aqueous extract obtained from mushrooms stored for 3 months with IC_{50}= 0.069 mg ml^{-1} which is lower than that of quercetin (P<0.05). All the extracts did not show significant difference (P<0.05) from the standard compound except for ethanol (Table 4).

The high contents of phenolic compounds and significant linear correlation between the values of the concentration of phenolic compounds and antioxidant activity indicated that these compounds in mushrooms contribute to the

Table 2. Effect of irradiation on flavonoid content of dried mushrooms stored in packaging materials for 12 months period

Time (month)	Package	Dose applied (kGy)	Extracts		
			Aqueous (mgQE/g)	Ethanol (mgQE/g)	Methanol (mgQE/g)
0	Polythene	0	7.67±0.8c	4.25±0.2b	3.93±0.2c
		0.5	8.92±0.6d	7.27±0.4c	3.81±0.2c
		1	8.07±0.7c	5.58±0.2c	4.61±0.4d
		1.5	3.70±0.2a	1.64±0.05a	3.51±0.2b
		2	6.73±0.5bc	7.88±0.4d	2.88±0.1b
	Polypropylene	0	3.09±0.2a	4.73±0.2b	4.18±0.2d
		0.5	8.75±0.8d	7.86±0.4c	5.37±0.5e
		1	7.92±0.6c	4.42±0.2b	2.50±0.2a
		1.5	7.92±0.6c	6.29±0.4c	2.41±0.1a
		2	3.46±0.3a	5.88±0.3c	4.90±0.4e
3	Polythene	0	7.53±0.7c	4.31±0.2b	3.84±0.2c
		0.5	8.88±0.6c	7.27±0.4c	3.81±0.2c
		1	8.00±0.7c	5.58±0.2b	4.58±0.4d
		1.5	3.74±0.2a	1.64±0.05a	3.72±0.2c
		2	7.03±0.5c	7.81±0.4c	2.88±0.1b
	Polypropylene	0	3.09±0.2a	4.69±0.2b	4.14±0.2d
		0.5	8.75±0.8d	7.86±0.4c	5.37±0.5e
		1	7.92±0.6c	4.42±0.2b	2.50±0.2a
		1.5	7.92±0.6c	6.29±0.4c	2.10±0.1a
		2	3.41±0.3a	6.02±0.3c	5.11±0.4e
6	Polythene	0	7.67±0.8c	4.33±0.2b	3.93±0.2c
		0.5	7.92±0.6c	7.27±0.4c	3.81±0.2c
		1	7.87±0.7c	5.51±0.2b	4.61±0.4d
		1.5	3.69±0.2a	1.69±0.05a	3.51±0.2bc
		2	6.73±0.5c	7.88±0.4d	2.88±0.1b
	Polypropylene	0	3.09±0.2a	4.57±0.2b	4.18±0.2d
		0.5	8.75±0.8d	7.86±0.4d	5.37±0.5e
		1	7.92±0.6c	4.42±0.2b	2.50±0.2a
		1.5	7.88±0.6c	6.35±0.4b	2.00±0.1a
		2	3.46±0.3a	5.78±0.3c	4.93±0.4e
12	Polythene	0	7.63±0.8c	4.25±0.2ab	3.93±0.2cd
		0.5	8.90 ± 0.6d	7.27±0.4c	3.81±0.2c
		1	8.00±0.7c	5.52±0.2c	4.61±0.4d
		1.5	3.7±0.2a	1.64±0.05a	3.51±0.2b
		2	6.73±0.5bc	7.82±0.4d	2.88 ±0.1b
	Polypropylene	0	3.05±0.2a	4.73±0.2b	4.18±0.2cd
		0.5	8.72±0.8c	7.86±0.4d	5.37±0.5a
		1	7.92±0.6c	4.42±0.2b	2.50±0.2a
		1.5	7.89±0.6c	6.29±0.4c	2.00±0.1a
		2	3.46±0.3a	5.81±0.3c	4.90±0.4d

Means with same letters in a column are not significantly (P>0.05) different

Table 3. Percentage inhibition (%) of DPPH in dried and irradiated mushrooms stored in packaging materials for 12 months storage period

Time (month)	Package	Dose applied (kGy)	Extracts Aqueous (%) (mgGAE/g)	Ethanol (%) (mgGAE/g)	Methanol (%) (mgGAE/g)
0	Polythene	0	7.02±0.10a	10.06±0.13bc	10.09±0.26b
		0.5	9.65±0.13bc	10.47±0.24c	13.03±0.04b
		1	11.60±0.05d	9.36±0.12bc	12.82±0.03e
		1.5	9.46±0.12bc	9.36±0.12bc	10.30±0.27b
		2	9.26±0.02b	8.31±0.04a	10.60±0.3b
	Polypropylene	0	9.65±0.13bc	8.95±0.05bc	10.40±0.30b
		0.5	8.24±0.02a	10.81±0.25d	11.21±0.04d
		1	11.12±0.05c	7.44±0.16a	9.09±0.12a
		1.5	12.71±0.02c	8.84±0.05bc	8.79±0.06a
		2	9.37±0.12bc	9.06±0.11bc	10.30±0.3b
3	Polythene	0	6.85±0.11a	9.12±0.05b	10.23±0.25b
		0.5	10.0±0.3b	11.11±0.05d	12.89±0.10e
		1	11.42±0.05c	9.36±0.12b	13.03±0.20e
		1.5	9.04±0.02b	9.27±0.03b	10.00±0.13b
		2	9.15±0.02b	8.30±0.04b	11.32±0.05d
	Polypropylene	0	10.00±0.02b	11.15±0.04de	10.40±0.30b
		0.5	8.02±0.01a	11.22±0.15d	11.21 ± 0.04d
		1	11.51±0.02bc	7.34±0.14a	9.12±0.14a
		1.5	11.60±0.02bc	9.12±0.04b	9.00±0.11a
		2	9.30±0.04b	9.11±0.12b	10.00±0.02b
6	Polythene	0	7.05±0.10a	10.06±0.13bc	10.09±0.26b
		0.5	9.65±0.13bc	10.47±0.24c	13.03±0.04e
		1	11.60±0.05d	9.36±0.12bc	12.82±0.03d
		1.5	9.46±0.12bc	9.36±0.12bc	10.30±0.27b
		2	9.26±0.02b	8.31±0.04a	10.60±0.3b
	Polypropylene	0	9.65±0.13bc	8.95±0.05bc	10.40±0.3b
		0.5	8.24±0.02a	10.81±0.25d	11.21±0.04d
		1	11.12±0.05c	7.44±0.16a	9.09±0.12a
		1.5	12.71±0.02d	8.84±0.05bc	8.79±0.06a
		2	9.37±0.12b	9.06±0.11bc	10.30±0.3b
12	Polythene	0	7.00±0.10a	10.06±0.13bc	10.09±0.26b
		0.5	9.65±0.13bc	10.47±0.24c	13.03±0.04e
		1	11.60±0.05d	9.36±0.12bc	12.82±0.03d
		1.5	9.46±0.12bc	9.36±0.12bc	10.30±0.27c
		2	9.26±0.02b	8.31±0.04a	10.60±0.3b
	Polypropylene	0	9.65±0.13bc	8.95±0.05bc	10.40±0.3c
		0.5	8.24±0.02a	10.81±0.25d	11.21±0.04d
		1	11.12±0.05c	7.44±0.16a	9.09±0.12a
		1.5	12.71±0.02d	8.84±0.05bc	8.79±0.06a
		2	9.37±0.12bc	9.06±0.11bc	10.30±0.3b

Means with same letters in a column are not significantly (P>0.05) different

strong antioxidant activity. Previous studies by Mujic et al. [53] revealed a range of 0.02- 0.198 mg/ml for *L. edodes*, *H. erinaceous* and *A. aegerita* which are comparable to *P. ostreatus*. Qusti et al. [67] also reported comparable values of 0.22, 0.47, 0.54, 0.73 mg/ml for figs, snake cucumber, banana and white grapes respectively which were ranked high in antioxidants.

Although gamma irradiation can damage biomolecules directly by rupturing covalent bonds as a result of transfer of photon energy, and indirectly, by producing free radicals and other non-radical reactive oxygen species [68] its adverse effect was not realized and so was evident in our results (Table 4).

Table 4. Effect of storage time on the half maximal inhibitory concentration (IC_{50}) of dried *P. ostreatus*

	Extracts (mg/ml)			
Time	Aqueous	Ethanol	Methanol	Quercetin (standard)
0 month	0.071a	1.038c	0.22a	0.00287a
3 month	0.069a	1.041c	0.25a	0.00287a
6 month	0.073a	1.020c	0.27a	0.00287a
12 month	0.072a	1.071c	0.26a	0.00287a

Means with same letters in a row are not significantly (P>0.05) different

4. CONCLUSION

Our study clearly demonstrates that over the twelve months storage period, gamma irradiation had significant effect on the total phenolic, total flavonoid contents and DPPH radical scavenging activities in the mushroom samples. But packaging materials had no effect. Preservation of these antioxidants is dose dependent, as high doses of gamma radiation has been shown to breakdown some of these compounds. In view of these observations, gamma irradiation could be used to extend shelf life of food products due to its ability to destroy microorganisms, insects and larvae which cause deterioration during storage.

CONSENT

All authors declare that 'written informed consent was obtained from the patient (or other approved parties) for publication of this case report and accompanying images.

ETHICAL APPROVAL

All authors hereby declare that all experiments have been examined and approved by the appropriate ethics committee and have therefore been performed in accordance with the ethical standards laid down in the 1964 Declaration of Helsinki.

ACKNOWLEDGEMENTS

Authors are most grateful to all laboratory technicians of the Applied Radiation and Biological Centre, Radiological and Medical Research Institute of the Ghana Atomic Energy Commission where the antioxidant analysis were carried out. We would also like to thank the staff of Mushroom Unit, Food Research Institute-Council for Scientific and Industrial Research, Ghana.

COMPETING INTERESTS

Authors have declared that no competing interests exist.

REFERENCES

1. Tel G, Apaydın M, Duru ME, Öztürk M. Antioxidant and cholinesterase inhibition activities of three tricholoma species with total phenolic and flavonoid contents: The edible mushrooms from Anatolia. Food Anal. Methods. 2012;5:495–504.
2. Oyetayo OV. Medicinal uses of mushrooms in Nigeria: Towards full and sustainable exploitation. African Journal of Traditional, Complement and Alternative Medicine. 2011;8 (3):267-274.
3. Ling TN, Okogun JI, Folk WR. 21st century natural product research and drug development and traditional medicines. Natural Product Reports. 2013;30(4):584-592.
4. Kortei NK. Growing oyster mushrooms (*Pleurotus ostreatus*) on composted agrowastes: An efficient way of utilizing lignocellulosic materials. Lambert Academic Publishing, Germany. 2011;9.
5. Dzomeku M, Apetorgbor AK, Apetorgbor MM, Obodai M. Ailments and application of Pleurotus tuber-regium (ptr) among indigenes of two regions in Ghana. 2014; 7(3):129-132.
6. Personal communication (Madam Grace Kessiwa Simpeh) Kwahu-East district, Eastern Region, Ghana; 2013.
7. Obodai M. An ethnobotanical study of mushroom gerplasm and its domestication in the Bia biosphere reserve. UNESCO-MBA document; 2001.
8. Apetorgbor MM, Apetorgbor AK, Obodai M. Indiginuous knowledge and utilization of edible mushrooms. Ghana Journal of Forestry. 2006;19-20:20-34.
9. Apetorgbor MM, Apetorgbor AK, Nutakor E. Utilization and cultivation of edible mushrooms for rural livelihood in Southern Ghana. 17th Commonwealth Forestry Conference, Colombo, Sri Lanka; 2005.

10. Personal communication (Nii Abban Kortei II, Chief of Ofankor) Ga West, Greater Accra Region, Ghana; 2014.
11. Osemwegie OO, Okhuoya JA, Dania AT. Ethnomycological conspectus of West African mushrooms: An awareness document. Advances in Microbiology. 2013;4:39-54.
12. Dzomeku M. Studies on the occurrence, ethnomycology and cultivation of pleurotus tuber-regium. An MPhil. Dissertation, Department of Theoretical and Applied Biology, Kwame Nkrumah University of Science and Technology, Kumasi. 2009; 152.
13. Kinge TR, Tabi EM, Mih AM, Egbe EA, Njouonkou LA, Nji TM. Ethnomycology studies of macrofungi (Mushrooms) in Mount Cameroon Region. International Journal of Medicinal Mushrooms. 2011;13: 299-305.
14. Gryzenhpout M, Jefwa MJ, Yorou SN. The Status of Mycology in Africa: A Document to Promote Awareness. IMA Fungus. 2012; 3(1):99-102.
15. Kortei NK, Odamtten GT, Obodai M, Appiah V, Akuamoa F, Adu- Bobi AK, Annan SNY, Armah JNO, Acquah AS. Evaluating the effect of gamma radiation on the total phenolic content, flavonoids and antioxidant activity of dried *Pleurotus ostreatus* (Jacq.ex.fr) kummer stored in packaging materials. Advances in Pharmaceutics. 2014;Article ID 262807:1-8.
16. Lima GPP, Vianello F, Correa CR, Campos RAS, Borguini MG. Polyphenols in fruits and vegetables and its effect on human health. Food and Nutrition Sciences. 2014;5:1065-1082.
17. Dolatabadi JEN, Kashanian S. A review on DNA interaction with synthetic phenolic food additives. Food Research International. 2010;43:1223-1230.
18. Okubo T, Yokoyama Y, Kano K, Cell I. Death induced by the phenolic antioxidant tert-butylhydroquinone and its metabolite tert-butylquinone in human Monocytic Leukemia U937 Cells. Food and Chemical Toxicology. 2003;41:679-688.
19. Iverson F. Phenolic antioxidants: Health protection branch studies on butylatedhydroxyanisole. Cancer Letters. 1995;93(1):49-54.
20. Chirumbolo S. The role of quercetin, flavonols and flavonone in modulating inflammatory cell function. Inflamm Allergy Drug Targets. 2010;9:263-285.
21. Selma MV, Esprin JC, Tomas-Barberan FA. Interaction between phenolics and gut microbiota: Role in human health. J Agric Food Chem, 2009;57:6485-6501.
22. Kemperman RA, Bolca S, Roger LC, Vaughan EE. Novel approaches for analyzing gut microbes and dietary polyphenols: Challenges and opportunities. Microbiology. 2010;156:3224-3231.
23. Rodriguez Vaquero MJ, AredesFerna´ndez PA, Manca de Nadra MC, Strasser de Saad AM: Phenolic compound combinations on Escherichia coli viability in a meat system. J Agric Food Chem. 2010; 58:6048-6052.
24. Jayaraman P, Sakharkar MK, Lim CS, Tang TH, Sakharkar KR. Activity and interactions of antibiotic and phytochemical combinations against Pseudomonas aeruginosa in vitro. Int J Biol Sci. 2010; 6:556-568.
25. Saavedra MJ, Borges A, Dias C, Aires A, Bennett RN, Rosa ES, Simoes M: Antimicrobial activity of phenolics and glucosinolate hydrolysis products and their synergy with streptomycin against pathogenic bacteria. Med. Chem. 2010; 6:174-183.
26. Daglia M. Polyphenols as antimicrobial agents. Current Opinion in Biotechnology. 2012;23:174-181.
27. Ferreira ALA, Salvadori DM, Nascimento MC, Rocha NS, Correa CR, Pereira EJ, Matsubara LS, Matsubara BB, Ladeira MSP. Tomato-Oleoresin Supplement Prevents Doxorubicin-Induced Cardiac Myocyte Oxidative DNA Damage in Rats. Mutation Research/ Genetic Toxicology and Environmental Mutagenisis. 2007; 631:26-35.
28. Yeum KJ, Russell RM, Krinsky NI, Aldini G. Biomarkers of Antioxidant Capacity in the Hydrophilic and Lipophilic Compartments of Human Plasma. Archives of Biochemistry and Biophysics. 2004;430:97-103.
29. Poli G, Schaur RJ, Siems WG, Leonarduzzi G. 4-Hydroxynonenal: A Membrane Lipid Oxidation Product of Medicinal Interest. Medicinal Research Reviews. 2008;28:569-631.
30. Ralser M, Wamelink MM, Kowald A, Gerisch B, Heeren G, Struys EA, Klipp E, Jakobs C, Breitenbach M, Lehrach H, Krobitsch S. Dynamic rerouting of the

carbohydrate flux is key to counteracting oxidative stress. Journal of Biology. 2007; 6:10.

31. McDonald S, Prenzler PD, Antolovich M, Robards K. Phenolic content and antioxidant activity of olive extracts. Food Chemistry. 2001;73:73–84.
32. Jang HD, Chang KS, Huang YS, Hsu CL, Lee SH, Su MS. Principal phenolic phytochemicals and antioxidant activities of three Chinese medicinal plants. Food Chemistry. 2007;103:749–756.
33. Aldini G, Dalle-Donne I, Facino RM, Milzani A, Carini M. Intervention strategies to inhibit protein carbonylation by lipoxidation-derived reactive carbonyls. Medicinal Research Review. 2007;27:817-868.
34. Brownlee M. The pathobiology of diabetic complications: A unifying mechanism. Diabetes. 2005;54:1615-1625.
35. De MeloVaz AF, de Souza MP, Argolo MACC, de Albuquerque Melo AMM, Oliva MLV, Xavier HS, Coelho LCBB, dos Santos Correia MT. Stability of the antioxidant activity of flavonoids after gamma irradiation. Food and Nutrition Sciences. 2011;2:490-493.
36. Obodai M, Okine JC, Vowotor KA. Comparative study on the growth and yield of *Pleurotus ostreatus* mushroom on different lignocellulosic by products. J. Industr. Microbial. Biotechnol. 2003; 30(3):146-149.
37. Parekh J, Chanda SV. *In vitro* antimicrobial activity and phytochemical analysis of some Indian medicinal plants. Turk J Biol. 2007;31:53-58.
38. Stankovic MS. Total phenolic content, flavonoid concentration and antioxidant activity of *Marrubium peregrinum* L. extracts. Kragujevac J. Sc. 2011;33:63-72.
39. Singleton VL, Orthofer R, Lamuela-Raventos RM. Analysis of total phenols and other oxidation substrates and antioxidants by means of Folin-Ciocalteu reagent. Methods Enzymol. 1999;299: 152-178.
40. Quettier DC, Gressier B, Vasseur J, Dine T, Brunet C, Luyckx MC, Cayin JC, Bailleul F, Trotin F. Phenolic compounds and antioxidant activities of buckwheat (*Fagopyrum esculentum* Moench) hulls and flour. J. Ethnopharmacol. 2000;72: 35-42.
41. Tekao T, Watanabe N, Yagi I, Sakata K. A simple screening method for antioxidant and isolation of several antioxidants produced by marine bacteria from fish and shellfish. Biosci. Biotechnol. Biochem. 1994;58:1780-1783.
42. Botchway SW, Crisostomo AG, Parker AW, Bisby RH. Near infrared multiphoton-induced generation and detection of hydroxyl radicals in biochemical system. Arch. Biochem. Biophysics. 2007;464:314.
43. Taheri S, Abdullah TL, Karimi E, Oskoueian E, Ebrahimi M. Antioxidant capacities and total phenolic contents enhancement with acute gamma irradiation in Curcuma alismatifolia (Zingiberaceae) leaves. Int. J. Mol. Sci. 2014;15(7):13077-13090.
44. Hirashima FK, Fabbri ADT, Sagretti JMA, Nunes TCF, Galvao NS, Lanfer Marquez UM, Sabato, SF. Influence of gamma irradiation on phenolic compounds of minimally processed baby carrots, International Nuclear Atlantic Conference, 2013; PE, Brazil.
45. Kumari N, Kumar P, Mitra D, Prasad B, Tiwary BN, Varshney L. Effects of ionizing radiation on microbial decontamination, phenolic contents and anti-oxidant properties of Triphala. Journal of Food Science. 2009;74 (3):M109-M113.
46. Obodai M, Ferreira ICFR, Fernandes A, Barros- L, Narh Mensah DL, Dzomeku M, Urben AF, Prempeh J, Takli RK. Evaluation of chemical and antioxidant properties of wild and cultivated mushrooms of Ghana. 2014; Molecules 19: 19532-19548.
47. Unekwu MR, Audu JA, Makun MH, Chidi EE. Phytochemical screening and antioxidant activity of methanolic extract of selected wild edible Nigerian mushrooms. Asian Pacific Journal of Tropical Disease, 2014;4(1):153-157.
48. Choi Y, Lee SM, Chun J, Lee HB, Lee J. Influence of heat treatment on the antioxidant activities and polyphenolic compounds of Shiitake (*Lentinus edodes*) mushroom. Food Chem. 2006;99:381-387.
49. Mau JL, Chao GR, Wu KT. Antioxidant properties of methanol extracts from several ear mushrooms. J. Agric. Food Chem. 2001;49:5461-5467.
50. Kho YS, Vikineswary S, Abdullah N, Kuppusamy UR, Oh HI. Antioxidant capacity of fresh and processed fruit bodies and mycelium of Auricularia auricula-judae (Fr.) Quél. J. Med. Food. 2009;12:167-174.

51. Kottoh ID, Agyekum AA, Akuamoah F, Asarel. Evaluating the effect of gamma irradiation and storage period on the phytochemical stability of some selected spices on the Ghanaian market. Int. J. Recent Trends in Sc. And Tech. 2014; 10(1):153-157.
52. USDA. The United States Development Agency-Nutrient Database for standard reference. Release. 1998;12:1.
53. Mujic I, Zekovic Z, Lepojevic Z, Vidovic S, Zivkovic J. Antioxidant properties of selected edible mushroom species. Journal of Central European Agriculture. 2013;11(4):387-392.
54. Tanaka M, Kuei CW, Nagashima Y, Taguchi T. Application of antioxidative Millard reaction products from histidine and glucose to sardine products. Nippon Suisan Gakkaishil. 1998;54:1409-1414.
55. Kortei NK, Odamtten GT, Obodai M, Appiah V, Akuamoa F, Adu-Bobi AK, Annan SNY, Armah JO, Acquah SA. Evaluating the effect of gamma radiation on the total phenolic content, flavonoids and antioxidants of dried *P. ostreatus* (Jacq.ex.Fr) Kummer stored in packaging materials. Advances in Pharmaceutics. 2014;article ID 262807:1-8.
56. Marfak A, Trouillas P, Allais DP, Champavier Y, Calliste CA, Duroux JL. Radiolysis of Kaempferol in Water/ Methanol Mixtures. Evaluation of Antioxidant Activity of Kaempferol and Products Formed. Journal of Agricultural and Food Chemistry. 2003;51(5):1270-1277.
57. Breitfellner F, Solar S, Sontag G. Effect of gamma irradiation on flavonoids in strawberries. European Food Research & Technology. 2002;215(1):28-31.
58. Pannala AS, Chan TS, O'Brien PJ, Rice-Evans CA. Flavonoid B-Ring Chemistry and Antioxidant Activity: Fast Reaction Kinetics, Biochemical and Bio-physical Research Communications. 2001;282(5): 1161-1168.
59. Lin Y, Wang C, Chen I, Jheng J, Li J, Tung C. TIPdb: A database of anticancer, antiplatelet and antituberculosis phytochemicals from indigenous plants in Taiwan. Scientific World J. 2013;4(2):148-154.
60. Obodai M, Owusu E, Schwinger GO, Asante IK, Dzomeku M. Phytochemical and mineral analysis of 12 cultivated oyster mushrooms (*Pleurotus* species). Advances in Life Sciences and Technology. 2014;26:36-42.
61. Iwalokun BA, Usen UA, Otunba AA, Olukoya DK. Comparative Phytochemical Evaluation, Antimicrobial and Antioxidant properties of *Pleurotus ostreatus*. Afr. J. Biotechnol. 2007;6(16):1732-1739.
62. Lele SS, Mali AB, Khedkar. Effect of gamma irradiation on total phenolic content and *in vitro* antioxidant activity of pomegranate (*Punica granatum* L) peels, Food and Nutrition Sciences. 2011;2428-433.
63. Molyneux P. Use of DPPH to estimate antioxidant activity. Journal of Science and Technology. 2004;26:2.
64. Internet: wikepedia.org/wiki/IC50
65. Chye FK, Wong JY. Antioxidant properties of selected tropical wild edible mushrooms. Journal of Food Composition and Analysis. 2008;22:269-277.
66. Pourmoradi F, Hosseinimehr SJ, Shahabimajd N. Antioxidant, phenol and flavonoid contents of some selected Iranian medicinal plants Afr. J. Biotechnology. 2006;5:1142-1145.
67. Qusti SY, Abo-Khatwa, Bin Lahwa. Screening of antioxidant activity and phenolic content of selected food items cited in the Holy Quran. EJBS. 2010;2(1): 41-51.
68. Kempner ES. Effects of high-energy electrons and gamma rays directly on protein molecules. Journal of Pharmaceutical Sciences. 2001;90(10): 1637-1646.

Experimental and Kinetic Studies on *Penicillin G* Adsorption by *Lemna minor*

Davoud Balarak[1], Ferdos Kord Mostafapour[1] and Ali Joghataei[2*]

[1]Department of Environmental Health, Health Promotion Research Center, School of Public Health, Zahedan University of Medical Sciences, Zahedan, Iran.
[2]Student Research Committee, Qom University of Medical Sciences, Qom, Iran.

Authors' contributions

This work was carried out in collaboration between all authors. All authors read and approved the final manuscript.

Article Information

Editor(s):
(1) Abdelwahab Omri, Department of Chemistry and Biochemistry and Departments of Biomolecular Sciences, Laurentian University, Canada.
Reviewers:
(1) Alejandro Córdova Izquierdo, Universidad Autónoma Metropolitana Unidad Xochimilco, Mexico.
(2) M. Angeles calvo torras, Autonomous University of Barcelona, Spain.

ABSTRACT

This study examined the ability of dried duckweed (*Lemna minor*) to remove soluble *Penicillin G* from aqueous solution. Batch experiments were conducted to investigate the effects of pH, contact time, initial *Penicillin G* concentration, biomass dose and temperature on penicillin G adsorption. Maximum adsorption capacity of the duckweed was 36.18 mg g^{-1} when 94.6% of the *Penicillin G* was removed. The adsorption equilibriums were analyzed by Langmuir, Freundlich, Temkin and BET isotherm models. It was found that he data fitted to Langmuir better than isotherm other models. Batch kinetic experiments showed that the adsorption followed pseudo-second-order kinetic model with correlation coefficients greater than 0.99. The adsorption capacity of *penicillin G* increased from 31.11 to 41.82 mg/g with increasing the temperature from 20 to 50℃, indicating that the process is endothermic. According to achieved results, it was defined that *Lemna minor* not only was an inexpensive absorbent, but also a quite effective factor in removal of *Penicillin G* from water and wastewater.

Keywords: Adsorption; Lemna minor; Penicillin G; antibiotic; kinetic.

**Corresponding author: Email: alijoghatayi69@gmail.com*

1. INTRODUCTION

Pharmaceuticals are not environmentally different from other chemicals, such as pesticides and herbicides, but they have not aroused attention as potential pollutants until fairly recently [1,2]. Antibiotics are designed specifically as a drug to treat or prevent infective diseases in human or animal body [3,4]. The use of antibiotics has become an indispensable in human life and the global market consumption of these drugs increase steadily every year [5,6]. For preventing or treating infections in humans or animals, only some parts of the antibiotics given dose are metabolized and the rest are excreted still as active compound [7,8]. *Penicillin* is an extremely important antibiotic, and *penicillin G* is the raw material of the semi synthetic penicillin's [9]. Over 20 countries manufacture over 11,000 tones of *penicillin* per year. Its wide usage is a result of its lack of toxicity and irritancy [10,11]. *Penicillin G* is commonly produced by submerged aerobic fermentation using strains of Penicillium chryogenum. Penicillin G is a weak monocarboxylic acid (pKa = 2.75) [12]. For several decades now antibiotics have been used in veterinary and human medicine, yet these compounds when released into the environment have potential risks for aquatic and terrestrial organisms [13]. High concentrations of antibiotics are now detected in drinking waters, reducing their quality [14]. They generally have a low biodegradability and high toxicity, and some are reported to have mutagenic and carcinogenic characteristics [15]. The removal of antibiotics from pharmaceutical wastewater is quite expensive, however this wastewater must be treated properly prior to the release into environment [16]. Among the available process for the treatment of wastewater containing antibiotics, the adsorption process is considered as the most effective and efficient method [17,18]. The main drawback of adsorption process for wastewater treatment is the cost of adsorbent [19]. Commercially available adsorbents such as activated carbon are expensive [20]. If inexpensive and abundantly available materials are found in nature as the alternative adsorbents, the adsorption process offers a very attractive method for environmental remediation [21,22]. Recently, various materials such as Azolla, wheat straw, fungus, orange peels, Rice straw, Wheat straw and Sawdust been applied to develop as low-cost and effective adsorbent [23,24]. The *Lemna minor* is one of wide-spread aquatic plant which is belonged to duckweed species with special characteristics including rapid growth, high nutritional value, and high water purification capabilities have been used to remove the pollutant from water and wastewater [25,26]. Therefore, the purpose of present study was to assess the *Lemna minor* ability as adsorbent for remove the *Penicillin G* antibiotic. Also, the effect of several parameters including contact time, pH, adsorbent dose and initial *Penicillin G* concentration was investigated.

2. MATERIALS AND METHODS

2.1 Chemicals

The *Penicillin G* used in the experiments was supplied by Aldrich Chemicals. Stock solutions of *Penicillin G* were prepared in distilled water. All chemicals used in this study were purchased from Merck Co. All solutions used in this study were diluted with distilled water as required.

In this study, the *Lemna minor* was used for *Penicillin G* removal from aqueous solutions. The *Lemna minor* were collected from *Anzali* wetland. The collected materials were then washed several times with distilled water to remove all dirt particles. The dried materials were then ground, using steel mill. The crushed particles were then treated with 0.5 M H_2SO_4 for 2 h followed by washing with distilled water and then kept for shaded dry [15].

The BET surface area of *Lemna minor* was measured using surface area analyzer (Micromeritics ASAP 2020 V3.04 H). Treated *Lemna minor* biomass before and after use were examined using an environmental scanning electron microscopy (ESEM) instrument (Philips XL30).

2.2 Adsorption experiments of synthetic *Penicillin G* solution

The Initial *Penicillin G* solutions with different concentrations were prepared by diluting a *Penicillin G* stock standard solution of 1000 mg/L with distilled water. The solution pH was adjusted using either diluted 0.1 M H_2SO_4 or 0.1 M NaOH solution. 100 ml of *Penicillin G* solution and 4 g biomass was placed in a Pyrex glass and stirred at constant speed for 90 hours using a magnetic stirrer (Remi Make, India). The equilibrium times at different temperatures (30℃, 40℃ and 50℃) were estimated by testing the samples collected at different time intervals until *Penicillin G* content in the sample was constant. At the end of the equilibration time, the solution was centrifuged (EBA21, Hettich) at 3600 rpm for 10 min. The equilibrium concentration of *Penicillin G* in solution was determined by *HPLC* (kenaver, Germany). In the HPLC analysis, the mobile phase was a mixture of 50 μm phosphoric acid and methanol (40:60,v/v). The flow rate was 1.0 ml/min, the detection wavelength was 215 nm, and the injection volume was 10 ml [12]. All batch experiments were carried out in triplicate.

The amount of *Penicillin G* adsorbed per was calculated by following mass-balance equation [27,28]:

$$q_e = \frac{(Co - Ce) \times V}{M}$$

Where C_0 and C_e are the initial and the equilibrium *Penicillin G* concentrations in liquid phase (mg/L) respectively, V is the volume of solution and m is the mass of adsorbent.

2.3 Adsorption Isotherms

The equilibrium adsorption isotherm is importance in the design of adsorption systems. Although several isotherm equations are available, but four important isotherms including Langmuir, Freundlich, Tekmin and BET isotherms were selected.

The Langmuir equation is given as follows [29,30]:

$$\frac{1}{q_e} = \frac{1}{q_{max}} + \frac{1}{q_{max}\, K_L} \times \frac{1}{C_e}$$

Where q_e (mg/g) and C_e (mg/L) are the amount of adsorbed *Penicillin G* per unit weight of adsorbent and unabsorbed *Penicillin G* concentration in solution at equilibrium, respectively. The constant K_L is the Langmuir equilibrium constant.

The Freundlich isotherm model equation is expressed as [12]:

$$\text{Ln } q_e = \ln K_F + \frac{1}{n} \ln Ce$$

Where q_e is the equilibrium *Penicillin G* concentration on the adsorbent (mg g^{-1}); Ce, the equilibrium *Penicillin G* concentration in solution (mg L^{-1}); and K_F is the Freundlich constant.

The Tempkin isotherm model equation is expressed as [29]:

$$q_e = B \ln A + B \ln Ce$$

Where B = RT/b, T is the absolute temperature in K, R the universal gas constant (8.314 JK^{-1} mol^{-1}), A the equilibrium binding constant and the constant B is related to the heat of adsorption.

The BET isotherm model in the linear form as used is represented as [20]:

$$\frac{C_e}{(C_i - C_e)q} = \left(\frac{1}{q_m A}\right) + \left(\frac{A-1}{q_m A}\right)$$

C_e is the equilibrium concentration (mg/L), C_i the adsorbate monolayer saturation concentration (mg/ L), A the BET adsorption isotherm relating to the energy of surface interaction (l/mg).

2.4 Adsorption Kinetics

The study of kinetic models was performed in contact time between 10-180 min with *Penicillin G* concentration of 25 and 200 mg/L and optimum amount of pH and adsorbent dose. To evaluate the differences in the biosorption rates and uptakes, the kinetic data were described with Elovich, Intraparticle diffusion, pseudo first, pseudo second order models.

The pseudo first order kinetics model in the linear form as used is represented as [31,32]:

$$\text{Log } (q_e - q_t) = \log q_e - \frac{K_1}{2.303} t$$

Where q_e and q_t are the amounts of *Penicillin G* (mg g^{-1}) adsorbed at equilibrium and time t, respectively, and k_1 is the rate constant of adsorption (min^{-1}) biosorption.

The pseudo-second-order kinetic model is expressed as [12]:

$$\frac{t}{q_t} = \frac{1}{k_2 qe^2} + \frac{1}{qe}t$$

Where q_e is the biosorbed *Penicillin G* amount at equilibrium (mg g^{-1}) for the pseudo-second-order biosorption, q_t is the amount of *Penicillin G* biosorbed at time t (mg g^{-1}) and k_2 is the pseudo-second-order kinetic rate constant (g mg^{-1} min^{-1}).

The intraparticle diffusion equation can be written as follows [13]:

$$q_t = k_{dif}\, t^{0.5} + c$$

where C is the intercept, and kdif is the intraparticle diffusion rate constant (mg g^{-1} min^{-1}).

The Elovich model equation is generally expressed as [20]:

$$q_e = (\frac{1}{\beta})\ln(\alpha\beta) + (\frac{1}{\beta})\ln t$$

where α is the initial adsorption rate (mg/g.min) and β is the adsorption constant (g/mg) during any experiment.

3. RESULTS AND DISCUSSION

The specific surface area is related to the number of active adsorption sites of dried *Lemna minor*. The adsorption was increased with the specific surface area and pore volume of the sorbent. The specific surface area of the modified *Lemna minor* was determined in the size of 32.5 m^2/g.

Dried *Lemna minor* was also examined before and after use using environmental scanning electron microscopy. Fig. 1(a) clearly shows the pore textural structure of dried *Lemna minor* before use. However, as shown in Fig. 1(b), clear pore textural structure is not observed on the surface of dried *Lemna minor* after use which could be due to either agglomeration on the surface or the incursion of *penicillin G* into the pores of dried *Lemna minor* biomass.

3.1 Effect of Contact Time and Initial *Penicillin G* Concentration

The adsorption of *penicillin G* onto *Lemna minor* was studied as a function of contact time in order to decide whether the equilibrium was reached. For, 10-200 mgL^{-1} of *penicillin G* solutions at pH 5 were contacted with 4 gL^{-1} of *Lemna minor* suspensions. The samples were taken at different periods of time and analyzed for their *penicillin G* concentration (Fig. 2). The *penicillin G* adsorption rate is high at the beginning of the experiment because initially the adsorption sites are more available and *penicillin G* ions are easily adsorbed on these sites [33]. The equilibrium can be reached within 75 min, and thus, further adsorption experiments were carried out for a contact time of 75 min.

3.2 Effect of pH

The surface charge of the adsorbent and the ionization degree of the adsorbate are strongly affected by the pH of the aqueous solutions, hence the uptake of *penicillin G* by the adsorbent depends on the solution pH. In order to evaluate the effect of pH on the adsorption of *penicillin G* onto *Lemna minor*, the adsorption experiments were carried out with initial *penicillin G* concentration of 50 mg L^{-1} and biomass dose of 4 gL^{-1} by varying the pH of the solutions over a range of 2–10 (Fig. 3). The uptake of *penicillin G* by the *Lemna minor* is almost constant in the pH range of 2–5. However when the pH value exceeds 5, the adsorption of *penicillin G* decreases abruptly. *Penicillin G* as a acid compound with p*K*a value of 2.8 is dissociated at pH>p*K*a [34]. At higher pH values, the ionization degree of *penicillin G* and the quantity of OH^- ions increase thereby the diffusion of *penicillin G* are hindered, and the electrostatic repulsion between the negatively charged surface sites of the adsorbent and *penicillin G* ions increases [35]. As a result, the removal of *penicillin G* is greater at lower pH compared to the higher pH. Similar results were reported by *Malakotian* [12]. From the experimental results, pH 5 was selected as an optimum pH value.

3.3 Effect of *Lemna minor* Concentration

The effects of *Lemna minor* dose on the removal of *penicillin G* from aqueous solutions were investigated by using different *Lemna minor* dose in the range of 0.5–8 g L^{-1} and initial *penicillin G* concentration of 100 mg L^{-1} at pH 5. As the *Lemna minor* dose was increased from 1 to 8 g L^{-1}, the equilibrium adsorption capacity of *Lemna minor* (q_e), decreased from 6.0 to 2.6 mg g^{-1}, whereas, the *penicillin G* removal efficiency increased from 5.5% to 58.5% (Fig. 4). The increase in adsorption percentage of *penicillin G* was probably due to the increased more availability of active adsorption sites with the increase in *Lemna minor* dose [36]. The decrease in equilibrium adsorption capacity of *Lemna minor* for *penicillin G* uptake could be attributed to two reasons. First, the *Lemna minor* particles aggregated with increasing the adsorbent dose hence total surface area of the adsorbent decreased and diffusion path length of *penicillin G* increased [37]. Secondly, the increase in *Lemna minor* dose at constant concentration and volume of *penicillin G* lead to unsaturation adsorption sites, so the equilibrium adsorption capacity of *Lemna minor* decreased [12].

The adsorption kinetics is one the most important data in order to understand the mechanism of the adsorption and to assess the performance of the adsorbents. For evaluating the kinetics of *penicillin G-Lemna minor* interactions, the pseudo-first-order, pseudo-second-order and intraparticle diffusion models were used to fit the experimental data. The pseudo-first-order rate constant k_1 and the value of q_e cal were calculated and the results are given in Table 1. The correlation coefficient (R^2) is relatively low which may be indicative of a bad correlation. In addition, q_e cal determined from the model is not in a good agreement with the experimental value of q_e exp. Therefore, the adsorption of *penicillin G* onto *Lemna minor* is not suitable for the first-order reaction.

From Table 1, the value of C obtained from intraparticle diffusion model is not zero, and the correlation coefficient is not satisfactory thereby intraparticle diffusion may not be the controlling factor in determining the kinetics of the process. The pseudo-second-order rate constant k_2 and the value of q_e cal were determined from the model and the results are presented in Table 1. The value of correlation coefficient is very high (R^2 >0.994) and the calculated q_e cal value is closer to the experimental q_e exp value. In the view of these results, the pseudo-second-order kinetic model provided a good correlation for the adsorption of *penicillin G* onto *Lemna minor* in contrast to the pseudo-first-order and intraparticle diffusion model.

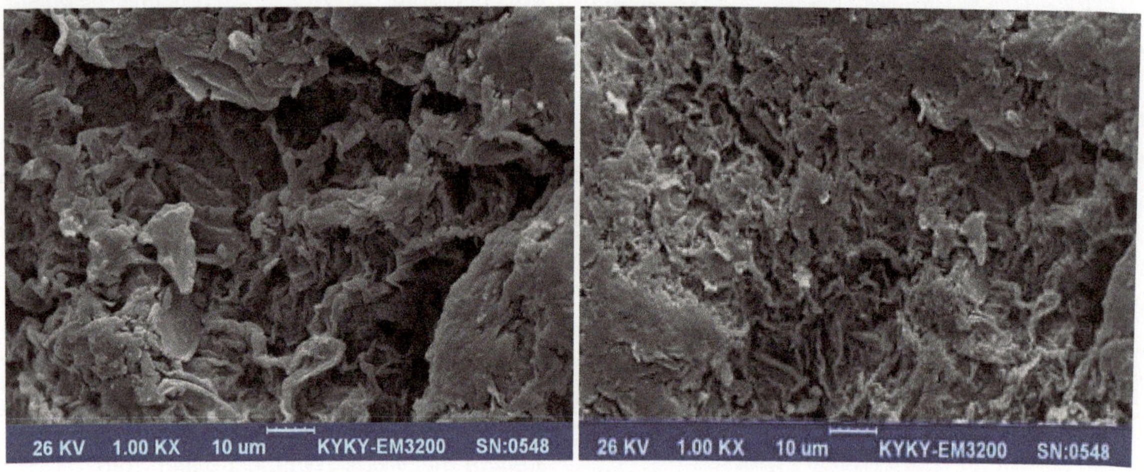

Fig. 1. The SEM image of modified *Lemna minor* before and after used

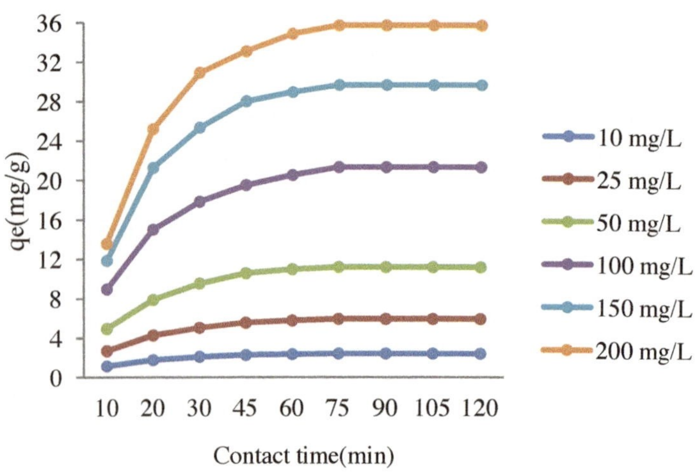

Fig. 2. Effect of contact time and initial *penicillin G* concentration (pH = 3, dose: 4 g/L and temp 30℃)

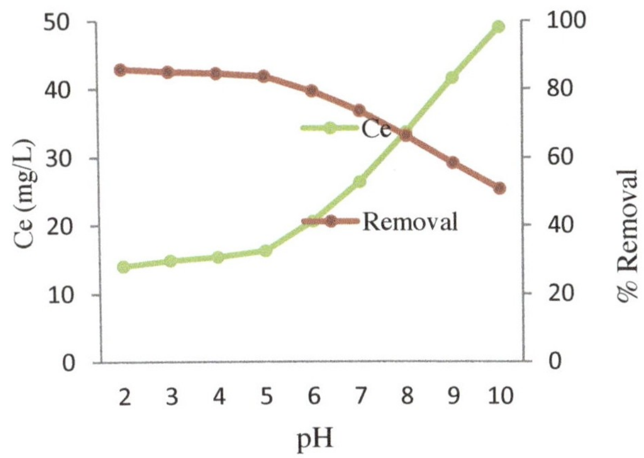

Fig. 3. Effect of pH on adsorption (Con = 100 mg/L, Contact time = 75 min, dose: 4 g/L and temp 30°C)

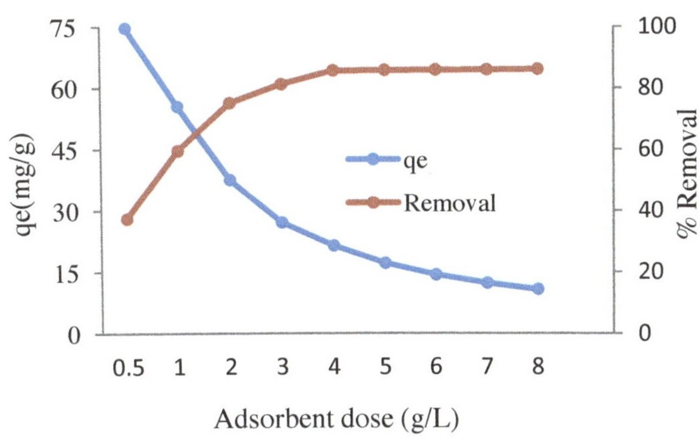

Fig. 4. Effect of adsorbent dose (Contact time = 75 min, pH = 5, Con: 100 mg/L and temp 30°C)

Table 3. Parameters of pseudo-first-order, pseudo-second-order and intraparticle diffusion models

C_0(mg/L)	q_e (mg/L)	Pseudo-first-order			Pseudo-second-order			Intraparticle diffusion		
		k_1	q_e (mg/g)	R^2	q_e (mg/g)	k_2	R^2	k	C (mg/g)	R^2
25	5.96	0.014	3.41	0.901	5.68	0. 32	0.994	0.128	2.17	0.845
50	11.45	0.0 22	7.65	0.916	11.39	0. 49	0.996	0.156	2.95	0.869
100	21.32	0.036	17.39	0.887	21.94	0. 67	0.999	0.194	3.64	0.837
200	35.71	0.044	29.76	0.877	36.42	0. 86	0.998	0.223	4.11	0.912

A study of the temperature dependence of adsorption reactions gave valuable knowledge about the enthalpy and entropy changes during adsorption. The removal of *penicillin G* onto *Lemna minor* was studied at 20, 30, 40 and 50°C to determine the adsorption isotherms and thermodynamic parameters. As seen in Fig. 5, adsorption ability of *Lemna minor* for *penicillin G* increased with increasing temperature. The adsorption capacity of *penicillin G* increased from 31.11 to 41.82 mg/g by increasing the temperature of the solution from 20 to 50°C, indicating that the process is endothermic.

The equilibrium adsorption isotherm is of importance in the design of adsorption systems. In general, the adsorption isotherm describes how adsorbate interacts with adsorbents and thus is critical in optimizing the use of adsorbents. Several isotherm equations are available, and four important isotherms were selected for this study: The Langmuir, Freundlich, Tekmin and BET isotherms. The Langmuir adsorption isotherm assumes that adsorption takes place at specific homogeneous sites within the adsorbent, and it has been used successfully for many adsorption processes of monolayer adsorption.

The values for q_m, K_L, k_F , B, k_t , A and n are summarized in Table 2. The isotherm data were calculated from the least square method and the related correlation coefficients (R^2 values) are given in the same table. As seen from Table 2, the Langmuir equation represents the adsorption process very well; the R^2 values were all higher than 0.99, indicating a very good mathematical fit. The fact that the Langmuir isotherm fits the experimental data very well may be due to the homogeneous distribution of active sites onto the *Lemna minor* surface, since the Langmuir equation assumes that the surface is homogenous. As seen in Table 4, the maximum adsorption capacities for *penicillin G* onto *Lemna minor* at 20, 30, 40 and 50°C were found to be 32.36, 36.18, 38.45 and 42.27 mg/g, respectively. Maximum adsorption capacities of *Lemna minor* increased with increasing temperature.

It is generally stated that the values of n in the range of 1 to 10 represent good adsorption. In the present work, the exponent was 1 <n <10, indicating favorable adsorption.

The essential features of the Langmuir isotherm can be expressed in terms of a dimensionless constant separation factor (R_L), which is defined by the following relationship [38].

$$R_L = \frac{1}{1+K_L C_0}$$

The value of R_L indicates the type of the isotherm; which is unfavorable (R_L >1), linear (R_L =1), favorable (0<R_L <1) or irreversible (R_L=0). The results given in Table 2 show that the adsorption of *penicillin G* onto *Lemna minor* is favorable.

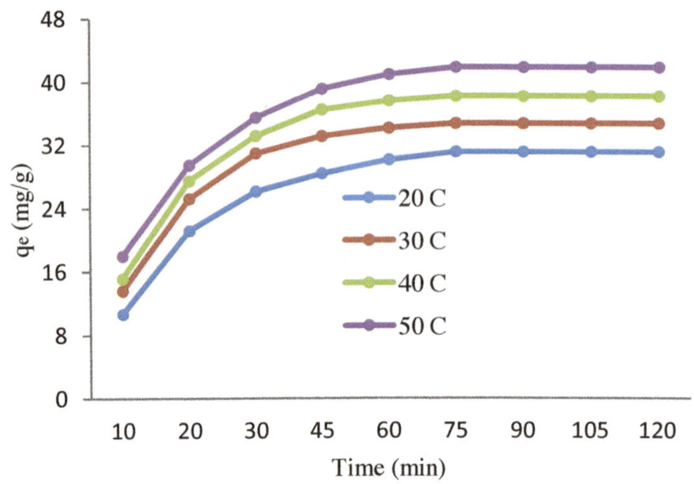

Fig. 5. Effect of contact time on the adsorption at different temperature

Table 4. The adsorption isotherms constants for the removal *penicillin G* onto *Lemna minor*

Tem	Langmuir model			Freundlich model			Temkin model			BET model		
(°C)	qm	KL	R2	n	KF	R2	B	A	R2	kt	B	R2
20	22.45	0.0014	0.994	2.65	6.14	0.812	31.71	7.41	0.804	14.4	0. 041	0.914
30	23.95	0.0039	0.995	2.17	7.39	0.845	37.45	6.52	0.781	17.7	0. 073	0.943
40	25.29	0.0063	0.997	3.09	7.85	0.791	41.12	4.36	0.768	21.2	0.095	0.904
50	26.17	0.0098	0.998	3.44	8.13	0.826	44.69	2.79	0.819	23.4	0.104	0.935

4. CONCLUSIONS

1. The present study shows that *Lemna minor*, can be used as an adsorbent for the removal of antibiotics from aqueous solutions.
2. The amount of *penicillin G* adsorbed was found to vary with adsorbent dosage, initial *penicillin G* concentration, pH, and temperature.
3. The amount of *penicillin G* uptake (mg/g) was found to increase with increase in contact time, temperature, and in initial *penicillin G* concentration, but decreased with an increase in adsorbent dosage.
4. The rate of adsorption was found to conform to pseudo-second-order kinetics with a good correlation.
5. Equilibrium data fitted very well in the Langmuir isotherm equation, confirming the monolayer adsorption capacity of *penicillin G* onto *Lemna minor* with a monolayer adsorption capacity of 36.18 mg/g at room temperature.
6. The dimensionless separation factor (R_L) showed that *Lemna minor* can be used for removal of *Lemna minor* from aqueous solutions.
7. *Lemna minor*, an inexpensive and easily available material, can be an alternative for more costly adsorbents used for antibiotics removal in wastewater treatment processes.

CONSENT

It is not applicable.

ETHICAL APPROVAL

It is not applicable.

COMPETING INTERESTS

Authors have declared that no competing interests exist.

REFERENCES

1. Hirsch R, Ternes T, Haberer K, Kratz KL. Occurrence of antibiotics in the aquatic environment. Sci Total Environ. 1999;225: 109–18.
2. Gulkowsk A, Leung HW, So MK, Taniyasu S, Yamashita N. Removal of antibiotics from wastewater by sewage treatment facilities in Hong Kong and Shenzhen, China. Water Reserch. 2008;42:395-403.
3. Adriano WS, Veredas V, Santana CC, Goncalves LRB. Adsorption of amoxicillin on chitosan beads: Kinetics, equilibrium and validation of finite bath models. Biochemical Engineering Journal. 2005;27: 132-7.
4. Polo M, Ferro-García MA, Medellín-Castillo NA. Kinetic study of the adsorption of nitroimidazole antibiotics on activated carbons in aqueous phase. J. Colloid Interf. Sci. 2010;345:481-490.
5. Zhao Y, Geng J, Wang X, Gu X, Gao S. Adsorption of tetracycline onto goethite in the presence of metal cations and humic substances. J. Colloid Interf. Sci. 2011; 361:247–251.
6. Yu A, Lin C, Yu T-H, Lateef SK. Removal of pharmaceuticals in secondary wastewater treatment processes in Taiwan. J. Hazard Mater. 2009;167:1163–9.
7. Kim SH, Shon HK, Ngo HH. Adsorption characteristics of antibiotics trimethoprim on powered and granular activated carbon. J. Ind. Eng. Chem. 2010;16:344-349.
8. Putra EK, Pranowo R, Sunarso J, Indraswati N. Performance of activated carbon and bentonite for adsorption of amoxicillin from wastewater: Mechanism, isotherms and kinetics. Water Res. 2009; 43:2419e2430.
9. Bi PY, Dong HR, Guo QZ. Separation and Purification of *Penicillin G* from fermentation broth by solvent sublation. Separation and Purification Technology. 2009;65:228–31.
10. Jonathan W, Peterson A, Laura J, Petrasky B. Adsorption and breakdown of penicillin antibiotic in the presence of titanium oxide nanoparticles in water. Chemosphere. 2012;87:911–7.
11. Yaghmaeian K, Moussavi Gh, Alahabadi A. Removal of amoxicillin from contaminated water using NH4Cl-activated carbon: Continuous flow fixed-bed adsorption and catalytic ozonation regeneration. Chemical Engineering Journal. 2014;236:538–544.
12. Malakootian M, balarak D, Mahdavi Y, Sadeghi SH, Amirmahani N. Removal of antibiotics from wastewater by azolla filiculoides: Kinetic and equilibrium studies. IJAPBS. 2015;4(7):105-113.
13. Aksu Z, Tunc O. Application of biosorption for *Penicillin G* removal: Comparison with

activated carbon. Process Biochemistry. 2005;40(2):831-47.
14. Ding R, Zhang P, Seredych M, Bandosz TJ. Removal of antibiotics from water using sewage sludge- and waste oil sludge-derived adsorbents. Water Research. 2012;90:40-6.
15. Bui TX, Choi H. Adsorptive removal of selected pharmaceuticals by mesoporous silica SBA-15. J. Hazard Mater. 2009; 168:602–8.
16. Choi K-J, Kima S-G, Kimb S-H. Removal of antibiotics by coagulation and granular activated carbon filtration. Journal of Hazardous Materials. 2008;151:38–43.
17. Ding R, Zhang P, Seredych M, Bandosz TJ. Removal of antibiotics from water using sewage sludge- and waste oil sludge-derived adsorbents. Water Research. 2012;90:40-6.
18. Crisafully R, Milhome MAL, Cavalcante RM, Silveira ER. Removal of some polycyclic aromatic hydrocarbons from petrochemical wastewater using low-cost adsorbents of natural origin. Bioresour. Technol. 2008;99:4515-4519.
19. Ali I. New generation adsorbents for water treatment. Chem. Revs. 2012;112:5073-509.
20. Zazouli MA, Mahvi AH, Mahdavi Y, Balarakd D. Isothermic and kinetic modeling of fluoride removal from water by means of the natural biosorbents sorghum and canola. Fluoride. 2015;48(1):15-22.
21. Zazouli MA, Balarak D, Mahdavi Y. Effect of *Azolla filiculoides* on removal of reactive red 198 in aqueous solution. J Adv Environ Health Res. 2013;1(1):1-7.
22. Zazouli MA, Yazdani J, Balarak D, Ebrahimi M, Mahdavi Y. Removal acid blue 113 from aqueous solution by canola. J Mazand Uni Med S. 2013;23(2):73-81.
23. Diyanati RA, Balarak D, Ghasemi SM. Survey of efficiency agricultural weast in removal of acid orang 7(AO7) dyes from aqueous solution: Kinetic and equilibrium study: Iranian Journal of Health Sciences. 2013;2(1):35-40.
24. Balarak D, Mahdavi Y. Survey of efficiency agricultural waste as adsorbent for removal of P-Cresol from aqueous solution. International Research Journal of Pure & Applied Chemistry. 2016;10(2):1-11.
25. Balarak D, Pirdadeh F, Mahdavi Y. Biosorption of acid red 88 dyes using dried *Lemna minor* biomass. Journal of Science, Technology & Environment Informatics. 2015;1(02):81–90.
26. Diyanati RA, Yousefi Z, Cherati JY, Balarak D. The ability of *Azolla* and *Lemna minor* biomass for adsorption of phenol from aqueous solutions. J Mazand Uni Med S. 2013;23(106):21-8.
27. Zazouli MA, Mahvi AH, Dobaradaran S, Barafrashtehpour M, Mahdavi Y, Balarak D. Adsorption of fluoride from aqueous solution by modified *Azolla filiculoides*. Fluoride. 2014;47(4):349-58.
28. Zazouli MA, Balarak D, Karimnezhad F, Khosravi F. Removal of fluoride from aqueoussolution by using of adsorption onto modified *Lemna minor*: Adsorption isotherm and kinetics study. J Mazand Uni Med S. 2014;23(109):208-17.
29. Ali I. The quest for active carbon adsorbent substitutes: Inexpensive adsorbents for toxic metal ions removal from wastewater. Sepn. & Purfn. Rev. 2010;39(3-4):91-171.
30. Ali I, Asim M, Khan TA. Low cost adsorbents for the removal of organic pollutants from wastewater. J. Environ. Manag. 2012;113:170-183.
31. Gupta V, Ali I, Mohan D. Equilibrium uptake and sorption dynamics for the removal of a basic dye (basic red) using low-cost adsorbents. J. of Colloid Interface Sci. 2003;265:257-264.
32. Gupta VK, Ali I, Saini VK, Gerven TV, Bruggen BV, Vandecasteele C. Removal of dyes from wastewater using bottom ash. J. Ind. & Eng. Chem. 2005;44:3655-64.
33. Zhang L, Song X, Liu X, Yang L, Pan F. Studies on the removal of tetracycline by multi-walled carbon nanotubes. Chem. Eng. J. 2011;178:26-33.
34. Mohammadi AS, Sardar M. The removal of *Penicillin G* from aqueous solutions using chestnut shell modified with H2SO4: Isotherm and kinetic study. Journal of Health & Environmental. 2012;6(1):497-508.
35. Rahardjo A, Susanto M, Kurniawan A, Indraswati N. Modified Ponorogo bentonite for the removal of ampicillin from wastewater. J. Hazard Mater. 2011;190: 1001–8.
36. Zhang CL, Qiao GL, Zhao F, Wang Y. Thermodynamic and kinetic parameters of ciprofloxacin adsorption onto modified coal fly ash from aqueous solution. Journal of Molecular Liquids. 2011;163:53–6.

37. Rivera-Utrilla J, Prados-Joya G, Sánchez-Polo M. Removal of nitroimidazole antibiotics from aqueous solution by adsorption/bioadsorption on activated carbon. J. Hazard Mater. 2009;170:298–305.

38. Balarak D, Bazrafshan E, Kord Mostafapour F. Equilibrium, kinetic studies on the adsorption of acid green 3 (AG3) dye onto *Azolla filiculoides* as adosorbent. American Chemical Science Journal. 2016;10(2):1-11.

24

Effect of Resveratrol on Some Haematological Parameters of Lead-intoxicated Male Wistar Rats

Salisu Muhammad Highab[1*], Danjuma Nuhu Muhammad[1], Musa Aliyu[2] and Bala Yauri Muhammad[3]

[1]Department of Pharmacology and Therapeutics, Faculty of Pharmaceutical Sciences, Ahmadu Bello University, Zaria, Nigeria.
[2]Department of Pharmacology, Faculty of Clinical Sciences, Bayero University Kano, Nigeria.
[3]Department of Pharmacology and Toxicology, Unaizah College of Pharmacy, Qassim University, Unaizah 51911, Al-Qassim Province, Saudi Arabia.

Authors' contributions

This work was carried out in collaboration between all authors. Author SMH performed the experiments, designed the study, managed the analyses of the study, performed the statistical analysis, wrote the protocol and wrote the first draft of the manuscript. Author DNM supervised the study and managed the literature searches. Author MA supervised the study and did all correction mentioned by the reviewers. Author BYM supervised and did some corrections on manuscript. All authors read and approved the final manuscript.

Article Information

Editor(s):
(1) R. Deveswaran, M.S. Ramaiah College of Pharmacy, Bangalore, India.
(2) Alyautdin Renad N, Chair of the Department of Pharmacology (Pharmaceutical Faculty), I. M. Sechenov MSMU, Moscow, Russia.
Reviewers:
(1) Carolina Baraldi Araujo Restini, University of Ribeirão Preto, SP, Brazil.
(2) Daniela Hanganu, Iuliu Haţieganu University of Medicine and Pharmacy, Romania.
(3) Juan Carlos Troiano, University of Buenos Aires, Argentina.
(4) Anonymous, Cairo University, Egypt.

ABSTRACT

The aim of this experiment was to investigate the effect of resveratrol on haematological parameters of lead-induced toxicity in male wistar rats. The study employed 36 male wistar rats (150 - 250 g) divided equally into six (6) groups. The first group (negative control) was administered carboxymethylcellulose (CMC) 10 g/L body weight (BW) daily for 19 days. The second group (positive control) was administered lead acetate solution (120 mg/kg BW) daily for 2 weeks. The third group was administered lead acetate solution (120 mg/kg BW) daily for 2 weeks then treated with succimer (10 mg/kg BW) daily for 5 days. The fourth group was administered lead acetate

**Corresponding author: E-mail: smhighab@gmail.com*

solution (120 mg/kg BW) daily for 2 weeks then treated with resveratrol (200 mg/kg BW) daily for 5 days. The fifth group was administered lead acetate solution (120 mg/kg BW) daily for 2 weeks then treated with resveratrol (400 mg/kg BW) daily for 5 days. The sixth group was pretreated with resveratrol (400 mg/kg BW) daily for 5 days then administered lead acetate solution (120 mg/kg BW) daily for 2 weeks and considered as prophylactic group. All treatments were administered orally by *gavage*. The animals were euthanized and blood sample were taken for heamatological analysis. In the result, there was significant ($P < 0.05$) increase in platelet counts in group 5 compared to both negative and positive control groups. No significant ($P > 0.05$) change was recorded for the other heamatological parameters, when the resveratrol-treated groups were compared to negative and positive control groups. No significant ($P > 0.05$) change was recorded for the other heamatological parameters, when the resveratrol-treated groups were compared to negative and positive control groups. Thus, the effect of resveratrol in platelet level is dose dependent. This study also observed that all the groups had normal levels of packed cell volume (absence of anemia).

Keywords: Resveratrol; lead acetate; succimer; male rats.

1. INTRODUCTION

Lead is a heavy, low melting, bluish-gray metal that occurs naturally in the Earth's crust. However, it is rarely found singly as a metal. It is usually found combined with two or more other elements to form lead compounds. For these reasons, lead has been used by humans for millennia and widespread today in products as diverse as pipes, storage batteries, pigments and paints, glazes, vinyl products, weights, and ammunition, cable covers, and radiation shielding. Tetra-ethyl lead was used extensively from the 1930s to the 1970s as a petrol additive to improve engine performance [1,2]. Tetra-ethyl lead has been eliminated from petrol in majority of countries, but is still used in about nine countries [3].

Lead inhibits the body's ability to make hemoglobin by interfering with several enzymatic steps in the heme pathway. Specifically, lead decreases heme biosynthesis by inhibiting *d*-aminolevulinic acid dehydratase (ALAD) and ferrochelatase activities. Ferrochelatase, which catalyzes the insertion of iron into protoporphyrin IX, is quite sensitive to lead. A decrease in the activity of this enzyme results in an increase of the substrate, erythrocyte protoporphyrin (EP), in the red blood cells (also found in the form of ZPP-bound to zinc rather than to iron). Also associated with lead exposure is an increase in blood and plasma d-aminolevulinic acid (ALA) and free erythrocyte protoporphyrins (FEP) [4,5].

Environmental Protection Agency (EPA) estimated the threshold BLL for a decrease in hemoglobin to be 50 μg/dL for occupationally lead exposed adults and approximately 40 μg/dL for children, although other studies have indicated a lower threshold (25 μg/dL) for children [4,5].

Recent data indicate that the erythrocyte protoporphyrin (EP) level, which has been used in the past to screen for lead toxicity, is not sufficiently sensitive at lower levels of blood lead and is therefore not as useful a screening test as previously thought.

Lead can induce two types of anemia, often accompanied by basophilic stippling of the erythrocytes [5]. Acute high-level lead exposure has been associated with hemolytic anemia. Frank anemia is not an early manifestation of lead exposure and is evident only when the BLL is significantly elevated for prolonged periods. In chronic lead exposure, lead induces anemia by both interfering with heme biosynthesis and by diminishing red blood cell survival. The anemia of lead intoxication is hypochromic and normo- or microcytic with associated reticulocytosis.

The heme synthesis pathway, on which lead has an effect, is involved in many other processes in the body including neural, renal, endocrine and hepatic pathways. There is a concern about the meaning of and possible sequelae of these biochemical and enzyme changes at lower levels of lead.

Resveratrol (3, 5, 4'-trihydroxystilbene) is a polyphenol that occurs naturally in foods and drinks, available in grapes and peanuts, and also in a number of herbal remedies, both alone and as part of plant extracts [6]. Resveratrol attracted little interest until 1992, when its use was postulated to explain some of its cardioprotective properties and was thought to account in part for the so-called 'French Paradox', that is, the finding that the rate of coronary heart disease mortality in France is lower than that observed in other industrialized countries with a similar risk factor profile [7]. Since then, reports have shown that resveratrol prevents or slows the progression of a wide variety of illnesses, including cancer, cardiovascular disease [8] and ischaemic injuries [9]. Resveratrol enhances stress resistance and extends the lifespan of various organisms from yeast to vertebrates [10]; it reduces the incidence of breast cancer [11-14], cardiovascular diseases [15,16], and possesses antioxidant property [17]. Resveratrol's antioxidant property has been demonstrated to ameliorate adverse effects of heat stress-induced toxicity [18-20]. Information on the ameliorative effect of resveratrol on heavy metals induced organ toxicity is however scanty. The present study was undertaken to assess the ameliorative effect of resveratrol on lead induced organ toxicity in rats.

Succimer is an analogue of dimercaprol (2, 3-dimercapto-1-propanol, British anti-lewisite, BAL), and has replaced dimercaprol as one of the main antidotes used in the management of poisoning by lead and other heavy metals. The advantages of succimer are that it is effective by oral administration because it is soluble in water; it is well-tolerated, has relatively low toxicity and can be given at the same time as iron supplements to treat iron deficiency anaemia. It does not cause significant increase in urinary excretion of essential minerals unlike the other widely used lead chelating agent, sodium calcium EDTA.

2. MATERIALS AND METHODS

2.1 Materials

2.1.1 Chemicals

Trans-resveratrol (60g) of analytical grade was purchased from Candlewood Stars Incorporated, Danbury, USA (Batch Number: MR 110218). Lead acetate (product No; 10142, BDH Laboratory chemicals limited Poole, England), Carboxymethylcellulose CMC (10 g) (Product No: 27929, BDH Laboratory chemicals limited Poole, England) were obtained from the Department of Pharmacology, Faculty of Pharmaceutical Sciences, Ahmadu Bello University, Zaria. *Trans*-Resveratrol, due to its low solubility in water, was suspended in 10 g/L CMC [21].

2.1.2 Equipment

Lead Care II User's Guide, Lead Care II blood analyser, Automated Haematology Analyzer (Sysmex model 2X-12N, USA). Automated Biochemistry Analyzer (Selectra XL, Vital Scientific, Netherlands) Dissecting sets, syringes, and needles, spatula, regent bottles, digital weighing balance, Sensors (2 containers of 24 each), Treatment Reagent tubes, Capillaries/plungers, Transfer droppers, Calibration button, Alcohol wipes, Gauze pads, Power free Gloves, High and low control

2.1.3 Experimental animals

Thirty six (36) male wistar rats (weighing 150 - 250 g) were used for this study. The animals were housed in the Department of Pharmacology and Therapeutics, Ahmadu Bello University, Zaria. They were given access to pelletized growers marsh and water *ad libitum*. The rats were acclimatized for two weeks in the home cages and environment before commencement of the experiment. All experimental protocols were in accordance with the Ahmadu Bello University research policy and regulations governing the care and use of experimental animals (NIH publication number 85-23, revised 1996). The experiments were conducted in a quiet environment between the hours of 900 and 1600.

2.2.4 Experimental Site

The experiments were carried out during the hot-humid (rainy) season (August- September, 2014) at the Department Pharmacology and Therapeutics, Ahmadu Bello University, Zaria (11° 10' N, 07° 38' E), at the elevation of 650 m above sea level, located in the Northern Guinea Savannah zone of Nigeria [22].

2.2 Experimental Procedure

2.2.1 Resveratrol preparation and administration

Trans-resveratrol (Batch Number: MR 110218), due to its low solubility in water, was suspended in 10 g/L Carboxymethylcellulose (CMC), and administered orally once daily for 14 days [23].

2.2.2 Lead acetate induction and resveratrol pretreatment

Male wistar rats were divided into six groups, of six (6) animals each. The first group servered as negative control and animals were given carboxymethylcellulose (CMC) (10 g/L body weight) orally. The second, third, fourth and fifth groups were given lead acetate (120 mg/kg) body weight orally for 14 days and the sixth group was pretreated with resveratrol (400 mg/kg body weight) [24,25] orally for 5 days serving as prophylaxis.

2.2.3 Treatments with succimer and resveratrol

After the lead acetate induction for 14 days and resveratrol pretreatment for 5 days, treatment with succimer and resveratrol commenced on the 15th day and lead acetate induction on the 5th day, where the second group was serving as the positive control (lead poisoned), the third group was treated with succimer (10 mg/kg body weight) [26,27], the fourth group was treated with Resveratrol (200 mg/kg body weight) [24,25], the fifth group was treated with resveratrol (400 mg/kg body weight) [24,25] orally for five (5) days and the sixth group was induced with lead acetate (120 mg/kg body weight) orally for 14 days serving as prophylactic group [24].

2.3 Methods

2.3.1 Determination of effect of resveratrol on haematological parameters in lead-induced toxicity in male wistar rats

Blood samples were collected at the end of treatment period. (3 – 4 mls) was collected into K^+ EDTA bottles for estimation of packed cell volume (PCV), platelets, white blood cell count (WBC) and differentials using Automated Haematology Analyzer (Sysmex model 2X-12N, USA).

2.3.2 Statistical analysis

Data obtained were expressed as mean ± SEM. Statistical analysis was carried out using SPSS version 20 and all the analysis were done using one way ANOVA followed by Tukey post *hoc* test for multiple comparisons. Values of $P < 0.05$ were considered significant.

3. RESULTS

3.1 Effect of Resveratrol on Haematological Parameters of Lead-induced Toxicity in Male Wistar Rats

There was a statistical significant (P < 0.05) increase in platelets count (392.33±31.81 L/L) in Lead acetate (120 mg/kg) + Resveratrol (400 mg/kg) group when compared to positive control (Lead acetate 120 mg/kg) (210.50±24.99 L/L) and negative control (carboxymethylcellulose 10 g/L) (219.50±30.50 L/L) group. There was no statistical significant (P > 0.05) difference in PCV, WBC, neutrophils, lymphocytes and monocytes in resveratrol-treated groups when compared to negative (carboxymethylcellulose 10 g/l) and positive control groups (lead acetate 120 mg/kg) (Table 3.1).

4. DISCUSSION

Lead is a ubiquitously found environmental and industrial pollutant that has been detected in nearly all phases of environment and biological system. Its persistence in human and animal tissues has quite often been associated with considerable health risks [28]. This study was to investigate the effects of resveratrol on some heamatological parameters lead induced organ toxicity in male wistar rats.

Blood platelet aggregation under physiological conditions is an important process that arrests bleeding, but excessive platelet aggregation causes thrombosis and atherosclerosis [29,30]. The haemopoietic system serves as important target for toxic chemicals and is a sensitive index of pathological conditions. In the present study, treatment with resveratrol did not cause any alteration in haematological parameters except in the platelet (PLT) level. Increase in platelets count observed in group 5 might be an indication of resveratrol non-toxic effects on the bone marrow and it is possible that prolonged consumption of resveratrol could prevent thrombocytopenia (reduced PLT level), preventing bleeding disorders, due to its ability to cause an increased platelet count at dose of 400 mg/kg. Although, this finding was actually in disagreement with the finding of [30] who demonstrated that resveratrol significantly reduced platelet count but in hyperhomocysteinaemia induced wistar rats as against the present study which used lead-induced toxicity in male wistar rats. Thus, the effect of resveratrol in PLT level is dose dependent. This study also observed that all the groups had normal levels of packed cell volume (absence of anemia). However, anemia has been reported following lead poisoning which was attributed to various inhibitory effects of Pb on heme biosynthesis [31]. Besides, excessive Pb exposure inhibits the body's ability to make hemoglobin by interfering with several enzymatic

Table 3.1 Effect of resveratrol on haematological parameters in lead-induced toxicity in male wistar rats

Treatments	Packed cell volumes (L/L)	White blood cells (L/L)	Platelets (L/L)	Neutrophils (%)	Lymphocytes (%)	Monocytes (%)
CMC(10 g/L)	0.95±3.53	12.83±5.51	219.50±30.50	25.17±7.29	70.67±6.71	4.60±1.01
LA(120 mg/kg)	0.42±0.03	14.33±4.18	210.50±24.99	22.83±3.90	76.33±3.98	3.00±0.00
LA(120mg/kg)+ S (10 mg/kg)	0.39±0.02	9.98±3.30	261.00±30.51	37.20±4.96	59.60±4.96	4.00±1.56
LA(120 mg/kg)+ R (200 mg/kg)	0.50±0.02	12.16±2.87	237.00±19.72	15.80±2.46	83.80±2.25	_
LA(120mg/kg)+ R (400 mg/kg)	0.40±0.02	19.18±5.25	392.33±31.81^{a*}	38.00±6.22	49.83±5.93	3.50±0.65
R(400mg/kg)+ LA(120 mg/kg)	0.44±0.02	6.87±0.41	181.67±47.57	18.67±2.91	81.33±2.91	_

Values are represented as means ± SEM ^{c*} = $P < 0.001$ compared to CMC (10 g/l) and Lead acetate (120 mg/kg) one way ANOVA followed turkey test. LA-Lead-acetate, R-Resveratrol, CMC-Carboxymethylcellulose, S-Succimer

steps in the heme pathway, through inhibiting aminolevulinic acid dehydratase and ferrochelatase activity, leading to anemia and erythrocytes degeneration or destruction [32].

5. CONCLUSION

In conclusion, intervention with resveratrol has significantly increased platelet counts (392.33±31.8) in the lead poisoned male wistar rats. Resveratrol's effectiveness in platelet count in this experimental group was found to be dose dependent.

CONSENT

It is not applicable.

ETHICAL APPROVAL

All authors hereby declare that "Principles of laboratory animal care" (NIH publication No.85-23, revised 1985) were followed, as well as specific national laws where applicable. All experiments have been examined and approved by the appropriate ethics committee.

COMPETING INTERESTS

Authors have declared that no competing interests exist.

REFERENCES

1. Rosner D, Markowitz G. A 'gift of God'? The public health controversy over leaded gasoline during the 1920s. American Journal of Public Health. 1985;75:344–352.
2. Landrigan PJ. Environmental pollutants and disease in American children: Estimates of morbidity, mortality, and costs for lead poisoning, asthma, cancer, and developmental disabilities. Environmental Health Perspectives. 2002;110(7):721–728.
3. UNEP. Target 2008: global elimination of leaded petrol. Nairobi, United Nations Environment Programme; 2008. Available:http://www.unep.org/pcfv/PDF/LeadReport-Brochure.pdf (Accessed 5 October 2009)
4. EPA. Air quality criteria for lead. Research Triangle Park, NC: U.S. Environmental Protection Agency, Office of Research and Development, Office of Health and Environmental Assessment, Environmental Criteria and Assessment Office. EPA600883028F; 1986.
5. ATSDR. Toxicological profile for mercury from agency for toxic substances and disease registry; 1999. Available:http://www.atsdr.cdc.gov/toxprofiles/tp46.pdf
6. Siemann EH, Creasy LL. Concentration of the phytoalexin resveratrol in wine. American Journal of Enology and Viticulture. 1992;43:49–52.
7. Bradamante S, Barenghi L, Villa A. Cardiovascular protective effects of resveratrol. Cardiovascular Drug Review. 2004;22:169–188.
8. Sinha K, Chaudhary G, Gupta YK. Protective effect of resveratrol against oxidative stress in middle cerebral artery occlusion model of stroke in rats. Life Science. 2002;71:655–665.

9. Valenzano DR, Terzibasi E, Genade T, Cattaneo A, Domenici L, Cellerino A. Resveratrol prolongs lifespan and retards the onset of age-related markers ina short-lived vertebrate. Current Biology. 2006;16: 296–300.
10. Whitsett TG, Lamartiniere CA. Genistein and resveratrol: Mammary cancer chemoprevention and mechanisms of action in the rat. Expert Review Anticancer Therapy. 2006;6(12):1699-1706.
11. Wesierska-Gadek J, Kramer MP, Maurer M. Resveratrol modulates roscovitine-mediated cell cycle arrest of human MCF-7 breast cancer cells. Food Chemcal Toxicology; 2007.
12. Ferry-Dumazet H, Garnier O, Mamani-Matsuda M, Vercauteren J, Belloc F, Billiard C, Dupouy M, Thiolat D, Kolb JP, Marit G, Reiffers J, Mossalayi MD. Resveratrol inhibits the growth and induces the apoptosis of both normal and leukemic haematopoietic cells. Carcinogenesis. 2002;23(8):1327-1333.
13. Joe AK, Liu H, Suzui M, Vural ME, Xiao D, Weinstein IB. Resveratrol induces growth inhibition, S-phase arrest, apoptosis, and changes in biomarker expression in several human cancer cell lines. Clinical Cancer Research. 2002;3:893-903.
14. Renaud S, de Lorgeril M. Wine, alcohol, platelets, and the French paradox for coronary heart disease. Lancet. 1992;339: 1523–1526.
15. Renaud S, Gueguen R. The French paradox and wine drinking. Novartis Foundation. Symptoms. 1998;216:208–217.
16. Giovannini L, Migliori M, Longoni BM, Das DK, Bertelli AA, Panichi V, Filippi C, Bertelli A. Resveratrol, a polyphenol found in wine, reduces ischaemia-reperfusion injury in rat kidneys. Journal of Cardiovascular Pharmacology. 2001;37(3): 262-70.
17. Putics A, Vegh EM, Csermely P, Soti C. Resveratrol induces the heatshock response and protects human cells from severe heat stress. Antioxidants and Redox Signaling. 2008;10(1):65-75.
18. Das A. Heat stress-induced hepatotoxicity and its prevention by resveratrol in rats. Toxicology Mechanisms and Methods. 2011;21(5):393–399.
19. Sahin K, Orhan C, Akdemir F, Tuzcu M, Iben C, Sahin N. Resveratrol protects quail hepatocytes against heat stress: Modulation of the Nrf2 transcription factor and heat shock proteins. Journal of Animal Physiology and Animal Nutrition. 2012; 96(1):66-74.
20. Lia ME, Juan M Pilar Vinardell, Planas JM. The daily oral administration of high doses of trans-resveratrol to rats for 28 days is not harmful. Journal of Nutrition. 2002; 132(2):257–260.
21. Akpa GN, Asiribo OO, Alawa JP, Dim NI, Osinowo OA, Abubakar BY. Milk production by agropastoral Red Sokoto goats in Nigeria. Tropical; 2002.
22. Juan ME, González-Pons E, Munuera T, Ballester J, Rodríguez-Gil JE, Planas JM. T*rans*-resveratrol, a natural antioxidant from grapes, increases sperm output in healthy rats. Journal of Nutrition. 2005;135: 757-760.
23. Magaji GM, Abolarin M, Opeyemi IA, Magaji AR. Modulatory effect of resveratrol on neuropsychiatric behavior in mice. Department of Pharmacology and Therapeutics, Ahamdu Bello University, Zaria Nigeria; 2014a.
24. Magaji RA, Magaji MG, Yusha'u Y, Faruk F, Muhammad UA, Fatihu MY. Book of proceedings of the world congress of pharmacology, Final abstract No. 1158. 2014b;65.
25. Joanne MA, Xiaomei L, Christopher QR, Brandi P, MinYou. Resveratrol alleviates alcoholic fatty liver in mice. American Journal of Physiology. Gastrointestinal and Liver Physiology. 2008;295(4):G833-G842.
26. POISINDEX. Succimer. In Klasco RK (Ed): POISINDEX® System. Thomson Micromedex, Greenwood Village, Colorado, USA; 2009.

    Available:http://www.thomsonhc.com (Accessed 7 April 2009)
27. TOXBASE. Lead chelation therapy in children. United Kingdom National Poisons Information Service; 2009.

    Available:www.toxbase.org (Accessed 17 August 2009)
28. Juberg DR, Kleiman CF, Simona CK. Position paper of the American Council on Science and Health: Lead and human health. Ecotoxicol Environ Saf. 1997;38: 162–80.
29. Olas B, Wachowicz B. Resveratrol, a phenolic antioxidant with effects on blood

platelet functions. Platelets. 2005;16(5): 251–260.

30. Malinowska J, Olas B. Response of blood platelets to resveratrol during a model of hyperhomocysteinaemia. Platelets. 2011; 22(4):277–283.

31. Kim Y, Yoo CI, Lee CR, Lee JH, Lee H, Kim SR, Chang SH, Lee WJ, Hwang CH, Lee YH. Evaluation of activity of erythrocyte pyrimidine 5-nucleotidase (P5N) in lead exposure workers, with focus on the effect on hemoglobin. Ind Health. 2002;40:23-27.

32. Patocka J, Cerný K. Inorganic lead toxicology. Acta Medica. 2003;46:65-72. Payton M, Hu H, Sparrow D, et al. Low-level lead exposure and renal function in the normative aging study. Am J Epidemiol. 1994;140(9):821-829.

25

Comparative Hepatic Effects of *Hippocratea africana* Root Bark Extract on Female and Male Albino Wistar Rats

Jessie Idongesit Ndem[1*] and Efosa Godwin Ewere[1]

[1] *Department of Biochemistry, Faculty of Basic Medical Sciences, University of Uyo, P.M.B. 1017, Uyo, Akwa Ibom State, Nigeria.*

Authors' contributions

This work was carried out in collaboration between both authors. Author JIN designed the study, wrote the protocol and wrote the first draft of the manuscript. Authors JIN and EGE managed the literature searches. Author JIN performed the spectroscopy and statistical analyses. Authors JIN and EGE managed the experimental process and author JIN identified the specie of plant. Both authors read and approved the final manuscript.

Article Information

Editor(s):
(1) Vasudevan Mani, Universiti Teknologi MARA (UiTM), Selangor, Malaysia.
Reviewers:
(1) M. Angels Calvo Torras, Universitat Autonoma de Barcelona, Spain.
(2) S. Aurasorn, Naresuan University, Thailand.
(3) Justin N. Kabera, Tianjin University of TCM, China.

ABSTRACT

Aim: To compare the effects of *Hippocretea africana* root bark extract on liver function biomarkers of female and male albino Wistar rats.

Study Design: 48 albino Wistar rats weighing 163-227 gms consisting 24 females and 24 males were randomly distributed into 4 groups of six animals each on sex basis. Group I served as normal control and were given 1 ml of distilled water. Groups II, III and IV were administered 100, 200 and 300 mg/kg body weight respectively of the extract by oral intubation.

Place and Duration of Study: Department of Biochemistry, Faculty of Basic Medical Sciences, University of Uyo, Uyo. The duration of the study was 14 days.

Methodology: Liver function biomarkers (AST, ALT, ALP and GGT) and Oxidative Stress markers (catalase (CAT), Superoxide dismutase (SOD) activities and MDA concentrations were assayed

**Corresponding author: Email: jessndem@yahoo.com*

using standard procedures. Histopathological examinations of liver organs were also carried out using standard methods.

Results: Generally, there were increases in ALT and AST activities for both female and male groups II and III extract treated rats while test group IV recorded decreased activities for the female compared with the control. AST and ALP activities were significantly ($p < 0.05$ and $p < 0.01$) higher in male rats with exception of AST for group IV and GGT for groups II and III compared with the control. Treatments with extract significantly ($p < 0.05$ and $p < 0.01$) increased the activities of SOD and CAT and also significantly ($p < 0.05$ and $p < 0.01$) increased MDA concentrations in female and male rats.

Conclusion: It can be concluded that *Hippocratea africana* root bark extract has a mild toxic effect on liver tissues as seen from the concentrations of liver function enzymes, and the histopathological examination. The increased activities of SOD and CAT and MDA concentrations may probably be a way of first line defence. Thus, long-term administration of the herb may not be advised in the males even with its good antiplasmodial property.

Keywords: Hippocratea africana; antiplasmodial activity; liver enzymes; catalase; superoxide dismutase; malondialdehyde.

1. INTRODUCTION

Different parts of plants; leaves, barks, roots and even latex are used medicinally by Traditional Medicine Practitioners (TMPs) for the treatment of various body ailments such as hypertension, diabetes mellitus, ulcer, malaria, typhoid fever, gonorrhea, syphilis, cancer etc [1].

Research interest is now focused on various herbs that possess hypoglycaemic, hypolipidaemic, antiplatelet, antihypertensive, antidiabetic, antitumour, immune stimulating or antimalarial properties etc. that may be useful in complementary properties or alternative medicine [2]. This interest is fuelled in Africa (Nigeria in particular) by the rising cost of prescription drugs in the maintenance of personal health and well-being. Available evidence also shows that some herbal remedies used in the treatment of ailments are affordable and efficacious [3]. Exploration of nature as a source of new active agents is thus essential for the discovery of bioactive chemical substances from natural product for the development of novel molecular diversity of efficacious drugs. Natural products from plants, used either alone or with combinatorial synthetic methodologies, constitute a multidisciplinary approach to the current drug productivity [4,5].

Hippocratea africana is a plant that inhabits green forests and is a perennial climber with hairs (glabrous) and reproduced from seeds [6]. The plant is widely distributed in tropical Africa and the roots are used traditionally in the treatment of various ailments such as fever, malaria, body pains, diabetes and diarrhea [7]. It has been reported to possess *in vivo* antiplasmodial activity with LD50 of 2.45 mg/kg body weight in mice [7]. Okokon et al. [7] also reported that *H. africana* possesses anti-inflammatory, analgesic and anti-pyretic properties which are probably mediated via inhibition of various autocoid formation and release. Other species of *Hippocratea* which possess anti- inflammatory activity are *Hippocratea excels* [8] and *Hippocratea indica* [9]. In the phytochemical study of *Hippocratea africana* Willd. (Loes). (Hippocrateaceae), Ndem et al. [10] reported that the plant contain significant quantities of phytochemicals such as alkaloids, cardiac glycosides, tannins, anthraquinonones and flavonoids. Alkaloids are known to exhibit emetic amoebicide, expectorant, anaesthetic, antipyretic, analgesic, antihelminthic properties and are used for the treatment of stomach problems [3]. The presence of cardiac glycosides in the *H. africana*, known to be useful in the treatment of diseases associated with the heart [11], further confirms the usefulness to the Traditional Medicine Practitioners (TMPs) in the treatment of hypertension. Flavonoids elicit a wide range of therapeutic activities such as antihypertensive, antimicrobial, anti-tumour and its usefulness by herbalist confirms the presence of phytochemical properties in *Hippocratea africana* [12,13].

The blood promising schizontocidal activity of *H. africana* both in early and established malaria infection at oral doses of 200 to 600 mg/kg/day in mice have been reported [7] and owing to the wide spread use of the root bark of this plant as an antiplasmodial herb by the Niger Delta people of Nigeria (Akwa Ibom State), its effect on the liver as the major organ of xenobiotic metabolism was studied to ascertain the possible toxic or adverse effects that may be associated with its use.

2. MATERIALS AND METHODS

2.1 Collection and Preparation of Plant Extract

The roots of *Hippocratea africana* (Willd) Loes were harvested from Afaha Etok Ibesikpo forest in Ibesikpo-Asutan, L.G.A of Akwa Ibom State in Nigeria. They were identified and authenticated by a Taxonomist in the Department of Botany, University of Uyo, Uyo. A voucher specimen of the root was deposited in the herbarium of Botany Department, University of Uyo, Uyo. The roots were washed using tap water and the bark scrapped with a knife, cut into very tiny pieces, air dried and pulverised using an electric blender. The powdered sample (2 Kg) was stored in a dried, airtight container at 37℃.

One kilogramme of the powdered *H. africana* was exhaustively macerated in 2000 ml of 80% ethanol. It was left overnight to allow for the solvent to interact with the extract and solubilise the active ingredients. The clear orange filtrate was carefully siphoned using a tube and concentrated in vacuum at 40℃ to obtain a dry orange crude extract. The dried crude extract was stored in the refrigerator at 4℃ until required for use.

2.2 Experimental Animals

Forty-eight mature albino Wistar rats consisting of twenty four males and twenty four females weighing 163 - 227 grams each were obtained from the animal house of the College of Health Sciences, University of Uyo, Uyo. The animals were divided into four groups of six rats each on sex basis. They were caged in plastic cages made of stainless steel bottom. Stainless steel mesh were placed at the bottom of the cages for collection of faeces and feed droppings. The males were caged separately from the females to prevent mating during the treatment period.

2.3 Administration of Plant Extract

The extract was administered orally once daily for fourteen (14) days by use of a canular attached to syringe. All the experimental animals were given normal rat chow and water *ad libitum* throughout the treatment period.

2.4 Collection of Blood Samples

At the end of the fourteen days treatment, the weights of animals were taken. The animals were denied feeds but still had water *ad libitum* for sixteen hours before they were chloroform anaesthetized and dissected. Blood sample was obtained by cardiac puncture using sterile syringes and needles and collected into plain sample bottles for serum separation. The serum was obtained by centrifugation of clotted blood in a MSE table top centrifuge at 4,000 rpm for 10 minutes. The separated sera were stored in a refrigerator at 4℃.

2.5 Assessment of Serum Activities of Oxidative Stress Biomarkers and Assay of Serum Activities of Liver Function Enzymes

Serum activities of superoxide dismutase (SOD), catalase (CAT), as well as lipid peroxidation (LPO) measured in terms of malondialdehyde (MDA) concentration was assessed.

Superoxide Dismutase and catalase activities were assayed based on the method by Wheeler et al. [14]. Assessment of lipid hydroperoxide (LPO) measured in terms of malonyldialdehyde (MDA) concentration was carried out based on method by Mihaljevic et al. [15]. They were all done using Cayman laboratory research kits.

Serum activities of aspartate aminotransferase (AST), alanine aminotransferase (ALT), alkaline phosphatise (ALP), and gamma glutamyl transferase (GGT), were assessed. ALT, AST and ALP activities were determined using Randox laboratory reagent kit, UK, BT 29 4QY based on method by Reitman and Frankel [16]. Serum activity of gamma-glutamyl-transferase (GGT) activity was estimated using Randox laboratory kit reagent, UK, BT294QY based on method by Szassz [17].

2.6 Histological Examinations

The liver tissues were extracted by the use of forceps and scissors. They were placed on clean filter paper to mop up excess blood, weighed and stored in screw tight containers containing 10% buffered formaldehyde solution. Histological analysis was carried out according to the procedure recommended by Drury and Wallington [18]. The slides were examined using a light microscope and the histopathological changes especially morphological changes were recorded. Photomicrographs of prominent pathological lesions were taken.

2.7 Statistical Analysis

The results of all determinations were expressed as Mean ± standard deviation. Data between treatment groups were analysed using one way analysis of variance (ANOVA). Pairwise comparison was done using the student's t-test. Values of $p < 0.05$ and $p < 0.01$ were regarded as being significant.

3. RESULTS

3.1 Effect of Extract on Serum Activities of Superoxide Dismutase (SOD), Catalase (CAT) and Concentration of Malonyldialdehyde (MDA) of Female and Male Albino Wistar Rats

Tables 1 and 2 shows the serum activities of superoxide dismutase (SOD), catalase and concentration of MDA of female and male rats administered 100, 200 and 300 mg/kg bw of *H. africana* root bark extract to test groups II, III and IV respectively against control group I rats administered distilled water.

For the female rats, the result in Table 1 depicts a dose- dependent significant ($p < 0.05$ and $p < 0.01$) increase in superoxide dismutase activity of 1.26±0.04, 1.88±0.07 and 2.23±0.08 U/ml for test groups II, III and IV respectively administered 100, 200 and 300 mg/kg bw respectively of *H. africana* root bark extract compared with the control group I activity of 1.17±0.04 U/ml. Catalase activity showed significant ($p < 0.05$ and $p < 0.01$) increases of 14.52±0.45, 18.35±0.54 and 17.58±0.04 nmol/min/ml for test groups II, III and IV respectively compared with the control group I activity of 12.49±0.5 nmol/min/ml, although test group III recorded a non-significant higher value than test group IV. MDA concentration also depicts significant ($p < 0.05$ and $p < 0.01$) increasing activities of 1.92± 0.01, 2.46±0.06 and 2.35±0.04 μM for test groups II, III and IV respectively compared with the control group I concentrations of 1.52±0.02 μM.

Table 2 depicts the serum activities of superoxide dismutase (SOD) and catalase and concentration of MDA for male albino rats. SOD activity against concentration doses of 100, 200 and 300 mg/kg bw *H. africana* root bark extract showed a significant ($p < 0.05$) dose dependent increases of 1.34±0.01, 1.40±0.01 and 1.73±0.10 U/ml for test groups II, III and IV respectively compared with the control group I activity of 1.11±012 U/ml. Test groups II, III, and IV rats showed significant ($p < 0.05$ and $p < 0.01$) increasing catalase activity of 23.18±0.03, 31.29±0.57 and 26.12±0.38 nmol/min/ml compared with the control group I activity of 20.80±0.39 nmol/min/ml. Although, test group III rats recorded higher value than test group II rats. Graded concentrations of 100, 200, 300 mg/kg

Table 1. Serum activities of superoxide dismutase (SOD) and catalase (CAT) and concentration of Malonyldiadehyde (MDA) of female albino Wistar rats administered graded doses of ethanol extract of *Hippocratea africana* root bark

Group/Dosage	Superoxide dismutase (SOD) (U/ml)	Catalase (nmol/min/ml)	Malonyldialdehyde (MDA) (μM)
Group I Control (distilled water)	1.17±0.04	12.49±0.53	1.52±0.02
Group II H.A (100 mg/kg body weight)	*,** 1.26±0.04	*,** 14.52±0.45	*,** 1.92±0.01
Group III H.A (200 mg/kg body weight)	*,** 1.88±0.07	*,** 18.36±0.54	*,** 2.46±0.06
Group IV H.A (300 mg/kg body weight)	*,** 2.23±0.08	*,** 17.58±0.04	*,** 2.35±0.04

*Results are presented as Mean ± SD, n = 6; H.A = Hippocratea africana root bark extract; *= Significantly different from control value at p < 0.05, ** =Significantly different from control value at p < 0.01*

Table 2. Serum activities of superoxide dismutase (SOD) and catalase (CAT) and concentration of malonyldiadehyde (MDA) of male albino Wistar rats administered graded doses of ethanol extract of *Hippocratea africana* root bark

Group/Dosage	Superoxide dismutase (SOD) (U/ml)	Catalase (nmol/min/ml)	Malonyldialdehyde (MDA) (μM)
Group I Control (distilled water)	1.11±0.12	20.80±0.39	1.19±0.05
Group II H.A (100 mg/kg body weight)	1.34±0.01 *	23.18±0.37 *,**	1.47±0.02 *,**
Group III H.A (200 mg/kg body weight)	1.40±0.01 *	31.29±0.57 *,**	1.55±0.02 *,**
Group IV H.A (300 mg/kg body weight)	1.73±0.10 *	26.12±0.38 *,**	1.52±0.01 *,**

Results are presented as Mean ± SD, n = 6, H.A= Hippocratea africana root bark extract
=Significantly different from control value at $p < 0.05$,=Significantly different from control value at $p < 0.01$*

bw administered to test groups II, III and IV rats respectively recorded significant ($p < 0.05$ and $p < 0.01$) increasing MDA concentrations of 1.47±0.02, 1.55±0.02, and 1.52±0.01 μM compared with the control group I concentration of 1.19±0.05 μM.

3.2 Effect of Extract on Activities of Serum Liver Enzymes and AST/ALT Ratio of Albino Wistar Rats

The effects of graded doses of ethanol extract of *H. africana* root bark on the activities of serum liver enzymes and AST/ALT ratio of female and male albino Wistar rats are depicted in Tables 3 and 4 respectively.

The female rats (Table 3) recorded Alanine aminotransferase (ALT) activities of 17.06±1.84, 22.84±3.56, 18.43±3.75, and 16.55±1.62 u/l for the control group I and test groups II, III and IV animals respectively. Only test group II increase activity was statistically significant ($p < 0.5$ and $p < 0.01$) compared with the control group I activity.

The aspartate aminotransferase (AST) activity for test groups II, III and IV were 191.43±1.96, 190.78±2.22 and 186.68 u/l respectively while the control group I rats recorded activity of 189.17±3.01 u/l. The result showed a non-significant ($p > 0.5$) dose-dependent reduction in AST activity compared with the control. Test groups II, III, and IV rats recorded dose-dependent decreases in Alkaline phosphatase (ALP) activity of 114.73±4.30, 111.29±3.74 and 109.18±4.67u/l that were all significant ($p < 0.5$ and $p < 0.01$) compared with the control group I activity of 125.71±1.16 u/l. Gamma glutamyl transferase (GGT) activity showed a non-significant ($p > 0.5$) decreasing values of 1.51 ±1.14, 2.28±0.88 and 1.93±0.55 u/l for test groups II, III and IV respectively compared with the control group I activity of 2.32 0.54u/l. The AST/ALT ratio were 8.38, 10.35 and 11.27 for test groups II, III and IV rats compared with control group rats ratio of 11.09.

The male rats (Table 4) recorded a significant ($p < 0.5$ and $p < 0.01$) increased ALT activities of 20.53±2.18 and 19.46±2.06 u/l for test groups II and III rats compared with the control group I activity of 14.14±1.68 u/l. Test group IV rats however recorded a non-significant ($p > 0.05$) decreased activity of 13.14±2.61 u/l compared with the control. The result shows increasing AST activities of 200.54±1.73, 186.33±4.06 and 205.55±2.91 u/l for test groups II, III and IV respectively compared with the control group I activity of 163.45 u/l. The increases though statistically significant ($p < 0.5$ and $p < 0.01$) were not dose-dependent. ALP activity depicts a dose-dependent significant ($p < 0.5$ and $p < 0.01$) increasing activities of 165.17±5.52, 185.53±8.04 and 207.00±8.59 u/l for test groups II, III and IV rats respectively compared with the control group I activity of 151.19±7.15 u/l. The GGT activity showed decreasing values of 2.32±0.02 and 2.70±1.08 u/l for test groups II and IV rats respectively compared with the control group 1 activity of 2.83±0.23 u/l. Test group III activity however showed a non-significant ($p > 0.05$) increase activity of 2.90±2.45 u/l compared with control group I activity. The decreases were only significant ($p < 0.5$ and $p < 0.01$) when test group II activity was compared with control group I activity. The AST/ALT ratio was 9.54, 9.58, 15.65 for test groups II, III and IV rats respectively and 11.56 for control group rats.

There were increases in ALT activity of female group II and III extract treated rats while test group IV recorded decrease activities. AST and ALP activity were significantly higher in male rats with exception of AST for group IV (300 mg/kg bw) and GGT for group II and III, enzyme activities in the male followed the same pattern as the female rats.

3.3 Histological Evaluations of the Liver Tissues of albino Wistar Rats Administered Graded Doses of *H. africana* Root Bark Extract

Sections from the liver were taken from all the animals used in this study after 14 days extract administration period and analysed for histopathological effects.

Table 3. Activities of serum liver enzymes and AST/ALT ratio of female albino Wistar rats administered graded doses of ethanol extract of *Hippocratea africana* root bark

Group/ Dosage	ALT (U/l)	AST (U/l)	ALP (U/l)	GGT (U/l)	AST/ALT
Group I Control (distilled water)	17.06±1.84	189.17±3.01	125.71±1.16	2.32±0.54	11.09
Group II H.A (100 mg/kg body weight)	*,** 22.84±3.56	191.43±1.96	*,** 114.73±4.30	1.51±1.14	8.38
Group III H.A (200 mg/kg body weight)	*,** 18.43±3.75	190.78±2.22	*,** 111.29±3.74	2.28±0.88	10.35
Group IV H.A (300 mg/kg body weight)	* 16.55±1.62	186.68±2.27	*,** 109.18±4.67	1.93±0.55	11.27

Results are presented as Mean ± SD, n = 6, H.A=Hippocratea africana root bark extract
*ALT = Alanine aminotransferase; AST = Aspartate aminotransferase; ALP = Alkaline phosphatise; GGT = Gamma glutamyl transferase; * = Significantly different from control value at p < 0.05; ** = Significantly different from control value at p < 0.01*

Table 4. Activities of serum liver enzymes and AST/ALT ratio of male albino Wistar rats administered graded doses of ethanol extract of *Hippocratea africana* root bark

Group/Dosage	ALT (U/l	AST (U/l)	ALP (U/l)	GGT (U/l)	AST/ALT
Group I Control (distilled water)	14.14±1.68	163.45±5.09	151.19±7.15	2.83±0.23	11.56
Group II H.A (100 mg/kg body weight)	*,** 20.53±2.18	* 200.54±1.73	*,** 165.17±5.52	*,** 2.32±0.02	9.54
Group III H.A (200 mg/kg body weight)	*,** 19.46±2.06	*,** 186.33±4.06	*,** 185.53±8.04	2.90±2.45	9.58
Group IV H.A (300 mg/kg body weight)	13.14±2.61	*,** 205.55±2.91	*,** 207.00±8.59	2.70±1.08	15.65

Results are presented as Mean ± SD, n = 6; H.A.= Hippocratea africana root bark extract
*ALT = Alanine aminotransferase; AST = Aspartate aminotransferase; ALP = Alkaline phosphatise; GGT = Gamma glutamyl transferase; * = Significantly different from control value at p < 0.05; ** = Significantly different from control value at p < 0.01*

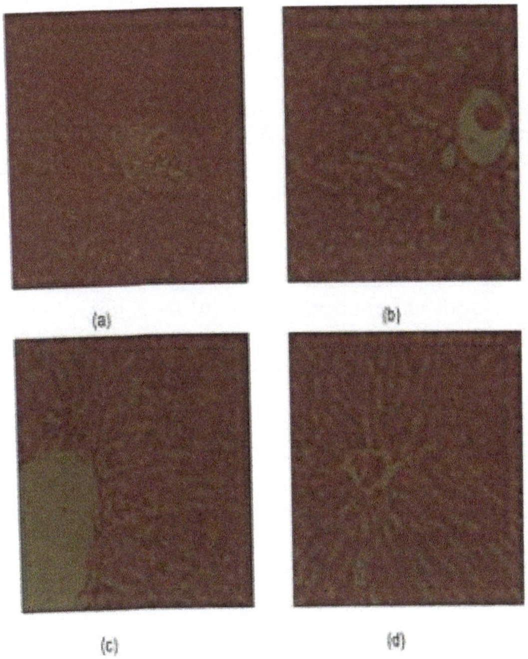

PLATE 1 : Photomicrographs of the liver tissue of adult female albino Wistar rats after administration of 100 (b), 200 (c) and 300 (d) mg/kg body weights of ethanol extract of *H. africana* root bark compared with the control group I (a)

(Mag. x 400)

(a)	Control group I	-	Normal hepatic tissue. No pathology.
(b)	Test group II	-	Marked diffuse atropy of hepatocytes with widening of the sinusoids. No inflammation is seen.
(c)	Test group III	-	Very mild fatty change. Diffuse periportal inflammation. Very mild hepatocyte death seen.
(d)	Test group IV	-	Very mild focal steatosis with the rest of the tissue being normal.

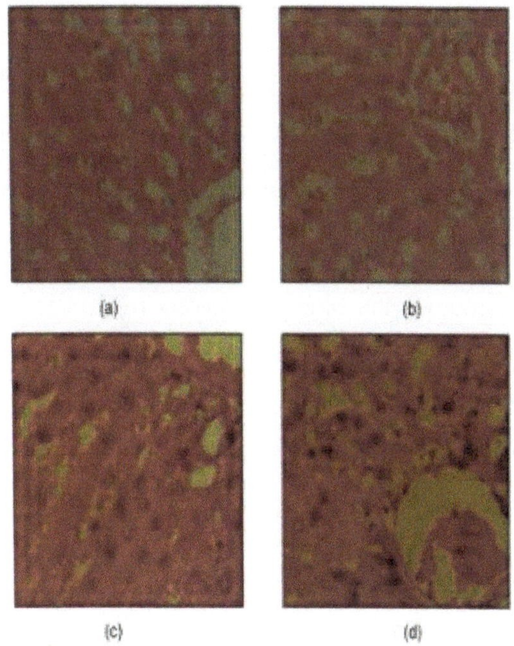

Plate 2: Photomicrographs of liver tissue of adult male albino Wistar rats after administration of 100(b), 200(c) and 300(d) mg/kg body weights of ethanol extract of *H. africana* root bark compared with control group I (a)

(Mag. x 400)

(a):	Control group I	-	Normal hepatic architecture. No pathology.
(b):	Test group II	-	Liver tissue displaying diffuse congestion of control veins which appear dilated with extravasation of blood into the sinusoids. Portal tracts appear normal and hepatocytes are viable and no pigment is seen.
(c)	Test group III	-	Hepatic congestion as seen in 6b.
(d)	Test group IV	-	Normal hepatic architecture showing radiating hepatocyte cords with limiting plates. The portal tracts sinusoids and central veins are normal

Fig. 1. Photographs of liver tissues of female and male experimental rats

4. DISCUSSION

Interest in medicinal plants as re-emerging health therapy have been fuelled by the rising costs of prescription drugs in the maintenance of personal health and well-being, and the bioprospecting of new plant-derived drugs [19]. One of such refocus interest in Africa, especially Nigerian (in both rural and urban areas) is herbal treatment for diseases. Despite the many orthodox drugs in the market, the upsurge in the number of people that rely on herbs for treating ailments has necessitated increased efforts to authenticating the efficacy and safety of some herbal claims. One of such herbs is *Hippocratea africana* root bark.

Biochemical and toxicological evaluations of crude drugs (herbs) and sometimes histopathological evaluations of tissue sections to compliment the changes that have occurred at the molecular level are necessary for the safety use of the drugs. The changes observed in these clinical biochemical indices may reveal the presence or absence of any tissue pathology. In the present study, biochemical and toxicological evaluations following administration of graded doses of *Hippocratea africana* root bark extract in both adult female and male albino Wistar rats, was undertaken.

Results obtained revealed increased activity of serum ALT for the female test rats at doses of 100 and 200 mg/kg bw of *H. africana* root bark extract. The dose of 300 mg/kg bw of the extract however had decreased ALT activity. The AST activity showed increases for 100 and 200 mg/kg bw of the extract treated groups. The 300 mg/kg bw of the extract treated group showed decrease activity. The slight increases in the ALT and AST activities at doses of 100 and 200 mg/kg bw of the extract observed indicate mild cellular damage in the female. ALT and AST are found in large amount in the liver and also small amount are found in the heart, kidney and muscles. When the liver is injured or inflamed as the case may be via its exposure to various forms of toxic substances, the level of ALT and AST in the blood is usually elevated. The level of these enzymes in the blood is directly related to the extent of the tissue damage [20-22]. The observed decrease in the activities of ALT and AST for 300 mg/kg bw treated group may be attributed to the dose-dependent protective effect of the antioxidant flavonoid phytochemical present in the herb Catechin, a flavonoid from *Uncaria gambri*, Roxbury and other plants used in the treatment of acute hepatitis have been reported to have a lowering effect on plasma aminotransferase activity compared with the control [23]. Vandenbergh et al. [24] have also reported a decrease in levels of transaminase in the liver of rats treated with bidisomide, an antiarrhythmic agent.

The male rats showed the same effects observed in the female rats for ALT and AST activities except that there was a significant increase and not decrease in AST activity following 300 mg/kg bw extract administration suggesting mild toxicity of the herb to males. Comparatively, sex appear to have impact on the enzyme activity with the increases in ALT and AST activities imposed by the herb affecting the male more than the female at 100 and 200 mg/kg bw dose of the extract and for all the test groups (100, 200 and 300 mg/kg bw of the extract) for AST activity.

The female rats recorded significant dose-dependent decreases in serum ALP activity. The male test groups' rats however, recorded dose-dependent increases in ALP activity. The ALPs are a group of enzymes that hydrolyse organic phosphate at alkaline pH. They are present in most tissues but are in particularly high concentration in the osteoblasts of bone and the cells of the hepatobiliary tract, intestinal wall, renal tubules and placenta [25]. In adults, plasma ALP is derived mainly from bone and liver in approximately equal proportions; the proportion due to the bone fraction is increased when there is increased osteoblastic activity that may be physiological [25]. Increased concentrations of vitamin C also elevate its concentration [25]. Serum ALP activity may also be raised due to primary neoplasm at site other than liver and non-neoplastic hepatobiliary diseases, as in the case of drugs and other chemically induced hepatoxicity [26]. Transient elevations may be found during healing of bone fractures and physiological bone growth elevates ALP in serum [27]. Low plasma ALP activity have been observed in arrested bone growth conditions (such as achondroplasia, hypothyroidism, and severe vitamin C deficiency), hypophosphatasia and treatment of hyperlipidaemia with a fibrate drug e.g. bezafibrate [25]. The significant dose-dependent decreases in ALP activity for the female rats observed in this study is likely due to the fact the phytochemicals present in the herb may have promoted bone growth and the herb may contain high concentration of vitamin C. while the significant increases in male may be attributed to disturbances in the tissue integrity of the experimental animals.

Non-significant ($p > 0.05$) decrease in GGT activity was observed in all the female treatment groups' rats in this study (Table 3). The male test rats also showed decrease in GGT activity for 100 and 300 mg/kg bw extract treatment. The 200 mg/kg bw extract treated group however, recorded a slight non significant ($p > 0.05$) increased activity (Table 4). GGT is the enzyme actively involved in the extracellular catabolism of glutathione, in the main mammalian [28]. GGT is present on the outer surface of plasma membrane of most cell types and in blood, where it forms complexes with several plasma components especially with albumin and lipoprotein [29]. The determination of serum GGT activity is a well-established diagnostic test for hepatobiliary diseases, and is used as a sensitive marker of liver damage. Increased serum GGT activity is associated with diseases of the liver, biliary system and pancreas [30,29]. The decrease in GGT activity in female suggest non toxicity, however, the slight non significant increase activity at 200 mg/kg bw of the extract for the male rats together with the significant increase in ALT and AST activities suggest toxicity. Long term administration is cautioned in males.

Administration of *H. africana* root bark extract at the different doses to both adult female and male albino Wistar rats significantly raised the serum activities of SOD and CAT and concentration of MDA in both sexes although the raised activities were not dose-dependent. The significantly ($p < 0.05$ and $p < 0.01$) raised activities of the serum oxidative stress enzymes (as shown in Tables 1 and 2) may be a way of the antioxidant defence systems of the rats attempting to combat the mild toxic effect of the extract by increasing the activities of the antioxidant enzymes. Xenobiotics have been reported as a source of reactive oxygen species because some of them can enhance the production of oxyradicals within the cells by inhibition of mitochondrial electron transport and subsequent accumulation of reduced intermediates [31], inactivation of antioxidant enzymes such as catalase and depletion of radical scavengers [32,33]. Massive oxidative stress, particularly in mitochondria induces necrosis [34]. No necrosis was observed in the histopathological analysis of the liver in both female and male Wistar rats which further support the mild toxic effect of the extract also indicating that long-term administration of the extract may be very toxic.

Administration of 100 mg/kg bw of the extract to female rats (Plate 1b) showed pronounced diffuse degeneration of the liver cells indicating possible toxicity, although no inflammation was seen. The liver is involved in about 8% of reports of adverse drug reactions, reflecting its central role in the metabolism and excretion of many drugs [35]. The pronounced diffuse degeneration of the liver cells observed at 100 mg/kg dose may be explained as first line effect of administration of foreign compound. The liver is usually the target of the immune system because of the production of drug metabolites that bind to proteins which are degraded to peptides presented on the surface with major histocompatibility complex class I [36]. Cell death is the crucial event leading to the clinical manifestation of drug-induced hepatoxicity. The pathogenesis of clinical drug hepatitis reflects either an immune-mediated attack on the liver or a biochemical effect of toxic metabolites leading to a loss of cell viability [37]. Plate 1 c of rats administered 200 mg/kg bw of the extract shows very mild fatty change. Diffuse periportal inflammation and very mild hepatocyte death is seen, indicating further mild toxic insult of the extract to the liver (Plate 1d) for test group IV rats administered 300 mg/kg bw shows mild focal steatosis with the rest of the tissue being normal.

The male, test groups II and III rats (Plates 2b and 2 c) administered 100 and 200 mg/kg bw of the extract liver tissues, depict diffuse congestion of central veins which appear dilated with extravasations of blood into the sinusoids. The dilation may obstruct the normal functioning at the liver of draining the blood i.e. carrying deoxygenated blood away from the liver. This may lead to accumulation of toxic materials and subsequently causing cell death [37]. However, the portal tracts appeared normal and the hepatocytes were viable with no pigment seen. Test group IV rats administered 300 mg/kg bw of the extract (Plate 2d) shows normal hepatic architecture showing radiating hepatocyte cords with limiting plates and the portal tract sinusoids and central veins appearing normal. Collectively, the overall results obtained from the histopathological examination of the liver tissues corroborate the results obtained for the liver enzyme activities.

5. CONCLUSION

The findings from this study show that *Hippocratea africana* root bark extract has a mild toxic effect on liver tissues as seen from the liver function enzyme results and from the liver histopathological examinations. Thus, long-term administration of this extract may be very toxic despite its blood promising schizontocidal activity and should be used with caution. Further study on its effect on the renal status is suggested.

CONSENT

It is not applicable.

ETHICAL APPROVAL

All authors hereby declare that the "Principles of laboratory animal care" (NIH publication No. 85-23, revised 1985) were followed as well as specific national laws where applicable. All experiments have been examined and approved by the appropriate ethics committee.

COMPETING INTERESTS

Authors have declared that no competing interests exist.

REFERENCES

1. Farombi EO. African indigenous plants with chemotherapeutic potentials and biotechnological approach to the production of bioactive prophylactic agents. African Journal of Biotechnology. 2003;2(12):662-671.
2. Borchers AT, Halkman RM, Keen CL, Steru JS, Gershwin ME. Complementary medicine a review of immunodilatory effects of Chinese herbal medicine. American Journal of Clinical Nutrition. 1997;66:1302-1321.

3. Fabricant DS, Farnsworth NR. The value of plants in traditional medicine for drug discovery. Environmental Health Perspectives. 2001;109(1):69-75.
4. Newman DJ, Cragg GM, Snader KM. Natural products as sources of new drugs over the period 1981-2002. Journal of Natural Products. 2003;66(7):1022-1037.
5. Cos P, Vlietinck AJ, Berghe DV. and Maes L. Anti-infective potential of natural products: How to develop a stronger *in* vitro 'Proof-of-Concept'. Journal of Ethno-pharmacology. 2006;106(3):290-302.
6. Dalziel JM. Useful plants of west tropical African. London: Crown Agents for Overseas Government; 1956.
7. Okokon JE, Ita BN, Udokpoh AE. The *in-vivo* antimalarial activities of *Uvariachamae* and *Hippocratea africana*. Annals of Tropical Medicine and Parasitology. 2006;100(7):585-590.
8. Perez RM, Zawala MA, Salazar M. Anti-inflammatory activity of the bark of *Hippocratea excelsa*. Journal of Ethno-pharmacology. 1995;47:85-90.
9. Ogbole OO, Ekor MN, Olumeri BB, Ajaiyeobu AA, Gbolade AA, Ayoola MA. and Adeyemi AA. Anti-inflammatory and anti-microial activities of *Hippocratea indica* root ark and *Poga oleosa* fruits. African Journal of Traditional and Complementry Alternative Medicine. 2007;4(3):372-380.
10. Ndem JI, Eteng MU, Uwah AF. Effect of *Hippocratea africana* root bark extract on the lipid profile of female and male albino Wistar rats. Journal of Scientific Research & Reports. 2014;3(19):2574-2583.
11. Trease A, Evans WC. Pharmacognosy 13th ed. London: Bailliere Tindall; 1989.
12. Latha PG, Panikkar KR. Inhibition of chemical carcinogenesis in mice by *Ixora coccineae* flowers. Pharmaceutical Biology. 2000;38(12):152-156.
13. Pieta PG. Flavanoids as antioxidants. Journals of Natural Product. 2000;63(7): 1035-1042.
14. Wheeler CR, Salzman JA, Elsayed N. Automated assays for superoxide dismutase, catalase, glutathione peroxidase and glutathione reductase activity. Analytical Biochemistry. 1990;184: 193-199.
15. Mihaljevic B, Katusin-Razen B, Razem D. The re-evaluation of the ferric thiocyanate assay for lipid hydroperoxides with special considerations of the mechanism aspects of the response. Free Radical Biology and Medicine. 1996;21:53- 63.
16. Reitman S, Frankel S. Serum-transaminase levels. American Journal of Clinical Pathology. 1957;28:56-63.
17. Szasz G, Bergmeyer HU. Method of enzymatic analysis. Weinheim: Verlag Chemie; 1974.
18. Drury RAB, Willington EA. Carleton's histological technique. 4th ed. London: Oxford University Press; 1967.
19. Hoareau L, Dasila EJ. Medicinal plants: A re-emerging health aid. Electronic Journal of Biotechnology. 1999;2:2-5.
20. Lum G, Gambino SR. Serum gamma-glutamyl transpeptidase activity as an indicator of disease of liver, pancreas, or bone. Clin Chem. 1972;18(4):358-362.
21. Halim A, El-Almady O, Hassab-Allah S, Abdel-Gelil F, Hafez Y, Derivis A. Biochemical effect of antioxidants on lipids and liver function in experimentally-induced liver damage. Annals of Clinical Biochemistry. 1997;34:656-663.
22. Udosen EO, Ojong AS. The biochemical, histological and hepatotoxic activity of the extract of *Sacoglothis gabonensis* in rats. Pharmaceutical Biology. 1998;36:467-469.
23. Thabrew MI, Hughes R. Phytogenic agents in the therapy of liver disease. Phytotherapy Research. 1996;10:461-467.
24. Vandenberghe Y, Mason, Palate B. and Roba J. Effects of folate supplementation on clinical chemistry and haematologic changes related to bidisomide administration in the rat. Drug Chemisty and Toxicology. 1995;18:L235-L270.
25. Crook MA. Clinical chemistry and metabolic medicine. 7th ed. New Delhi: Edward Arnold; 2006.
26. Bodansky O. Enzymes in cancer: The phosphohydrolases. In: Bodansky O. (Ed.), Biochemistry of human cancer. New York: Academic Press. 1995;61-92.
27. Burtis CA, Ashwood ER. Tietz textbook of clinical chemistry. 3rd ed. Tokyo: W. B. Saunders; 1999.
28. Huseby NE. Multiple forms of gamma-glutamyltransferase in normal human liver, bile and serum. Biochim Biophys Acta. 1978;522(2):354-362.
29. Huseby NE. Multiple forms of serum gamma-glutamyltransferase. Association of the enzyme with lipoproteins. Clin Chim Acta. 1982;124(1):103-112.
30. Betro MG, Oon RC, Edwards JB. Gamma-glutamyl transpeptidase and other liver

function tests in myocardial infarction and heart failure. Am J Clin Pathol. 1973; 60(5):679-683.

31. Nohl H. and Hegner D. Identification of free hydroxyl radicals in respiring heart mitochondria by spin trapping with nitrone. DMPO Federation of European Biochemical Societies Letter. 1981;123: 241-244.
32. Hasspieler BM, Behar JV, DiGiulio RT. Glutathione-dependent defense in channel catfish (*Ictalurus punctatus)* and brown bullhead *Ameriurus neblosus*). Ecotoxicology and Environmental Safety. 1994;28:82-90.
33. Kano Y, Fridovich I. Inhibition and reactivation of Mn-catalase. Implications for valence changes at the active site manganese. Journal of Biology and Chemistry. 1983;258:13646-13648.
34. Kaplowitz N. Mechanisms of liver cell injury. Journal of Hepatolog. 2001;32: 39-47.
35. Graffin JP. Manual of adverse drug reactions. 3rd ed. Bristol: J. Wright; 1988.
36. Robin M, LeRoy M, Descatoire V, Pessayre D. Plasma membrane cytochromes P450 as neoantigens and autoimmune target in drug-induced hepatitis. Journal of Hepatology. 1997;26: 23-30.
37. Kaplowitz N. Cell death at the millennium: Implications for liver diseases. Clinical Liver Disease. 2002;4:1-23.

26

Evaluation of the Physicochemical and *in vitro* Dissolution Properties of Metformin Hydrochloride Tablet Brands Marketed in Five Cities in Ghana

Akwasi Sougi[1], Kwabena Ofori-Kwakye[1*], Noble Kuntworbe[1], Samuel Lugrie Kipo[1] and Mariam El Boakye-Gyasi[1]

[1]Department of Pharmaceutics, Faculty of Pharmacy and Pharmaceutical Sciences, College of Health Sciences, Kwame Nkrumah University of Science and Technology (KNUST), Kumasi, Ghana.

Authors' contributions

This work was carried out in collaboration between all authors. Author AS performed the experimental work and wrote the first draft of the manuscript. Author KOK designed the study and reviewed the manuscript. Authors NK, SLK and MEBG were involved in data analysis and review of the manuscript. All authors read and approved the final manuscript.

Article Information

Editor(s):
(1) Mohamed Fathy, Assiut University, Assiut, Egypt.
Reviewers:
(1) Antonello Santini, University of Napoli Federico II, Italy.
(2) Panna Thapa, Kathmandu Unviersity, Nepal.

ABSTRACT

Aim: A comparative evaluation of the physicochemical and *in vitro* dissolution properties of metformin hydrochloride tablet brands sampled in five cities in Ghana was undertaken to assess their pharmaceutical equivalence.
Place and Duration of Study: Department of Pharmaceutics, KNUST, Kumasi, Ghana, between August 2012 and December 2012
Methodology: Fourteen brands of metformin tablets plus the innovator brand, Glucophage, purchased from retail pharmacies were studied. The genuineness of the samples was determined using Fourier transform infra-red (FTIR) spectroscopy and thin layer chromatography (TLC). Pharmacopoeia tests such as uniformity of weight, hardness, friability, disintegration and assay were used to assess the physicochemical equivalence of the tablet brands. *In vitro* dissolution testing was conducted and the dissolution data subjected to analysis involving dissolution

**Corresponding author: Email: koforikwakye@yahoo.com*

efficiency (DE), similarity factor (f_2) and Biopharmaceutics classification system (BCS)-based biowaiver conditions, as a surrogate for bioequivalence studies.

Results: All the tablet brands complied with the official specifications for identification, uniformity of weight hardness and disintegration. Brand M9 failed the friability test while brands M5, M9 and M12 failed the assay test. Dissolution efficiency (DE) and similarity factor (f_2) of the brands varied with pH of dissolution media with M4 (in 0.1 M HCl) having the highest DE and M9 (in phosphate buffer pH 6.8) the lowest.

Conclusion: Eleven of the fifteen tablet brands passed all the official tests and could be regarded as pharmaceutically equivalent but f_2 analysis showed only six brands were similar to the reference brand (with f_2 values ≥50 in the three dissolution media used). None of the metformin brands satisfied the criteria for BCS-based biowaiver for rapidly dissolving tablets. The study has shown that not all the metformin tablet brands sampled in five cities in Ghana are pharmaceutically equivalent.

Keywords: Metformin hydrochloride; physicochemical properties; in vitro dissolution; bioequivalence; biowaiver.

1. INTRODUCTION

Diabetes mellitus is a metabolic disease with characteristic chronic hyperglycaemia and defective protein, fat and carbohydrate metabolism due to deficient insulin secretion and/or action [1,2]. There are two main types of diabetes mellitus (type 1 and type 2 diabetes mellitus) though there are other rare forms of diabetes mellitus. Globally, 347 million people have diabetes [3]. Data on the prevalence of diabetes in Ghana is scanty and unreliable. The incidence of diabetes in Ghana among an urban outpatient population in Accra was estimated at 0.5% in the late 1950's [4]. However, a recent study reported a significant prevalence rate of 6.3% [5].

Metformin is an oral hypoglycaemic agent which belongs to the class of drugs called biguanides. It is the first line drug for the management of Type 2 diabetes mellitus. Metformin functions as an antihyperglycaemic agent through reduced gluconeogenesis and by enhancing the action of insulin in skeletal muscles. There are many generics of metformin hydrochloride tablets available in community pharmacies and hospitals in Ghana and other developing countries. Generic products are generally readily available and less expensive compared to the innovator products. The high prevalence of generic products is the major means through which people from developing countries are able to access important life-saving medicines [6]. However, generics are more likely to be of spurious and substandard quality than their innovator products. Also many generic products have been found to be fake or counterfeit products [7-10].

In addition to the obvious advantages of availability and low cost, generics are expected to demonstrate comparable quality with the innovator products before they could be clinically interchangeable. Thus, generics must exhibit equivalent pharmaceutical and therapeutic properties with the innovator products to make them acceptable substitutes. An important step in determining the therapeutic equivalence of a product is to establish whether they are chemically and biopharmaceutically equivalent [11].

Dissolution testing is an important quality control and drug development procedure employed in the pharmaceutical industry to evaluate the *in vitro* drug release profiles of solid dosage forms. Dissolution testing is used to establish the pharmaceutical quality of a product and it is also used as a surrogate for in vivo drug dissolution. The drug release profiles of a product and drug quality as a whole could be affected by the type and amount of API and excipients used in the manufacturing process as well as the manufacturing techniques employed. Dissolution testing is an important tool used to evaluate the pharmaceutical quality of generics and innovator products and to determine their possible equivalence. Thus pharmaceutically equivalent products would exhibit similar or equivalent drug release profiles. It should therefore be possible to select from a myriad of generic products one or more products which are pharmaceutically and therapeutically equivalent to the innovator drug. This is to prevent the situation whereby different products of the same API (generics) would demonstrate distinct differences in their therapeutic effects [12].

The aim of the current study was to ascertain the quality and drug release proficiency of commercial metformin hydrochloride tablet brands marketed in five cities in Ghana. This will allow prescribers to select appropriate generic metformin tablet brands as substitutes for the innovator brand, Glucophage.

2. MATERIALS AND METHODS

Pure metformin hydrochloride (RS) was obtained from the Department of Pharmaceutics, KNUST, Ghana. Hydrochloric acid fuming GR (Merck, Germany), sodium hydroxide, absolute ethanol, sodium nitroprusside, acetonitrile, glacial acetic acid (BDH, PROLABO), potassium dihydrogen orthophosphate (Fisons Laboratory), butanol, potassium ferricyanide, potassium bromide (BDH, Poole, England), ortho-phosphoric acid (Phillip Harris, England). All other reagents used were of analytical grade and were obtained from the Chemical store of the Department of Pharmaceutical Chemistry, KNUST, Kumasi, Ghana. Fourteen generic brands of metformin hydrochloride tablets plus the innovator brand Glucophage, each having label strength of 500 mg were purchased from retail pharmacies in five cities in Ghana, namely: Kumasi, Accra, Sunyani, Sekondi-Takoradi and Koforidua. General information on the metformin tablet brands is reported in Table 1.

2.1 Extraction of Metformin Hydrochloride from Tablets

A quantity of the powdered tablet equivalent to 60 mg of metformin hydrochloride was shaken with 60 ml of ethanol and filtered with Whatman filter paper (No 5). The filtrate was evaporated to dryness on a water bath and the residue dried at 105°C for one hour [13]. The procedure was repeated for the other tablet brands and the residue of each brand used for subsequent infra-red and thin layer chromatography analysis.

2.2 Identification of Extracted Metformin Hydrochloride Using TLC

TLC silica gel G plate was used and the solvent system consisted of a mixture of glacial acetic acid, butanol and water (10:40:50). Twenty milligram of the extracted residue of each metformin tablet brand as well as 20 mg of reference metformin hydrochloride powder was dissolved in distilled water and diluted to 5 ml with same solvent. The test solutions and the reference were spotted on the plate and immersed in the solvent system contained in the chromatank. The plate was removed when the solvent had moved three-fourths of the length of the plate. The solvent front was marked, allowed to evaporate from the plate and the spots detected by spraying with a mixture of equal volumes of sodium nitroprusside, potassium ferricyanide and sodium hydroxide solution all of 100 g/L. The Rf value of each spot was then determined [13].

2.3 Identification of Extracted Metformin Hydrochloride Using FTIR

Twenty milligram of the test sample (extracted residue) was triturated with 200 mg of dry, finely powdered KBr of spectroscopic grade using agate pestle and mortar. The mixture was ground thoroughly, spread uniformly in a suitable die and compressed into a disc using a pressure of 10 tons. A reference disc was similarly prepared with KBr alone. The resultant disc was mounted in a suitable holder in an Interspectrum Fourier Transform infra-red spectrophotometer and the IR spectrum was obtained at 600-4000 cm^{-1}. The infra-red spectrum of each brand of metformin tablet was then compared with the reference spectrum.

2.4 Thickness Test

A digital vernier caliper was used to measure the thickness of ten tablets from each brand and the mean (±S.D) determined.

2.5 Weight Uniformity Test

Twenty (20) tablets from a particular brand were randomly selected and weighed collectively to obtain a mean weight. The tablets were then weighed individually and the percentage deviation of each tablet from the mean was then calculated [13]. The procedure was repeated for the other brands.

2.6 Friability Test

Ten tablets were randomly selected from a particular brand, dusted and weighed together and then placed in the Erweka friabilator (Type TA 20, Germany) and operated for 4 minutes at 25 rpm. The tablets were dedusted and reweighed and the percentage weight loss calculated. The procedure was repeated for the other brands.

Table 1. Profile of metformin hydrochloride tablet brands studied

Sample code	Coating	Country of origin	Batch number	Mfg. date	Expiry date
M1	Film-coated	Ghana	2909m	*	09/16
M2	Film-coated	United kingdom	MEAG016	*	06/14
M3	Film-coated	Germany	81R	08/12	07/16
M4	Uncoated	Ghana	12018	05/12	05/16
M5	Film-coated	Germany	BS1579	05/12	05/16
M6	Film-coated	Malaysia	BC06712	06/12	06/15
M7	Film-coated	India	MH008	12/10	11/13
M8	Uncoated	India	NP11061	05/11	04/14
M9	Film-coated	Ghana	1012	-	11/14
M10	Film-coated	India	B344	12/11	12/14
M11	Film-coated	France	108007	04/12	03/17
M12	Film-coated	United Kingdom	BUH022139	*	11/16
M13	Film-coated	United Kingdom	RM1001	*	12/13
M14	Film-coated	United Kingdom	RM1286	*	07/14
M15	Uncoated	India	E07515	01/11	12/13

**, not provided*

2.7 Hardness Test

Ten tablets were selected at random from each brand to perform this test using a DBK hardness tester (India). A tablet was placed between the spindle and anvil of the tester and the calibrated scale adjusted to zero. Compression force was applied on the tablet and the position on the calibrated scale at which the tablet broke was recorded in Kgf units. A mean hardness (±S.D) was calculated for each brand.

2.8 Disintegration Test

Six tablets selected randomly from a brand were placed individually in each of the six cylindrical tubes of the basket rack of an Erweka disintegrating test apparatus (Type ZT 3/1, GmbH Heusenstamm, Germany) at 37±0.5°C. The disintegration time was taken to be the time no tablet fragment with firm core was left on the mesh.

2.9 Assay of Metformin Hydrochloride Tablets by HPLC

The content of metformin in each of the fifteen tablet brands was determined with a reverse phase chromatographic technique developed and validated by Kar and Choudhury [14] with minor modifications. A 100 μg/ml stock solution of metformin hydrochloride was prepared in a mobile phase of acetonitrile and phosphate buffer (65:35, pH 5.75). A series of 10 ml volumetric flasks containing 0.25-2.5 ml of the stock solution were made up to volume with the mobile phase. Each solution was filtered with a sintered glass filter and loaded in the injector of a Shimadzu HPLC (LC-10A Shimadzu pump with programmable absorbance detector and Shimadzu CR50 Chromatopac. Column used was Agilent Zorbax SB C-18 4.6 x 250 nm) fitted with 20 µl fixed volume loop, injected by rheodyne at a flow rate of 1.0 ml/min and the chromatogram for each injection was recorded. The calibration curve was plotted between concentration of drug and peak area of metformin hydrochloride.

A quantity of powdered metformin tablets equivalent to 10 mg metformin hydrochloride was accurately weighed into a 100 ml volumetric flask containing about 75 ml of mobile phase. The powder mixture was dissolved in the mobile phase with the aid of sonication and then made up to the 100 ml mark with the mobile phase. The solution was filtered through Whatman filter paper (No 5) and 1 ml was taken and made up to 10 ml with the mobile phase and filtered using sintered glass filters. The sample solution was analysed with a Shimadzu HPLC consisting of LC-10A Shimadzu pump with programmable absorbance detector and Shimadzu CR50 Chromatopac. The column used was Agilent Zorbax SB C-18 (4.6 x 250 nm). Flow rate employed was 1.0 ml/min, an injection volume of 20 µl and the detection of eluent was carried out at 232 nm. The injection was repeated three times and the peak area of metformin hydrochloride was recorded. The average peak area and calibration curve were used to calculate the amount of drug present [14]. The experimental procedure was repeated for the other metformin tablet brands.

2.10 *In vitro* Dissolution Study

Nine hundred milliliters each of 0.1 M HCl, phosphate buffer pH 4.5 and phosphate buffer pH 6.8 were used based on the FDA Guidance for Industry and the need to meet the criteria for biowaiver [15]. Nine hundred millilitres of 0.1 M HCl was placed in each of the six vessels of an Erweka dissolution apparatus (Type DT6, GmbH Heusenstamm, Germany) (USP Apparatus 2) rotating at 50 rpm and equilibrated to 37±0.5℃. One tablet was placed in each of the dissolution vessels and at 10, 15, 20, 30, 45, and 60 min, 10 ml samples were withdrawn and replaced with 10 ml of fresh dissolution medium. The withdrawn samples were filtered with Whatman filter paper (No 5) and diluted appropriately with distilled water. The diluted filtrates were analysed by UV spectrophotometer at 232 nm. The amount of drug released was determined from regression data obtained from calibration plot of metformin in distilled water (0.2-0.9 mg/100 ml) and the percentage drug released calculated. A plot of mean cumulative percentage drug release against time was established. The experiments were repeated using phosphate buffer pH 4.5 and phosphate buffer pH 6.8 as dissolution media.

2.11 Dissolution Data Comparison

Dissolution data obtained from the dissolution studies were fitted into a model-independent equation to determine the similarity factor (f_2) of the various brands compared to the reference drug (Glucophage)

$$f_2 = 50x\log \{[1+ (1/n) S\ t=1n\ (Rt-Tt)\ 2] - 0.5x100\}$$

where, f_2 = similarity factor, n = time points, Rt = cumulative percentage dissolved at time t for the reference, and Tt = cumulative percentage dissolved at time t for the test.

The similarity factor falls between 0 and 100. If $f_2 \geq 50$, it implies the two dissolution profiles are equivalent or similar therefore the two products could be interchanged. If $f_2 < 50$, it means the dissolution profiles are different or dissimilar hence the products cannot be interchanged.

The dissolution efficiency (DE) was estimated for each brand [16-18]. The dissolution efficiency was calculated using the equation:

$$DE = \{(0\int t\ Y.dt) / Y100.\ (t_2-t_1)\}\times 100$$

Where, (0∫t Y.dt) = area under the dissolution curve (AUC), Y= the percentage dissolved at t_2, t_2= time for all active ingredient to dissolve, and t_1= time at which first sample was withdrawn.

The dissolution data of metformin tablets (BCS class 3 drug) in the three dissolution media were subjected to BCS-based biowaiver under WHO criteria (i.e. very rapidly dissolving). The percentage drug dissolved at 15 minutes in 0.1 M HCl (pH 1.2), phosphate buffer pH 4.5 and phosphate buffer pH 6.8 were estimated and compared to the specification of ≥85% drug release at 15 min in all the three dissolution media.

3. RESULTS

Each of the fifteen metformin hydrochloride tablet brands purchased had at least 6 months left on the shelf-life and all analytical procedures were carried out before product expiration dates. Twelve brands were imported while three were manufactured in Ghana and this suggests the high prevalence of foreign brands of metformin tablets in Ghana. Twelve of the fifteen metformin tablet samples studied were film coated while three were uncoated.

In identification test employing thin layer chromatography (TLC), the principal spot in the chromatogram obtained for each brand of metformin tablet was similar in position, colour and size to the principal spot in the chromatogram obtained with the pure metformin hydrochloride. A retention factor (Rf) of 0.24 was obtained for ten tablet brands, 0.25 for three brands and 0.23 for two brands. These values are similar to the Rf value of pure metformin hydrochloride (0.25) (Table 2). The IR spectrum obtained for metformin extracted from each metformin tablet brand showed absorption bands at 740, 935, 1075, 1063, 1620 and 1580 cm^{-1} similar to the reference spectrum of pure metformin hydrochloride [13]. Fig. 1 presents a sample IR spectrum of metformin for tablet brand M1.

The physicochemical properties of the metformin tablet brands are shown in Table 3. The metformin tablet brands generally possessed good physicochemical properties. The tablets passed the uniformity of weight test and friability test except brand M9 (1.24%, friable). All twelve film-coated tablet brands disintegrated in aqueous medium <30 min and passed the disintegration test but one uncoated tablet brand (M8) disintegrated >15 min and hence failed the test. The drug content of the tablet brands was in the range 99.52-110.99%. Twelve metformin tablet brands passed the assay test while three (M5, M9, M12) were overdose hence failed the test. The amount of drug dissolved in 45 min (D_{45}), in all the tablet brands was >80%, thus passed the dissolution test for immediate release tablets.

Table 2. Rf values of various metformin hydrochloride tablet preparations

Sample code	Rf value
M1	0.24
M2	0.24
M3	0.24
M4	0.24
M5	0.24
M6	0.24
M7	0.23
M8	0.24
M9	0.24
M10	0.25
M11	0.23
M12	0.24
M13	0.24
M14	0.25
M15	0.25

Rf = Retention factor; Rf value of pure metformin hydrochloride powder (reference standard) = 0.25

The dissolution profiles of metformin hydrochloride tablet brands in 0.1 M HCl (pH 1.2), phosphate buffer pH 4.5 and phosphate buffer pH 6.8 are presented in Figs. 2, 3 and 4, respectively. The tablets showed similar dissolution profiles and achieved >80% drug release in 45 min in the three dissolution media. The dissolution efficiencies (DE) and similarity factors (f_2) of the various metformin tablet brands are presented in Table 4. Generally, both the DE and f_2 of the tablet brands varied with pH of the dissolution medium employed. Metformin tablets exhibited high dissolution efficiencies with 13 brands >90% DE in 0.1 M HCl, 14 brands > 90% DE in phosphate buffer pH 4.5, and 14 brands >90% DE in phosphate buffer pH 6.8. The f_2 values were ≥50 for ten brands in 0.1 M HCl, ten brands in phosphate buffer pH 4.5, and seven brands in phosphate buffer pH 6.8. Also, f_2 values were ≥50 for seven brands in both 0.1 M HCl and phosphate buffer pH 4.5, seven brands in 0.1 M HCl and phosphate buffer pH 6.8, and six brands in both phosphate buffer pH 4.5 and phosphate buffer pH 6.8. Six metformin tablet brands (M2, M5, M6, M12, M13 and M14) had f_2 values ≥50 in all the three dissolution media. All the tablet brands failed the BCS-based biowaver specifications for rapidly dissolving tablets as none of the brands achieved ≥85 % drug release in 15 minutes in the three dissolution media. However, eight tablet brands, M2, M3, M5, M6, M11, M12, M13 and M14 attained ≥85 % drug release in 30 min in the three media.

4. DISCUSSION

Fifteen metformin hydrochloride tablet brands were subjected to both FTIR and TLC analysis to ascertain the identity of the active pharmaceutical ingredient (API). Results from the identification tests indicated that all the metformin tablet brands contained metformin hydrochloride as API hence were not fake or counterfeit products. The capacity to identify fake and substandard pharmaceutical products on the market is a crucial component of a drug quality assurance system.

Metformin hydrochloride tablet brands sampled were subjected to pharmacopoeia and other tests to assess their quality and pharmaceutical equivalence. The assessment tests involved uniformity of weight, thickness, hardness, friability, disintegration, drug content and dissolution. These parameters are used to assess the consistency in quality among different batches of tablets and capsules during production. The nature of formulation of a drug product, the physicochemical properties of the API and excipients and the procedures used in manufacturing have marked effect on quality parameters of tablets [19]. The quality parameters are interrelated and have profound effect on drug absorption and bioavailability [20,21]. The tablet brands studied passed most of the quality evaluation tests undertaken. The thickness of a tablet can vary with no change in weight due to the difference in density of the granulation and the force of compression applied to the tablets. The uniformity of weight test is performed to assure constant dosing among tablets within a batch to prevent the incidence of overdosage or underdosage. The weight variation of a tablet directly affects the change in drug content of the tablet [22]. All the brands of metformin hydrochloride tablets weighed more than 350 mg, hence to pass the weight uniformity test, not more than two of the individual weight of the tablets should deviate from the average weight by more than ±5% and none of the tablets should deviate by more than twice the permissible percentage deviation [23]. All metformin tablet brands studied satisfied this specification and therefore passed the uniformity of weight test. This could be attributed to good flow properties of the granules and even feeding of granules into the die.

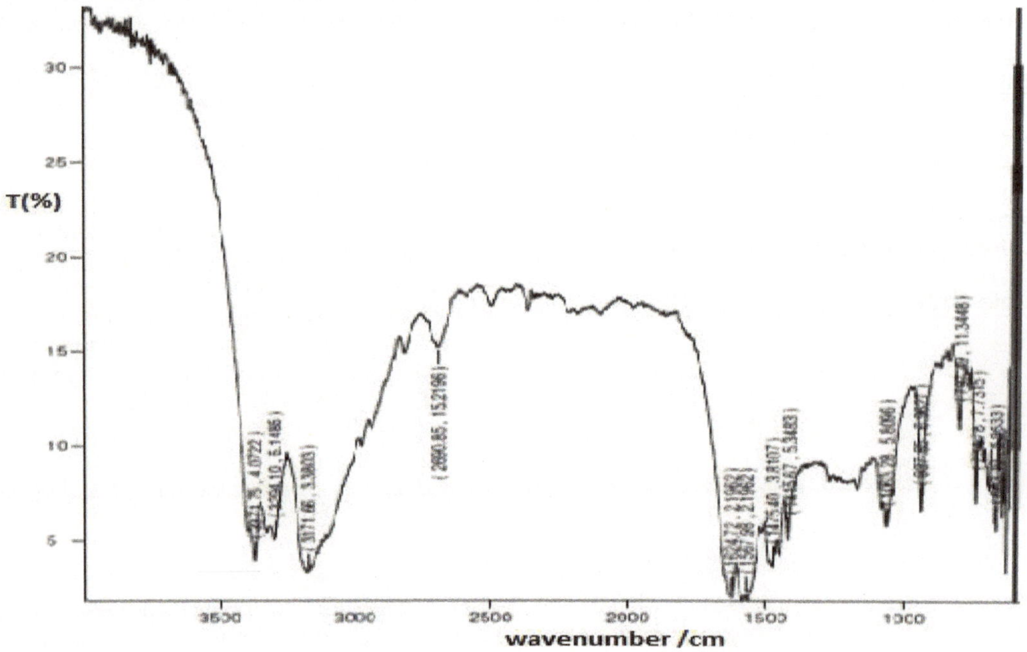

Fig. 1. Sample infra-red spectrum of one of the metformin tablet brands

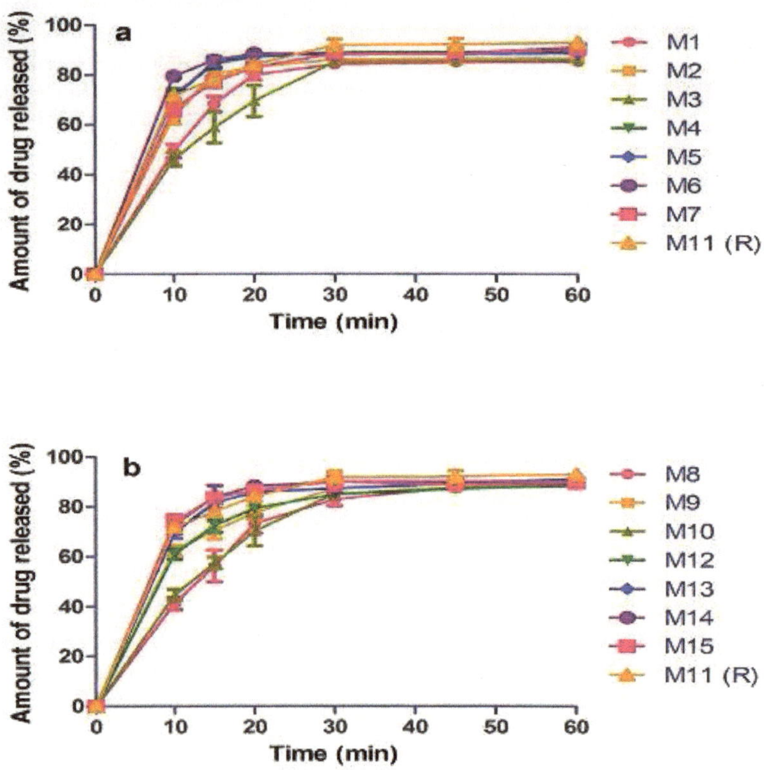

Fig. 2. Dissolution profiles of metformin hydrochloride tablet brands in 0.1 M HCl (pH 1.2), a) Brands M1-M7, M11 (R), b) Brands M8-M15, M11 (R) (mean ± S.D., *n* = 6)

Table 3. Evaluated physicochemical properties of metformin hydrochloride tablet samples

Sample code	Average weight g (S.D) n=20	Thickness mm (S.D) n=10	Hardness kg (S.D) n=10	Friability % n=10	Disintegration time (min)	Content of metformin	
						mg	*(%)
M1	0.6315(0.013)	5.80(0.02)	12.16(0.85)	0.63	13.12	498.7	99.74
M2	0.5916(0.008)	6.14(0.01)	18.76(0.04)	0.93	11.87	497.6	99.52
M3	0.6496(0.006)	6.08(0.02)	14.64(0.73)	0.15	17.14	521.1	104.21
M4	0.6117(0.015)	5.60(0.04)	8.24(0.97)	0.66	7.36	505.1	101.01
M5	0.6482(0.006)	5.88(0.01)	11.26(0.77)	0.15	9.22	539.2	107.84
M6	0.5679(0.008)	5.88(0.02)	18.78(0.05)	0.48	8.31	510.3	102.05
M7	0.6158(0.009)	5.67(0.02)	8.34(0.90)	0.16	16.74	512.0	102.39
M8	0.5949(0.006)	5.18(0.01)	15.52(1.44)	0.15	22.32	504.7	100.93
M9	0.6394(0.070)	5.25(0.01)	6.22(0.45)	1.24	21.09	554.9	110.99
M10	0.6366(0.009)	4.74(0.02)	14.62(0.79)	0.94	16.15	516.3	103.26
M11	0.5314(0.004)	5.62(0.02)	17.08(0.92)	0.94	7.81	517.4	103.47
M12	0.5986(0.007)	6.00(0.01)	13.64(0.52)	0.15	8.78	543.3	108.65
M13	0.5893(0.011)	5.93(0.01)	12.20(0.42)	0.16	8.82	502.5	100.49
M14	0.5810(0.010)	6.05(0.05)	10.62(0.47)	0.16	8.10	499.7	99.93
M15	0.6093(0.009)	5.33(0.01)	14.88(0.30)	0.66	9.30	494.9	98.99

**Percentage of the labelled amount*

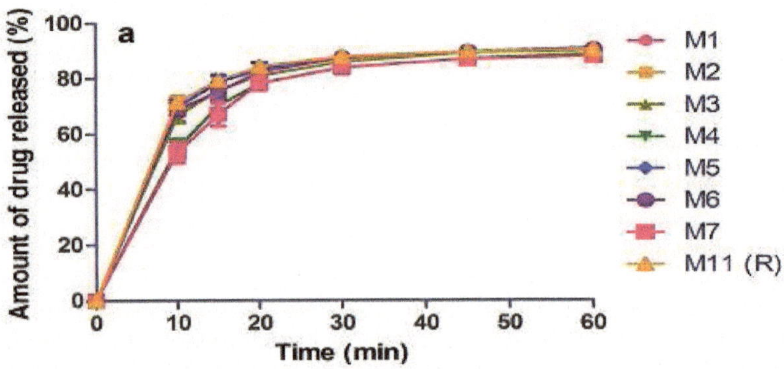

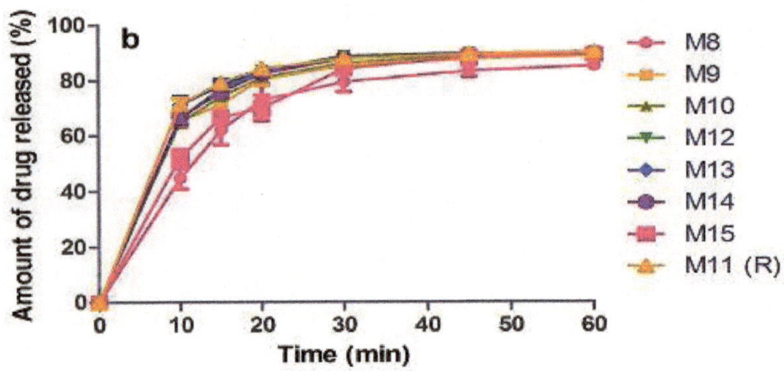

Fig. 3. Dissolution profiles of metformin hydrochloride tablet brands in phosphate buffer pH 4.5, a) Brands M1-M7, M11 (R), b) Brands M8-M15, M11 (R) (mean ± S.D., *n* = 6)

Friability test is used to assess the ability of a tablet to withstand abrasion associated with handling, packaging, transportation and shipping. This property of tablets is influenced by the nature and amount of binder used and the force of compression applied. A weight loss of not more than 1% of the weight of tablet being tested is generally considered acceptable for pharmaceutical products [13]. From the results, all the brands passed the friability test with the exception of M9 which had a percentage weight loss of 1.24%. The failure of M9 could be due to application of inappropriate compaction force and the use of insufficient binder. Tablet hardness determinations are made during tablet compression and are used to determine the need for pressure adjustment on tablet machines. A very hard tablet may fail to disintegrate in the required period in aqueous medium while a very soft tablet may not withstand handling processes such as coating, packaging and shipping operations. The hardness of a tablet depends on the force of compression and the nature and amount of the binder used. A 4 Kgf diametric crushing force is the minimum force for a satisfactory tablet. All the metformin hydrochloride tablet brands had optimal ability to withstand fracture as they exceeded the minimum 4 kgf.

Disintegration is an important step prior to drug release from immediate or conventional release dosage forms. The disintegration time of uncoated and coated tablets should not exceed 15 and 30 min, respectively [13]. From the results (Table 3), all the film coated and uncoated tablets, except M8 (uncoated) exhibited good disintegration properties. The poor disintegration properties of M8 could probably be due to the use of high amount of binder, inadequate amount of disintegrant and high compression force [24]. According to the British pharmacopoeia, metformin hydrochloride tablets should contain 95% - 105% of the label claim of the drug upon assay [13]. Results obtained from the HPLC analysis (Table 3) showed that all the brands, except M5, M9 and M12, satisfied this pharmacopoeia specification. Brands M5, M9 and M12 had percentage drug content above the upper limit of 105% and can be considered as of substandard quality. The failure of the assay test of M5, M9 and M13 could be attributed to inaccuracy in weighing the API, poor mixing during granulation and the use of excess amount of API during tablet formulation. This particular problem has also been reported in a recent study in Nigeria in which one out of eight brands of metformin hydrochloride tablets tested showed unacceptable quantity of the drug against the label claims [25].

Oral solid dosage forms only become available for absorption following disintegration and dissolution. Dissolution testing is therefore employed to predict product behavior *in vivo* and also to establish the influence of manufacturing variables, including binder effect, mixing effect, granulation procedure and excipients type on solid dosage forms [26]. Dissolution testing is employed as an *in vitro* bioequivalence test to determine the equivalence/similarity or otherwise of solid dosage forms [27]. Conventional or immediate release tablets should release ≥70 % of the prescribed amount in 45 min [13]. Results from the study revealed that all the brands exhibited good dissolution profiles as immediate release tablets.

The comparison of therapeutic performance of two medicinal products containing the same API is a critical means of assessing the possibility of interchangeability of the products. In the US Food and Drug Administration (FDA) guidance on Immediate Release, the similarity factor (f_2) was adopted in comparing profiles of a Reference and a Test drug and f_2 comparison has been the focus in various regulatory policies [28]. When two profiles are identical, f_2 is equal to 100. Conventionally, a test brand is considered similar to a reference brand if the f_2 value of the two profiles is between 50 and 100 [29]. From the results (Table 4), brands M2, M5,

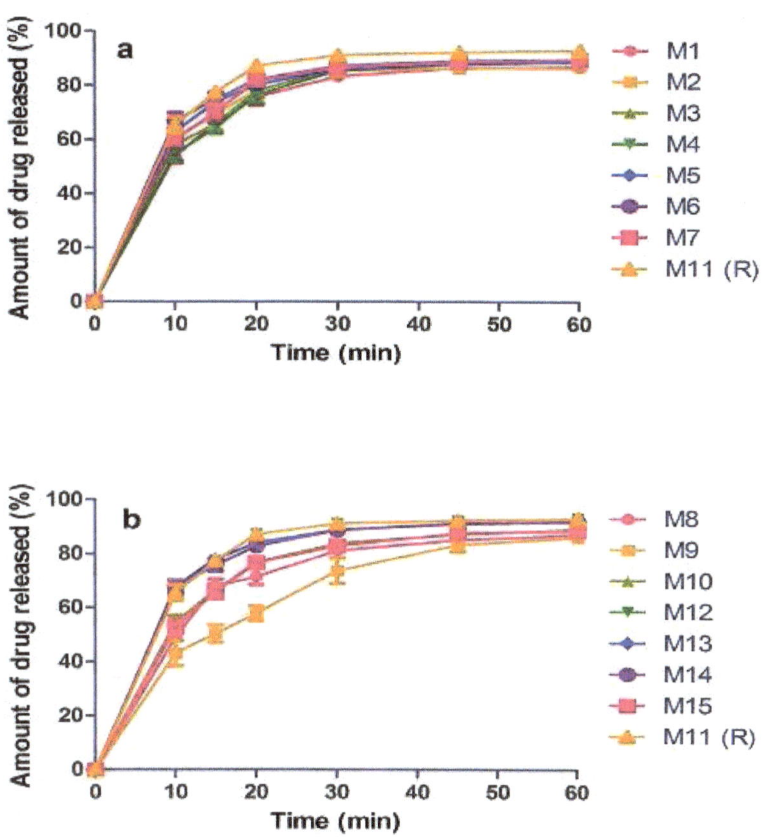

Fig. 4. Dissolution profiles of metformin hydrochloride tablet brands in phosphate buffer pH 6.8, a) Brands M1-M7, M11 (R), b) Brands M8-M15, M11 (R) (mean ± S.D., *n* = 6)

Table 4. Dissolution efficiencies (DE) and similarity factors (f_2) of metformin hydrochloride tablet samples in different dissolution media

Sample code	0.1 M HCl (pH 1.2)		Phosphate buffer pH 4.5		Phosphate buffer pH 6.8	
	DE (%)	f_2	DE (%)	f_2	DE (%)	f_2
M1	94.5	28	93.8	69	92.9	39
M2	97.1	55	95.1	86	94.1	51
M3	91.3	33	94.3	69	93.1	49
M4	98.1	63	92.5	42	91.8	45
M5	98.0	60	95.0	89	94.5	59
M6	96.8	56	94.3	75	95.0	65
M7	94.8	66	92.6	39	93.7	57
M8	88.7	27	90.4	30	90.6	35
M9	88.5	53	89.9	60	83.9	15
M10	93.5	33	94.0	64	91.4	41
M11	95.2	ND	95.8	ND	95.0	ND
M12	93.6	52	95.6	73	93.5	76
M13	95.2	69	95.8	94	93.7	70
M14	97.7	66	95.2	72	94.2	72
M15	97.8	66	90.5	36	91.5	40

ND= Not determined (reference sample)

M6, M12, M13 and M14 had f_2 values within the range specified by the FDA (50-100) in all the three dissolution media. These brands can therefore be considered to have the same drug release performance or bioequivalence with the reference brand, M11 in the three media. However, brands M1, M3, M4, M7, M8, M9, M10 and M15 had f_2 values outside the accepted range or within the accepted range in only one or two of the dissolution media used and therefore cannot be considered to be similar to the reference brand in terms of drug release performance in simulated gastrointestinal media. A study conducted by Akinleye and others found four out of seven brands of metformin hydrochloride tablets tested to have similar dissolution profiles as the innovator brand based on f_2 analysis [25].

The dissolution efficiency was determined for the tablet brands to ascertain their efficiency in releasing the drug to achieve their therapeutic activity. According to Anderson and others, the higher the dissolution efficiency, the more efficient the tablet is at releasing its embedded drug [18]. DE was generally higher in 0.1 M HCl (pH 1.2) than in phosphate buffers (pH 4.5 and 6.8). Brand M4 (in 0.1 M HCl) exhibited the highest dissolution efficiency of 98.1% while M9 (in phosphate buffer pH 6.8) had the least value of 83.8%. Based on this analysis, brand M4 could be considered the most efficient brand in the release of the API whereas M9 was the least efficient.

Two oral dosage forms are said to be bioequivalent if they demonstrate the same rate and extent of drug absorption. The bioequivalence of products are usually established through *in vivo* bioequivalence (human pharmacokinetic) studies. However, these *in vivo* bioequivalence studies are generally expensive and involve the use of invasive procedures [30]. *In vitro* dissolution studies have been shown to be as useful as and sometimes better than *in vivo* pharmacokinetic studies in demonstrating the bioequivalence of some products. Other advantages of *in vitro* dissolution studies in establishing product bioequivalence include low cost, better assessment of product performance and better ethical considerations [31].

Metformin hydrochloride is a Biopharmaceutics Classification System (BCS) class III drug which is characterized by high solubility and low permeability. The very rapid dissolution of metformin and other BCS class III drugs in aqueous media will facilitate their absorption *in vivo.* BCS class III drugs are therefore suitable for biowaiver under WHO criteria, thus exempt from *in vivo* bioequivalence studies, if a solid dosage form achieves ≥ 85% dissolution in 15 minutes using 0.1 M HCl (pH 1.2), phosphate buffer pH 4.5 and phosphate buffer pH 6.8) as dissolution media [32,33].

In the current study, none of the tablet brands met this biowaiver requirement of attaining ≥

85% dissolution in 15 minutes in all three dissolution media. Even though dissolution of metformin tablets was relatively slow in the three dissolution media used, a high *in vivo* drug absorption and bioavailability could still be achieved [34,35]. Thus, generic metformin tablets with different dissolution profiles could still exhibit similar therapeutic effect *in vivo* because of the relatively high dissolution of the drug in physiological media.

5. CONCLUSION

Fifteen metformin hydrochloride tablet brands sampled complied with the official specifications for identification, disintegration, uniformity of weight, hardness and dissolution rate test for immediate release tablets. One brand failed the friability test, while three failed the assay test. The dissolution efficiencies of the tablets were generally high (>83%) and varied with pH of dissolution media. Similarity factor, f_2 analysis, showed the dissolution profiles of M2, M5, M6, M12, M13 and M14 were similar to the reference brand (M11) in three physiological media. None of the brands satisfied the criteria for WHO BCS-based biowaiver for rapidly or very rapidly dissolving drugs. There is the need for drug regulatory authorities in Sub-Saharan Africa to intensity post-market inspection and surveillance on metformin and other life-saving medicines on the market to assure their quality and therapeutic efficacy.

CONSENT

It is not applicable.

ETHICAL APPROVAL

It is not applicable.

ACKNOWLEDGEMENTS

The authors gratefully acknowledge the technical assistance of technicians in the Department of Pharmaceutics, KNUST, Kumasi, Ghana.

COMPETING INTERESTS

Authors have declared that no competing interests exist.

REFERENCES

1. American Diabetes Association. Report of the expert committee on the diagnosis and classification of diabetes mellitus (2003). Diabetes Care. 2003;26(Suppl.1):S5-20.
2. World Health Organization Consultation Group. Definition, diagnosis and classification of diabetes mellitus and its complications. Part 1: Diagnosis and classification of diabetes mellitus. Provisional report of a WHO Consultation. Diabetic Medicine. 1998;15:539-553.
3. World Health Organization. Fact Sheet No 312 reviewed in October; 2013.
4. Dodu SR. The incidence of diabetes mellitus in Accra (Ghana); a study of 4,000 patients. West Afr. Med. J. 1958;7(3): 129-34.
5. Amoah AG, Owusu SK, Adjei S. Diabetes in Ghana: A community based prevalence study in Greater Accra. Diabetes Res. Clin. Pract. 2002;56(3):197-205.
6. Adegbolagun OA, Olalade OA, Osumah SE. Comparative evaluation of the biopharmaceutical and chemical equivalence of some commercially available brands of ciprofloxacin hydrochloride tablets. Trop. J. Pharm. Res. 2007;6(3):737-45.
7. Mackey TK, Liang BA. The global counterfeit drug trade: Patient safety and public health risks. J. Pharm. Sci. 2011; 100:4571-79.
8. Newton PN, Amin AA, Bird C, Passmore P, Dukes G, Tomson G, et al. The primacy of public health considerations in defining poor quality medicines. PloS Med. 2011; 8(12):e1001139.
   DOI: 10.1371/journal.pmed.1001139
9. Kelesidis T, Kelesidis I, Rafailidis PI, Falagas ME. Counterfeit or substandard antimicrobial drugs: A review of the scientific evidence. J. Antimicrob. Chemother. 2007;60:214-36.
10. Newton PN, Green MD, Fernandez FM. Impact of poor-quality medicines in the 'developing' world. Trends Pharmacol. Sci. 2010;31(3):99-101.
11. Olaniyi AA, Babalola CP, Oladehinde FO, Adegoke AO. Towards better quality assurance of drugs. Proceedings of 4th National Workshop, Department of Pharmaceutical Chemistry, University of Ibadan, Ibadan, Nigeria. 2001;59-60.
12. Fujii A, Yasui-Furukori N, Nakagami T, Niioka T, Saito M, Sato Y, et al. Comparative *in vivo* bioequivalence and in vitro dissolution of two valproic acid sustained-release formulations. Drug Des. Devel. Ther. 2009;2:139-44.

13. British Pharmacopoeia. Her Majesty‘s Stationery Office, London. 2013;2.
14. Kar M, Choudhury PK. HPLC method for estimation of metformin hydrochloride in formulated microspheres and tablet dosage form. Indian J. Pharm. Sci. 2009; 71(3):318-20.
15. FDA. Waiver of *in vivo* bioequivalence and bioequivalence studies for immediate-release solid oral dosage forms based on a Biopharmaceutics Classification System; Guidance for industry. U. S. Department of Health and Human Services, Center for Drug Evaluation and Research; 2000.
16. Khan KA, Rhodes CT. Effect of compaction pressure on the dissolution efficiency of some direct compression systems. Pharm. Acta Helv. 1972;47:594-607.
17. Khan KA. The concept of dissolution efficiency. J. Pharm. Pharmacol. 1975;27: 48-9.
18. Anderson NH, Bauer M, Boussac N, Khan-Malek R, Munden P, Sardaro M. An evaluation of fit factors and dissolution efficiency for the comparison of *in vitro* dissolution profiles. J. Pharm. Biomed. Anal. 1998;17(4-5):811-22.
19. Ofori-Kwakye K, Osei-Yeboah F, Kipo SL. Formulation and quality evaluation of two conventional release tablet formulations. Int. J. Pharm. Sci. Rev. Res. 2010;4(1): 94-9.
20. Awofisayo SO, Awofisayo OA, Eyen N, Udoh IE. Comparative assessment of the quality control measurements of multisource ofloxacin tablets marketed in Nigeria. Dissolution Technol. 2010;17(2): 20-5.
21. Jain N, Mandal S, Banweer J, Jain S. Effect of superdisintegrants on formulation of taste masked fast disintegrating Ciprofloxacin tablets. International Current Pharmaceutical Journal, 2012;1(4):62-7.
22. Rawlins EA. Bentley‘s textbook of pharmaceutics, 8th ed., Bailliere Tindal. 1977;289-90.
23. USP-NF. United States Pharmacopoeial Convention Inc. 2007;1:1480.
24. Sougi A. Physicochemical and in vitro dissolution properties of some metformin tablet preparations on the Ghanaian market. MPhil thesis, Kwame Nkrumah University of Science and Technology, Kumasi, Ghana. 2014;116.
25. Akinleye MO, Adelaja IA, Odulaja JO. Comparative evaluation of physicochemical properties of some commercially available brands of metformin hydrochloride tablets in Lagos, Nigeria. J. Appl. Pharm. Sci. 2012;02(02): 41-4.
26. Papadopoulou V, Valsami G, Dokoumetzidis A, Macheras P. Biopharmaceutics classification systems for new molecular entities (BCS-NMEs) and marketed drugs (BCS-MD): Theoretical basis and practical examples. Int. J. Pharm. 2008;361(1-2):70-7.
27. Amidon GL, Lennernäs H, Shah VP, Crison JR. A theoretical basis for a biopharmaceutic drug classification: The correlation of *in vitro* drug product dissolution and *in vivo* bioavailability. Pharm. Res. 1995;12:413-20.
28. FDA. Center for Drug Evaluation and Research, Guidance for Industry: Immediate release solid oral dosage forms. Scale-Up and post-approval changes, chemistry, manufacturing and controls, *in vitro* dissolution testing and *in vivo* bioequivalence documentation; 1995.
29. Gohel MC, Sarvaiya KG, Mehta NR, Soni CD, Vyas VU, Dave RK. Assessment of similarity factor using different weighting approaches. Dissolution Technol. 2005; 22-7.
30. Cook JA, Bockbrader HN. An industrial implementation of the Biopharmaceutics Classification System. Dissolution Technol. 2002;9(2):6-8.
31. Polli JE. *In vitro* studies are sometimes better than conventional human pharmacokinetic *in vivo* studies in assessing bioequivalence of immediate-release solid dosage forms. The AAPS Journal. 2008;10(2):289-99.
32. Löbenberg R, Amidon GL. Modern bioavailability, bioequivalence and Biopharmaceutics classification system. New scientific approaches to international regulatory standards. Eur. J. Pharm. Biopharm. 2000;50(1)3-12.
33. World Health Organization. Expert Committee on specifications for pharmaceutical preparations, proposal to waive *in vivo* bioequivalence requirement for WHO model list of essential medicines immediate-release, solid oral dosage forms; WHO Technical Report Series, no. 937, Annex 7; WHO: Geneva, Switzerland; 2006.

34. Blume HH, Schug BS. The biopharmaceutics classification system (BCS): Class III drugs - better candidates for BA/BE waiver? Eur. J. Pharm. Sci. 1999;9(2):117-21.
35. Kortejärvi H, Yliperttula M, Dressman JB, Junginger HE, Midha KK, Shah VP, et al. Biowaiver monographs for immediate release solid oral dosage forms: Ranitidine hydrochloride. J. Pharm. Sci. 2005;94(8): 1617-25.

Antioxidant Activity of the Fruit and Stem Bark of *Tetrapleura tetraptera* Taub (Mimosaceae)

O. E. Famobuwa[1*], L. Lajide[2], B. J. Owolabi[2], I. B. Osho[3] and U. E. Amuho[1]

[1]*Department of Chemistry, Adeyemi Federal University of Education, Ondo, Nigeria.*
[2]*Department of Chemistry, Federal University of Technology, Akure, Nigeria.*
[3]*Department of Animal Production and Health, Federal University of Technology, Akure, Nigeria.*

Authors' contributions

This work was carried out in collaboration between all authors. Author OEF designed the study, wrote the protocol and wrote the first draft of the manuscript. Author LL managed the literature searches. Author BJO designed and wrote part of the protocol. Author IBO managed the experimental process and author UEA identified the species of plant. All authors read and approved the final manuscript.

Article Information

Editor(s):
(1) Rafik Karaman, Bioorganic Chemistry, College of Pharmacy, Al-Quds University, USA.
(2) Ali Nokhodchi, Professor of Pharmaceutics and Drug Delivery, School of Life Sciences, University of Sussex, UK.
Reviewers:
(1) I. P. Tripathi, Tropical Forest Research Institute (TFRI), Jabalpur, India.
(2) Ines Maria Costa Brighente, Universidade Federal de Santa Catarina, Brazil.
(3) Anonymous, Lagos State University, Nigeria.
(4) Abdullahi M. Nuhu, College of Science and Technology, Kaduna Polytechnic, Kaduna, Nigeria.
(5) Upendarrao Golla, Indian Institute of Science Education and Research Bhopal (IISERB), India.

ABSTRACT

The present investigation was carried out to evaluate the antioxidant activity of ethanol extracts of *Tetrapleura tetraptera* stem bark and fruit. 1,1-diphenyl-2-picrylhydrazyl (DPPH) radical scavenging assay and ferric reducing antioxidant property (FRAP) assay were carried out to determine the antioxidant activity of the extracts. The antioxidant activity of the extracts which was determined by DPPH increases with a corresponding increase in concentration. The percentage DPPH radical inhibition ability of the stem bark ranged from 28.74% to 85.26% while that of fruit ranged from -10.56% to 66.01%. The percentage antioxidant activity of the stem bark extract is almost at par with that of ascorbic acid while that of fruit extract is about 75%. But at 25 mg/ml, the fruit extract showed a pro-oxidant activity. The reductive ability of the stem bark extract ranged from 0.393 to 1.641 mg ascorbic acid equivalent per mL of extract (about two-fifth of the reference drug) while that of fruit extract ranged from 0.342 to 1.325 mg ascorbic acid equivalent/mL of extract (one-third

**Corresponding author: Email: edyniyi@yahoo.com*

that of reference drug). The efficacy of the fruit and stem bark extracts of *T. tetraptera* in some of its bioactivities may be attributed to its favourable antioxidant potential.

Keywords: Tetrapleura tetraptera; DPPH radical scavenging assay; Fe^{+3}*reducing assay.*

1. INTRODUCTION

Tetrapleura tetraptera Taub (Mimosaceae) popularly called Aridan, in the Yoruba speaking area of South West Nigeria. It is a perennial, single-stemmed plant with dark green leaves. It is found in the rain forest belt of West Africa. The plant has many ethno-medicinal and non-medicinal uses such as anti-ulcer, anti-microbial, anti-convulsant, emulsifying, contraceptive, and as a nutritive agent [1,2]. Due to the foaming ability of the fruit, it is used in the production of black soap. The dry fruit has a pleasant aroma that is insect-repellant in nature [3]. The use of the fruit as spices in foods is as a result of its medicinal value. There is wide acceptance of medicinal plants in preference to synthetic drugs nowadays, because they are cheaper and of little or no adverse effect. Thus, there is great demand for natural antioxidants, because of lack of any undesirable effect. The ethnomedicinal activity of the fruit extract of *T. tetraptera* have been investigated by many authors with little or no work on the the stem bark of the plant. The objective of the present investigation therefore, was to evaluate, comparatively, the antioxidant potential of different concentrations of the ethanolic extracts of the stem bark and fruit of *T. tetraptera.*

2. MATERIALS AND METHODS

2.1 Collection of Plant Material

Fresh fruits and stem bark of *T. tetraptera* were collected from a plantation in Ondo, South-west, Nigeria. Identification and authentication were carried out by Mr. R.A. Sanni of the Department of Biology, Adeyemi College of Education, Ondo, Nigeria, with voucher number ACH 2614. Fresh plant material was washed under running tap water, air dried and then homogenized to fine powder and stored in airtight bottles.

2.2 Solvent Extraction

The solvent and chemicals used for this work were of analytical grade.

Thoroughly washed plant parts were dried in shade for five days and then powdered with the help of blender. The powdered plant parts were extracted successively with ethanol in Soxhlet extractor for 48 h. A brownish colour extracts were obtained. The fruit extract has a yield value of 15.94% while the stem bark extract has a yield value of 11.43%. The solvent extracts were concentrated under reduced pressure and preserved at 5°C in airtight bottle until further use.

2.3 Antioxidant Property

The ferric reducing property was determined by assessing the ability of extracts to reduce $FeCl_3$ solution as described [4]. Briefly, extracts (0-250 μL of stock) were mixed with 250 μL 200 mM sodium phosphate buffer (pH 6.6) and 250 μL of 1% potassium ferrocyanide, the mixture was incubated at 50°C for 20 min, thereafter 250 μL of 10% trichloroacetic acid was added, and subsequently centrifuged at 650 rpm for 10 min, 1000 μL of the supernatant was mixed with equal volume of water and 100 μL of 0.1g/100 mL ferric chloride, the absorbance was later measured at 700 nm. A higher absorbance indicates a higher reducing power.

1,1-diphenyl-2 picrylhydrazyl free radical scavenging ability: The free radical scavenging ability of the extracts against DPPH (1,1-diphenyl-2- picrylhydrazyl) free radical was evaluated as described by Halliwell et al [5]. Briefly, appropriate dilution of the extracts (1 mL) was mixed with 1 mL of 0.4 mM methanol solution containing DPPH (20 mg/L) free radicals, the mixture was left in the dark for 30 min and the absorbance was measured at 516 nm. The DPPH free radical scavenging ability was subsequently calculated.

$$\text{Scavenging ability} = A - B / A \times 100$$

Where A is absorbance of DPPH and B is absorbance of DPPH and extract combination.

3. RESULTS AND DISCUSSION

Studies have shown that the reactive oxygen species of low reactivity can be converted to a highly reactive species. Reaction of hydrogen peroxide (H_2O_2) with low valence forms of the transition metal ions iron (Fe^{2+}) and copper (Cu^{2+}) ion lead to the formation of $^{\cdot}OH$ (Fenton reaction) or species of comparable reactivity such as Fe^{2+}(Ferryl ion) or $Cu(OH)_2^+$ a copper III complex. The hydroxyl radical ·OH, abundant under physiological conditions are quite reactive, reacts rapidly with any type of biological molecules in living cells, such as sugars, amino acids, phospholipids and nucleobases (the components of nucleic acids) [6].

The antioxidant activities have been reported to be the concomitant development of reducing power [7].

The reductive ability of the stem bark extract ranged from 0.393 to 1.641 mg ascorbic acid equivalent per mL of extract (about two-fifth of the reference drug) while that of fruit extract ranged from 0.342 to 1.325 mg ascorbic acid equivalent/mL of extract (about 33% of that of reference drug) as shown in Fig. 1.

The antioxidant activity of the extracts which was determined by DPPH increases with a corresponding increase in the concentration of the extracts. The decrease in absorbance of DPPH is proportional to concentration of free radical scavenger added to DPPH reagent solution. Decrease in the DPPH solution absorbance indicates an increase in the DPPH scavenging activity. The percentage DPPH radical inhibition ability of the stem bark ranged from 28.74% to 85.26% while that of fruit ranged from -10.56% to 66.01%. The percentage antioxidant activity of the stem bark extract is almost at par with that of ascorbic acid while that of fruit extract is about 75% (Fig. 2). But at

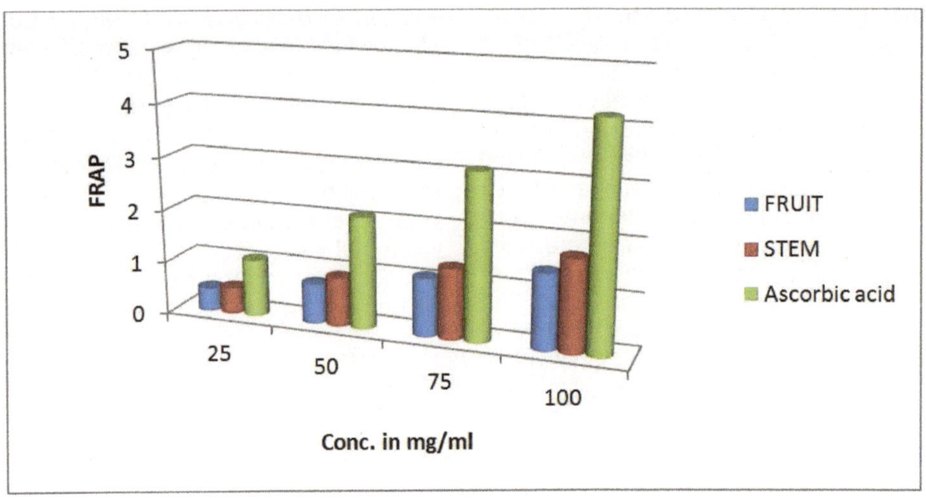

Fig. 1. Ferric reducing antioxidant property (mg/mL)

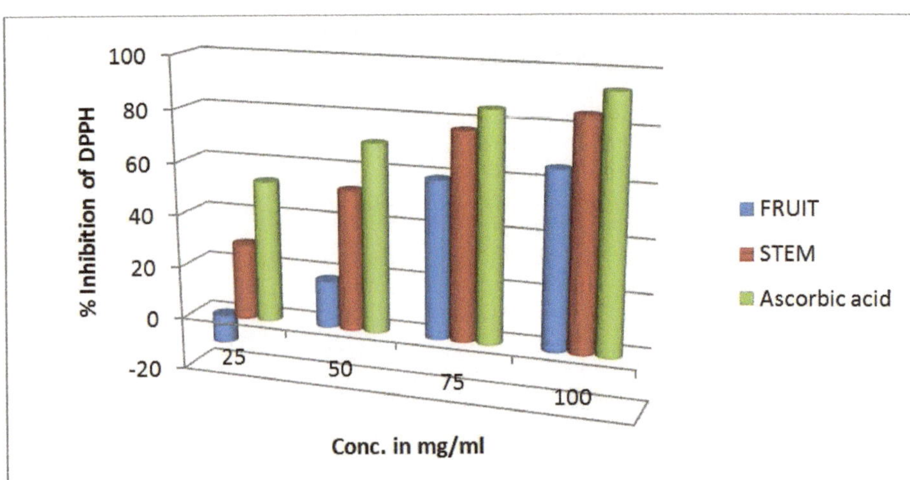

Fig. 2. % inhibition of DPPH

25 mg/mL, the fruit extract did not show any anti-oxidant but pro-oxidant activity. This implies that 25 mg/mL or lower concentration of the fruit extract is not safe as an anti-oxidant agent. The results indicate that the ethanolic extracts possess hydrogen donating capabilities and act as an antioxidant. The efficacy of the fruit and stem bark extracts of *T. tetraptera* in some of its bioactivity may be attributed to its favourable antioxidant potential.

Though the scavenging activity of the standard was higher than those of ethanolic extracts, they are potential antioxidant drugs.

4. CONCLUSION

The efficacy of the fruit and stem bark extracts of *T. tetraptera* in its bioactivities may be attributed to its potential antioxidant activity. From the results, the stem bark performed better as an anti-oxidant agent. Further studies on isolation of active constituents and their biological activities are to be carried out.

CONSENT

It is not applicable.

ETHICAL APPROVAL

It is not applicable.

ACKNOWLEDGEMENT

We are very grateful to the Tertiary Education Trust Fund (TETFUND), Nigeria for providing us with the fund to carry-out this research.

COMPETING INTERESTS

Authors have declared that no competing interests exist.

REFERENCES

1. Essein EU, Izunwane BC, Aremu CY, Eka OU. Significance for humans of the nutrient contents of the dry fruit of *Tetrapleura tetraptera*. Plant Food Human Nutrition.1994;45(1):47–51.
2. Okwu DE. The potentials of *Ocimum gratissimum, Penrgularia extensa* and *Tetrapleura tetraptera* as spice and flavouring agents. Nig Agric J. 2003;35: 143–148.
3. Aladesanmi JA, Molluscicidal activity and chemical constituents of *Tetrapleura tetraptera*. A review. Afr. J. Trad. Comp. Alter. Med. 2007:4(1):23–36.
4. Pulido R, Bravo L, Sauro-Calixo F. Antioxidant activity of dietary polyphenols as determined by a modified ferric reducing/antioxidant power assay. J. Agric. Food chem. 2000;48:3396-3402.
5. Halliwell B, Gutteridge JM, Cross CE. Free radicals, antioxidant and human disease: Where are we now? J. Laboratory and Clinical Medicine. 1992;119:598-620.
6. Meir S, Kanner J, Akiri B, Hadas SP. Determination and involvement of Aqueous reducing compounds in Oxidative Defence systems of various senescing leaves. J. Agric. Food Chem. 1995;43: 1813-1817.
7. Amzal H, Alaoni K, Tok S, Errachidi A, Charof R, Cherrah Y, Benjouad A. Protective effects of Saponins from *Argania spinosa* against free radical induced oxidative haemolysis. Fitoptera. 2008;79:337-344.

28

Phytochemical and Antimicrobial Analysis of Banana Pseudo Stem (*Musa acuminata*)

C. T. Onyema[1*], C. E. Ofor[1], V. C. Okudo[1] and A. S. Ogbuagu[1]

[1]Department of Pure and Industrial Chemistry, Faculty of Physical Sciences, Nnamdi Azikiwe University, Awka, Anambra State, Nigeria.

Authors' contributions

This research was carried out through joint collaboration of all authors. Their responsibilities spanned through the design of the study, literature survey, experimental, writing protocols, preparation of manuscript, financing and proof reading of approved manuscript.

Article Information

Editor(s):
(1) Sami Nazzal, College of Pharmacy, University of Louisiana at Monroe, USA.
(2) Faiyaz Shakeel, King Saud University, Riyadh, Saudi Arabia.
(3) Ke-He Ruan, Director of the Center for Experimental Therapeutics and Pharmacoinformatics (CETP), Professor of Medicinal Chemistry & Pharmacology Dept. of Pharmacological and Pharmaceutical Sciences University of Houston, USA.
Reviewers:
(1) Ayona Jayadev, All Saints' College, Trivandrum, Kerala, India.
(2) Anonymous, Universidad de Los Andes, Merida, Venezuela.
(3) Charu Gupta, Amity University, UP, India

ABSTRACT

Preliminary phytochemical screening of extracts of banana pseudo stem and antimicrobial activities revealed the presence of phenolic compounds, flavonoids, terpenoids, alkaloids, protein, tannins, saponins, cardiac glycosides. The phytochemical constituents were: Alkaloid (8.16%), Flavonoids (4.02%), Saponin (3.5%), Phenols (5.5743 mg/kg, Tannin (9.13%), Oxalate (0.162%), Heamaglutinin (1.8814 mg/kg), Phytate (1.2967 mg/kg), and Cardiac Glycoside (1.6%). Some of the extracts inhibited the growth of pathogens while some did not. Water extract notably had a high Zone Inhibition Diameter of 21 mm to *Streptococcus aureus* and 17 mm to *Pseudomonas aerugenosa*. The results obtained indicated that the pseudo stem of banana plant have pharmaceutical values and can be utilized in treatment of some ailments.

Keywords: Phytochemical constituents; antifungal; antimicrobial activity and banana pseudo stem.

**Corresponding author: Email: ct.onyema@unizik.edu.ng*

1. INTRODUCTION

Banana is the common name for herbaceous plants of the genus Musa. Binomial nomenclature of banana plant is *Musa acuminata*. Locally known as '*unere*', bananas come in a variety of sizes and colours when ripe, including yellow, purple, and red. The banana plant is the largest herbaceous flowering plant. Bananas and plantains constitute the fourth most important global food commodity (after rice, wheat and maize) grown in more than 100 countries over a harvested area of approximately 10 million hectares, with an annual production of 88 million tonnes [1]. The all year round fruiting habit of bananas puts the crop in a superior position in bridging the 'hunger gap' between crop harvests. It therefore contributes significantly to food and income security of people engaged in its production and trade, particularly in developing countries. In Africa they provide more than 25% of the carbohydrate requirements for over 70 million people [2]. Eastern and Southern Africa produces over 20 million tonnes of bananas which accounts for 25.58% of the total World output [3]. The Great Lakes region covering parts of Uganda, Rwanda, Burundi, Tanzania, Kenya and DRC is the largest producer and consumer of bananas in Africa [4] where per capita consumption has been estimated at more than 250 kg; the highest in the world [5].

2. MATERIALS AND METHODS

2.1 Sample Collection and Preparation

Matured banana pseudo stem was obtained on 30th July, 2015 during the rainy season from a humus farmland in Amawbia, Awka, South L.G.A of Anambra State. The banana pseudo stem was washed under running tap to remove debris; it was sliced and then air dried. After drying, the sample was ground into powder and stored in an airtight container for future use.

2.2 Preliminary Phytochemical Screening

Phytochemcial screening (quantitative and qualitative) was carried out on water, 50% ethanol, 90% ethanol, 50% methanol and 90% methanol extract of banana pseudo stem using Harbone [6] method for plant analysis. 150 ml of each solvent was used to extract the banana pseudo stem separately and the presence of the phytochemicals: alkaloids, saponins, flavonoids, phenol, steroids, glycosides and tannins were tested. The phytochemicals present were estimated quantitatively.

2.2.1 Qualitative analysis

10 g of the ground sample was weighed into three (3) different labelled conical flasks. 100 ml of the three (3) different solvents (distilled water, 50% methanol and 90% methanol) were poured into the three different conical flasks to extract the phytochemicals. After 24 hrs, the mixtures were filtered into conical flasks using whatmann filter paper (No.1). The filtrates were concentrated by placing the flasks into water bath at 100℃. The resulting filtrate were cooled to room temperature, Qualitative test was then carried out on the cool solution (extract) using [6,7] to ascertain the presence of the different phytochemicals in banana pseudo stem.

2.2.1.1 Test for alkaloids

1.0 ml of the above extract was pipetted into a test tube followed by 5.0 ml of 2% HCl and heated on a waterbath (Memmert) for 10 minutes. The solution was filtered using Whatmann No 1 filter paper and used for Wagner's reagent test.

For the test, 1.0 ml of filtrate was pippetted into a test tube followed by 1.0 ml of Wagner's reagent. A reddish brown precipitate indicated the presence of alkaloids.

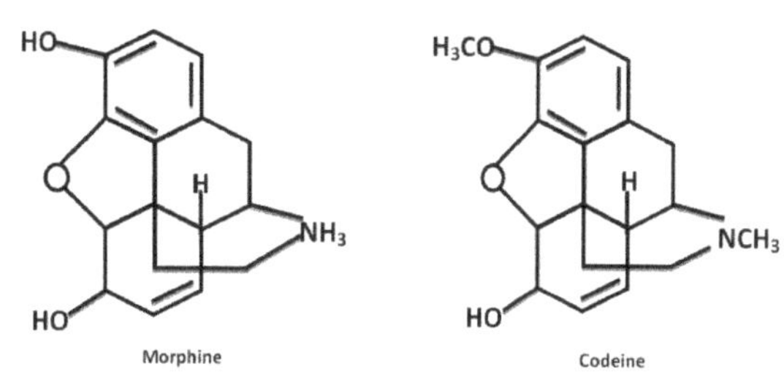

Fig. 1. Basic structures of some pharmacologically important plant derived alkaloids

2.2.1.2 Test for flavonoids

1.0 ml of filtrate was pippetted into a test tube followed by 1.0 ml 10% ferric chloride. Greenish brown or black colour/precipitate is an indication of presence of phenolic nucleus an indicator of the presence of flavonoids.

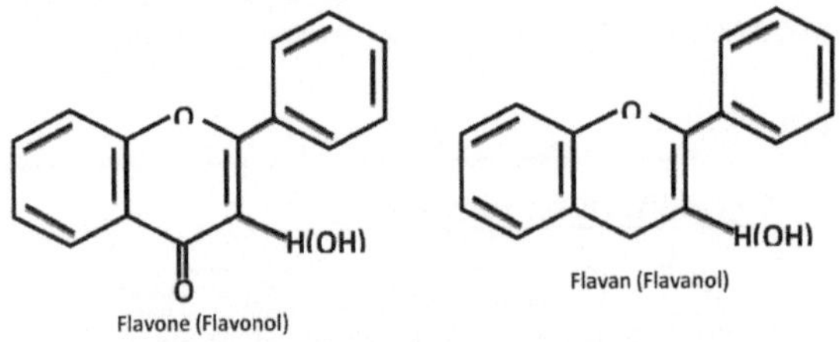

Fig. 2. Basic structures of some pharmacologically important plant derived flavonoids

2.2.1.3 Test for tannins

2.2.1.3.1 Acid test

3.0 ml of the extract was added to 2.0 ml of 1% HCl. The observation of a red colour or precipitate indicated the presence of phlobotannins.

2.2.1.3.2 Lead acetate test

To 2 ml of the extract was added 3 drops of 5% lead acetate solution to the extract. A dark blue to black precipitate indicated presence of phlobotannins.

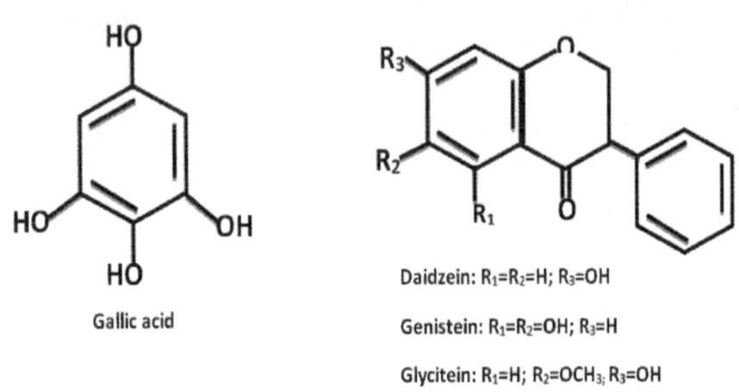

Fig. 3. Basic structures of some pharmacologically important plant derived tannins

2.2.1.4 Test for proteins

To a little portion of the filtrate in a test tube, 2 drops of Million's reagent were added. A white precipitate indicated the presence of protein.

2.2.1.5 Test for saponins

2 g of the powdered sample was boiled in 20 ml of distilled water in a water bath and filtered. 10 ml of the filtrate was mixed with 5 ml of distilled water and shaken vigorously for a stable persistent froth. The frothing was mixed with 3 drops of olive oil and shaken vigorously, then observed for the formation of emulsion.

2.2.1.6 Test for cardiac glycosides

1 ml of the extract was added to 10 cm^3 of 50% H_2SO_4 and was heated in boiling H_2O for 5 minutes. 10 cm^3 of Fehling's solution (5 cm^3 of each solution A and B) was added and boiled. A brick red precipitate indicating presence of glycosides was observed.

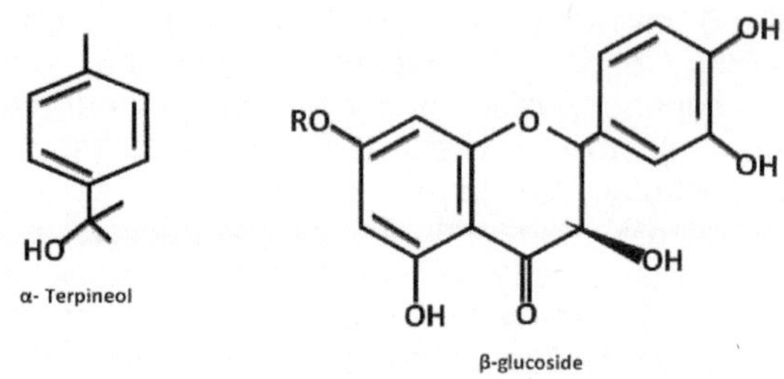

Fig. 4. Basic structures of some pharmacologically important plant derived glycosides

2.2.1.7 Test for steroids

To 0.5 ml of the chloroform, 1 ml concentrated H_2SO_4 was added to form a lower layer. Then the colour at the interface was observed and recorded.

2.2.1.8 Test for terpenoids

5 ml of each extract was mixed in 2 ml of chloroform (Numex, India), and concentrated H_2SO_4 (3 ml) was carefully added to form a layer. A reddish brown coloration of the inner face was formed to show positive results for the presence of terpenoids.

2.2.2 Quantitative analysis

Quantitative analysis were done using various procedures as follows: [8] (phytate), [9] (Tannin), [10] (Saponin), [11] (Flavonoids), [8,10] (Alkaloids and Oxalate).

2.2.2.1 Oxalate determination by titration method

This determination involved 3 major steps digestion, oxalate precipitation and permanganate titration.

2.2.2.1.1 Digestion

2 g of sample was suspended in 190 ml of distilled water in a 250 ml volumetric flask followed by the addition of 10 ml (6 M) HCl. The suspension was digested at 100°C for 1 hour, Cooled, and then made up to 250 ml mark before filtration.

2.2.2.1.2 Oxalate precipitation

Duplicate portions of 125 ml of the filtrate were measured into beakers and four drops of methyl red indicator added. This was followed by the addition of NH_4OH solution (drop wise) until the test solution changed from salmon pink colour to a faint yellow colour (pH 4-4.5). Each portion was then heated to 90°C, cooled and filtered to remove precipitate containing ferrous ion. The filtrate is again heated to 90°C and 10 ml of 5% $CaCl_2$ solution was added while being stirred constantly. After heating, it was cooled and left overnight at 25°C. The solution was then centrifuged at 2500 rpm for 5 minutes. The supernatant is decanted and the precipitate completely dissolved in 10 ml of 20% (v/v) H_2SO_4 solution.

2.2.2.1.3 Permanganate titration

At this point, the total filtrate resulting from the digestion was made up to 300 ml. Aliquots of 125 ml of the filtrate was heated until near boiling and then titrated against 0.05 M standardized $KMnO_4$ solution to a faint pink colour which persists for 30 seconds. The calcium oxalate content was calculated using the formula

$$\frac{T \times (Vme)(Df)}{(ME) \times Mf} \ (mg/100\ g)$$

Where T is the titre of KMnO4 (ml), Vme is the volume-mass equivalent (i.e. 1 ml of 0.05 M $KMnO_4$ solution is equivalent to 0.00225 g anhydrous oxalic acid). Df is the dilution factor Vt/A (2.4) where Vt is the total volume of titrate (300 ml) and A is the aliquot used (125 ml), ME is the molar equivalent of $KMnO_4$ in oxalate ($KMnO_4$ redox reaction) and Mf is the mass of sample used [6].

2.2.2.2 Alkaloid determination

5 g of the sample was weighed into a 250 ml beaker and 200 ml of 20% acetic acid in ethanol was added and covered and allowed to stand for 4 hours at 25°C. This was filtered with filter pape r No. 42 and the filtrate was concentrated using a water bath (Memmert) to one quarter of the original volume. Concentrated NH_4OH was added drop wise to the extract until the precipitate was complete. The whole solution was allowed to settle and the precipitate was collected and washed with dilute NH_4OH (1% NH_3 solution), then filtered with pre-weighed filter paper. The residue on the filter paper (alkaloid) was dried in the oven (precision electrothermal model BNP 9052 England) at 80°C. The alkaloid content was calculated and expressed as a percentage of the weight of the sample analysed [7,10].

Calculation: %weight of alkaloid = (Weight of filter paper with residue – weight of filter paper / Weight of sample analysed) ×100

2.2.2.3 Flavonoids determination

10 g of the plant sample was extracted repeatedly with 100ml of 80% aqueous methanol at room temperature. The whole solution was filtered through Whatmann filter paper No. 42 (125mm). The filtrate was later transferred into a crucible and evaporated into dryness over a water bath and weighed to a constant weight [11].

Calculation: % flavonoids = {(weight of crucible + residue) – (weight of crucible) / Weight of sample analysed}× 100

2.2.2.4 Determination of saponin

5 g of the sample was put into 20% acetic acid in ethanol and allowed to stand in a water bath at 50°C for 24 hours. This was filtered and the extract was concentrated using a water bath to one-quarter of the original volume. Concentrated NH_4OH was added drop wise to the extract until the precipitate was complete. The whole solution was allowed to settle and the precipitate was collected by filtration and weighed. The saponin content was weighed and calculated in percentage [10].

Calculation: % saponin content = {(Weight of filter paper + residue) – (weight of filter paper) / Weight of sample analysed ×100}

2.2.2.5 Cardiac glycosides determination

Wang and Filled method was used. To 1 ml of extract was added 1 ml of 2% solution of 3,5-DNS (Dinitro Salicylic acid) in methanol and 1 ml of 5% aqueous NaOH. It was boiled for 2 minutes (until brick-red precipitate was observed) and the boiled sample was filtered. The weight of the filter paper was weighed before filtration. The filter paper with the absorbed residue was dried in an oven at 50℃ till the dryness and weight of the filter paper with residue was noted. The cardiac glycoside was calculated in %.

Calculation: % cardiac glycoside= {(Weight of filter paper + residue) – (weight of filter paper) / Weight of sample analysed × 100}

2.2.2.6 Tannin determination by titration

The Follins Dennis titration method as described by Pearson [9] was used. To 20 g of the crushed sample in a conical flask was added 100 ml of petroleum ether and covered for 24 hours. The sample was then filtered and allowed to stand for 15 minutes allowing petroleum ether to evaporate. It was then re-extracted by soaking in 100 ml of 10% acetic acid in ethanol for 4 hours. The sample was then filtered and the filtrate collected.

25 ml of NH_4OH were added to the filtrate to precipitate the alkaloids. The alkaloids were heated with electric hot plate to remove some of the NH_4OH still in the solution. The remaining volume was measured to be 33 ml. 5 ml of this was taken and 20 ml of ethanol was added to it. It was titrated with 0.1 M NaOH using phenolphthalein as indicator until a pink endpoint is reached. Tannin content was then calculated in % ($C_1V_1=C_2V_2$) molarity.

Calculation:

Data

C_1= concentration of tannic acid
C_2= concentration of base
V_1= volume of tannic acid
V_2= volume of base

Therefore $C_1 = \frac{C_2V_2}{V_1}$

$$\% \text{ of tannic acid content} = \frac{C_1 \times 100}{\text{Weight of sample analysed}}$$

2.2.2.7 Phytate determination

Phytate contents were determined using the Young and Greaves method. 0.2 g of the sample was weighed into different 250 ml conical flasks. Each sample was soaked in 100 ml of 2% concentrated HCl for 3 hours, the sample was then filtered. 50 ml of each filtrate was laced in 250 ml beaker and 100 ml distilled water added to each sample. 10 ml of 0.3% ammonium thiocynate solution was added as indicator and titrated with standard iron (III) chloride solution which contained 0.00195 g iron per 1 ml.

$$\text{Phytic acid} = \frac{\text{Titre value} \times 0.00195 \times 1.19 \times 100}{\text{Weight of sample}}$$

2.2.2.8 Phenol determination

The quantity of phenols is determined using the Spectrophotometer method. The plant sample was boiled with 50 ml of $(CH_3CH_2)_2O$ for 15 minutes. 5 ml of the boiled sample was then pipetted into 50 ml flask and 10 ml of distilled water added. After the addition of distilled water, 2 ml of NH_4OH solution and 5 ml of concentrated $CH_3(CH_2)_3CH_2OH$ was added to the mixture. The samples was made up to the mark and left for 30 minutes to react for colour development and measured at 505 nm wavelength using a spectrophotometer (Apel PD-3000UV spectrophotometer).

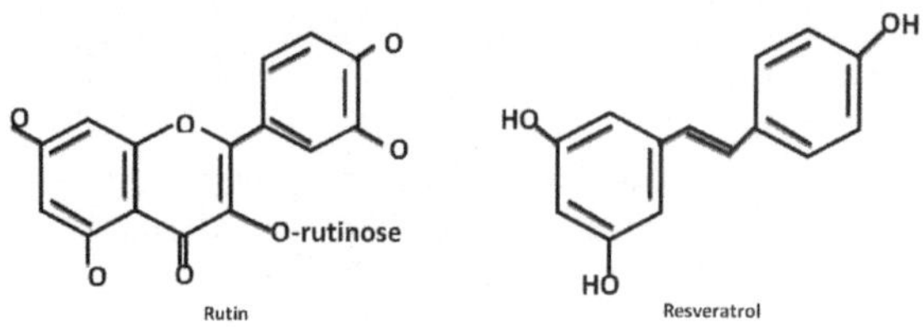

Fig. 5. Basic structures of some pharmacologically important plant derived phenolics

2.2.2.9 Heamaglutinin determination

To 2 g of the sample was added 20 ml of 0.9% NaCl and suspension shaken vigorously for 1 minute. The supernatant were left to stand for 1 hour, the samples were then centrifuged at 2000 rpm for 10 minutes and the suspension filtered. The supernatants in each were collected and used as crude agglutination extract. Absorbance was read at 420 nm.

2.3 Antimicrobial Susceptibility Test

The sensitivity of the various banana pseudo stem extracts against selected test organisms (*Streptococcus sp., Staphylococcus aureus, Escherichia coli, Pseudomonas aeruginosa, Aspergillus niger & Candida albican*) was carried out using the agar well diffusion method.

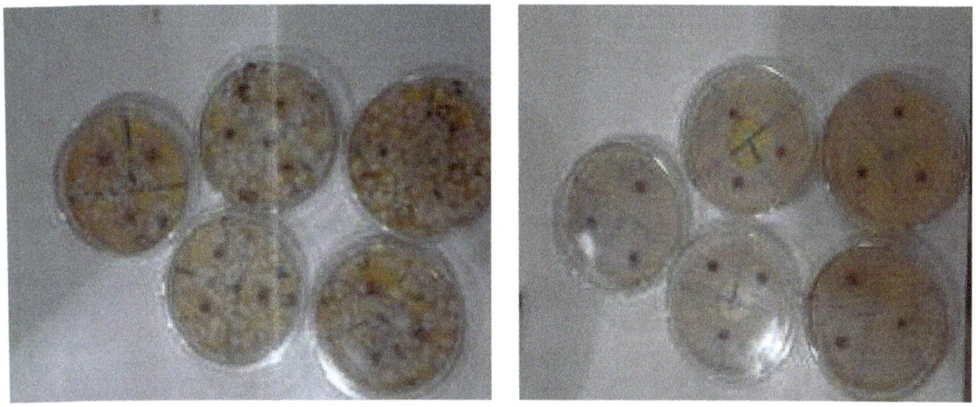

Fig. 6. Zone of inhibition for antifungal organisms

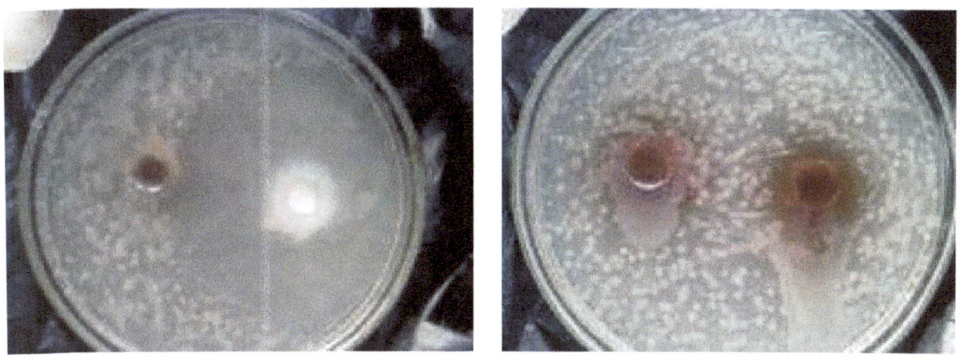

Fig. 7. Zone of inhibition for antibacterial organisms

3. RESULTS AND DISCUSSION

3.1 Phytochemical Screening Result

From Table 1 generally, water extract fared better with respect to amount of phytochemicals found in it except for Cardiac glycoside where it was notably absent. The presence of virtually all the phytochemicals in the water extract connotes that water could be used as the main solvent for the extraction of the metabolites for pharmaceutical purposes. The lapses observed by the absence of cardiac glycoside in the water extract should not be a problem as cardiac glycosides which serve as flavoring agents in pharmaceuticals [12] could be replaced by other flavorings.

Worthy of note also is the efficiency difference between methanol and ethanol. 50% methanol and 50% ethanol showed better efficiency than 90% methanol and 90% ethanol extract as all the phytochemicals were extracted by it unlike 90% methanol and 90% ethanol where alkaloids, tannins and saponins were conspicuously absent in the extract.

Also of interest is the extraction trend associated with the various extracting solvents wherein both 50% and 90% methanol and ethanol had the same Phytochemical constituents. This goes to show that there is the possibility of obtaining the same Phytochemical constituents in different alcohols of the same concentration.

The results in Table *2* show that the banana pseudo stem contain*s* phytochemicals in relative abundance with percentage comparative measure following the trend Tannin>Alkaloids>Flavonoids>Saponins>Cardia c glycosides while weight by weight comparison shows that Phenol> Haemaglutinin>Phytate>Oxalate.

Phytochemicals are known to occur in various parts of plants with diverse functions which include provision of strength to plants, attraction of insects for pollination and feeding, defence against predators, provision of colour, while

Table 1. Result of qualitative analysis of various solvent extracts of banana pseudo stem

S/N	Phytochemical	50% Methanol	90% Methanol	Water extract	50% Ethanol	90% Ethanol
1	Alkaloid	+	-	+	+	-
2	Cardiac glycoside	+	++	-	+	++
3	Flavonoid	++	+	+++	++	+
4	Phenol	+	+	+	+	-
5	Protein	++	++	++	+	+
6	Saponin	+	-	+	+	-
7	Steroid	++	+	+	++	+
8	Tannin	+	-	+	-	-
9	Terpenoid	++	+	+	+	+

Key: - Absent
+ Present in low concentration
+ + Present in moderate concentration
+ + +Present in high concentration

some are simply waste products [13]. When ingested by animals these secondary metabolites exhibit varied biochemical and pharmacological actions [14]. The presence of tannins in diets for livestock have been reported to have anti-nutritional and toxic effects including reduced fed intake, growth, feed efficiency and net metabolizable energy [15].

Table 2. Result of quantitative analysis of various fractions of banana pseudo stem

S/N	Phytochemical	Quantity
1	Alkaloids	8.16%
2	Cardiac glycosides	1.6%
3	Flavonoid	4.02%
4	Heamaglutinin	1.8814 mg/kg
5	Oxalate	0.1620 mg/Kg
6	Phenol	5.5743 mg/kg
7	Phytate	1.2976 mg/kg
8	Saponin	3.5%
9	Tannin	9.13%

Tannins in plants have been shown to confer antidiarrhoeic and anti-haemorrhagic properties on plants [16]. This is consistent with the traditional use of the pseudo stem of *Musa acuminata* for the treatment of diarrhoea, fresh wounds, cuts and insect bites as they have shown to contain these phytochemicals. Saponins have been reported to have antifungal properties [17] as well as serve as an expectorant and emulsifying agent [18]. Alkaloids, flavonoids and tannins have been known to show medicinal activity as well as exhibiting physiological activity [19]. Flavonoids are known to have antioxidant effects and have been shown to inhibit the initiation, promotion and progression of tumours [20]. The presence of these phytochemicals in the banana pseudo stem confers medicinal properties on the plant and this explains the use of this plant for treatment of different ailments. The findings of this study are consistent with reports of the presence of these phytochemicals in various parts of the banana plant as documented by [21].

3.2 Antimicrobial Test Results

The results of the antibacterial activity of the aqueous and methanolic extracts of banana pseudo stem against the test organisms are shown in Table 3. The zone of inhibition of the growth of the isolates was found to be a function of the relative antibacterial potency of the extracts. Thus zones of inhibition decreased as the concentration of the extracts decreased. Higher growth inhibition was obtained with the water extract compared with methanol extracts. In Table 3 the antibacterial activity of the aqueous extract of banana pseudo stem revealed the highest zone of inhibition to be 21 mm against *Streptococcus sp.* compared to 14 mm of methanolic extract. The bacteria *Staphylococcus aureus and Escherichia coli* were not inhibited with the water extract and thus showed no zone of inhibition.

Microorganisms vary widely in their degree of susceptibility to anti-microbial agents. A high MIC value indicates low activity and vice versa. In this study the gram- negative organisms had the lowest MICs and MBCs. This suggests their higher susceptibility to the extract of the banana pseudo stem. On the basis of the result obtained in this investigation it can be concluded that water extract of *Musa acuminata* pseudo stem had significant *in vitro* broad spectrum antimicrobial activity although do not really compete with the standard drug. Nevertheless,

Table 3. Result of the antibacterial activity of various fractions of banana pseudo stem extract

	Banana extracts IZD (mm)			
Extract	***Pseudomonas aerugenosa***	***Escherichia Coli***	***Staphylococcus aureus***	***Streptococcus spp.***
Water	*17*	*0*	*0*	*21*
50% Methanol	0	0	16	14
90% Methanol	0	0	0	13
50% Ethanol	0	0	0	18
90% Ethanol	0	18	0	13
Ampicillin	-	-	27	28
Ciprofloxacin	54	26	-	-

the extracts from the plant can be used to control infections caused by *Pseudomonas aerugenosa & Streptococcus sp.* for water extract and *Escherichia coli and Staphylococcus aureus* for 50% methanol.

Table 4. Result of the antifungal activity of various fractions of banana pseudo stem extract

	Banana extracts/IZD (mm)	
Extract	***Candida albicans***	***Aspergilus niger***
Water	0	0
50% Methanol	0	0
90% Methanol	0	7
50% Ethanol	0	0
90% Ethanol	0	2
Ketoconazole 50 μg/mL	30	0

According to Ibeh et al. [22], an inhibitory zone diameter of 11-15 mm shows intermediate effect while 26 mm and above indicated that the organism was susceptible to the compound. Therefore with the extracts having an inhibitory zone of 0-7 mm, we could infer that these extracts do not have any antifungal effect on the test organisms.

4. CONCLUSION

The aqueous, ethanol and methanolic extracts of banana pseudo stem have been found to contain significant amount of phytochemicals. Water, ethanol and methanol (50%) extracts were effective against some of antibacterial organisms. All the extracts however did not show any activity against fungal test organisms.

5. RECOMMENDATION

Further work could be done to isolate specific secondary metabolites present in this plant and structurally elucidate them.

CONSENT

It is not applicable.

ETHICAL APPROVAL

It is not applicable.

COMPETING INTERESTS

Authors have declared that no competing interests exist.

REFERENCES

1. Frison E, Sharrock S. The economic, social and nutritional importance of banana in the world. In: Picq C, Foure E, Frison EA, (Eds). Banana and Food Security International Symposium, Douala, Cameroon; 1999.
2. IITA (International Institute of Tropical Agriculture), Plantain and Banana Improvement Program-Annual Report for 1997. International Institute of Tropical Agriculture, Onne, Nigeria; 1998.
3. Karamura E, Frison E, Karamura DA, Sharrock S. Banana production systems in Eastern and Southern Africa. In: Banana and Food Security by Picq C, Foure E, Frison EA, (Eds.) International Symposium, Douala, Cameroon; 1999.
4. Smale M. Assessing the impact of crop genetic improvement in Sub-Saharan Africa: Research context and highlights. In: Melinda S, Edmeades S, De Groote (Eds.). Promising crop biotechnologies for smallholder farmers in East Africa: Bananas and Maize. Genetic Resources Policies Briefs. 2006;19.
5. F.A.O (Food and Agriculture Organization of the United Nations). Report of the Workshop on production and marketing

constraints on roots, tubers and plantains in Africa. 1985;1:1.

6. Harbone JB. Phytochemical Methods, A Guide to Modern Techniques of Plant Analysis, 3rd edn. Chapman & Hall, London; 1998.
7. Trease GE, Evans WC. Pharmacognosy, 13th edition, Brailiere Ttindal book publishing by Cassel and Collins, Macmillian Pub. Ltd; 1989.
8. Young SM, Greaves JP. Influence of variety and treatment on phytic acid content of wheat. J. Food Res. 1940;5: 103-105.
9. Pearson D. The chemical analysis of foods. 6th edn. Churchill Livingstone, Edinburgh; 1974.
10. Obadoni BO, Ochuko PO. Phytochemical studies and comparative efficacy of the crude extracts of some homostatic plants in Edo and Delta States of Nigeria. Global Journal of Pure Applied Sciences. 2001;8: 203-208.
11. Boham BA, Kocipai. Flavonoids and condensed tannins from leaves of hawaiian vaccinium vaticulatum and V. calycinium. Pacific Science. 1974;48:458-463.
12. Sarker SD, Nahar L. Chemistry for pharmacy students general, organic and natural product chemistry, England, John Wiley and Sons; 2007.
13. Ibegbulem CO, Ayalogu EO, Uzoho MN. Photochemical, anti nutritional contents and hepatotoxicity of zobo (*Hibiscus sabdariffa*) drink. Journal of Agricultural Food Science. 2003;1(1):35-39.
14. Amadi BA, Ibegbulem CO, Egbebu AC. Assessment of the effect of aqueous extract of *Asimina triloba* root on organ weights and liver function of albino rats. International Journal of Natural and Applied Science. 2006;2:79-81.
15. Acamovic T, Brooker JD. Biochemistry of plant secondary metabolites and their effects in animals. Proc. Nut. Soc. 2005;4: 403-412.
16. Asquith TN, Butler LG. Interaction of condensed tannins with selected proteins. Photochemistry. 1986;25(7):1591-1593.
17. Osuagwu GGE, Okwulehie IC, Emenike JO. Photochemical and mineral content of the leaves of four Nigerian *Pterocarpus* species. Int. J. Mol. Med. Adv. Sci. 2007; 3(1):6-11.
18. Edeoga HO, Okwu DE, Mbaebie BO. Mineral and nutritive value of some nigerian medicinal plants. Journal of Medicinal and Aromatic Plant Science. 2003;25:689-694.
19. Sofowora A. Medicinal plants and traditional medicine in Africa. Spectrum Books Ltd., Ibadan, Nigeria; 1993.
20. Kim SY, Kim JH, Kim SK, Ohandy MY, Jung. Antioxidant activities of selected oriental herb extracts. Journal Am. Oil Chem. Soc. 1994;71:633-640.
21. Akpuaka MU, Ezem SN. Preliminary photochemical screening of some Nigerian dermatological plants. Journal of Basic Phys. Res. 2011;2(1):1-5.
22. Ibeh IN, Uraih N. Practical Microbiology, Arabik press, Nigeria. 2003;1.

29

In vitro Antioxidant Activity and Hypolipidemic Effects of an Ethanol Extract of *Amaranthus viridis* Leaves on Hyperlipidemic Wistar Albino Rats

O. D. Omodamiro[1*], M. A. Jimoh[2] and P. U. Ezurike[1]

[1]*Department of Biochemistry, College of Natural Sciences, Michael Okpara University of Agriculture, Umudike, Abia State, Nigeria.*
[2]*Department of Plant Science and Biotechnology, College of Natural Sciences, Micheal Okpara University of Agriculture, Umudike, Abia State, Nigeria.*

Authors' contributions

This work was carried out in collaboration between all authors. Author ODO designed the study, wrote the protocol and wrote the first draft of the manuscript. Author PUE managed the literature searches, analyses of the study performed the spectroscopy analysis and author MAJ managed the experimental process and identified the species of plant. All authors read and approved the final manuscript.

Article Information

Editor(s):
(1) Syed A. A. Rizvi, Department of Pharmaceutical Sciences, College of Pharmacy, Nova Southeastern University, USA.
(2) Ali Nokhodchi, Professor of Pharmaceutics and Drug Delivery, School of Life Sciences, University of Sussex, UK.
Reviewers:
(1) Abdullahi M. Nuhu, Kaduna Polytechnic, Kaduna, Nigeria.
(2) Arhab Rabah, Universite de Tebessa, Algeria.
(3) Orapin Wongsawatkul, Srinakharinwirot University, Bangkok, Thailand.

ABSTRACT

Amaranthus viridis Linn. (AV), communally known as 'Slender or Green Amaranth' in English, is a multinational genus of herbs. Several species of *Amaranthus* are often considered as weeds, as leaf vegetables, cereals and ornamentals. Traditionally, an infusion of the plant (leaves and roots) is used to treat dysentery and epilepsy in children, purify blood, reduce inflammation, hemorrhoids, reduce labour pain and improve appetite in parts of Africa and India. The present study was designed to evaluate the In vitro antioxidant activity and hypolipidemic effect of an ethanol extract of AV leaves (EEAVL) in Wistar albino rats and mice using experimental models. Acute toxicity (LD_{50}) of EEAVL were studied in mice using standard method. The result showed a LD_{50} of 353.6 mg/kg of

---

**Corresponding author: Email: majekdamiro@yahoo.com*

the extract. Fourteen (14) Wistar albino rats of both sexes were divided randomly into seven (7) groups of two animals, each subjected to different treatment for 14 days. Group A was the non-high fat diet control; Group B was the high fat diet-induced control; Group C received 20 mg/kg of Simvastatin, a standard lipid lowering drug; Group D to G received 250 mg/kg, 125 mg/kg, 62.25 mg/kg and 31.13 mg/kg BW respectively of EEAVL of which all were still maintained on their induced diet. At the end of the treatment, the lipid profile and body weight were estimated and compared with the Simvastatin treated control group. The result showed a significant ($p < 0.05$) decrease in T-Cholesterol, Triglyceride and LDL-C ($p > 0.05$) while HDL-C was increased at the doses studied. EEAVL also caused a decrease in the rate of weight gain. In the in-vitro antioxidant test, there was a concentration dependent increase in the (%) Scavenging activity when compared with the Vitamin C (control) for 1,1-diphenyl-2-picrylhydrazyl (DPPH), Nitric oxide and anti-lipid peroxidation activity of AVL. The results showed no significant difference at higher concentrations when compared to the control. On a comparative basis, the measure of the antioxidant effectiveness of the extract showed better activity in quenching Nitric oxide radical with an IC_{50} values of 72 mg/ml compared to Lipid peroxidation radicals (78mg/ml) and DPPH radicals (108 mg/ml). The result have shown that *Amaranthus viridis* L, a traditional folklore medicinal plant has in vitro antioxidant potentials and hypolipidemic effect which may provide therapeutic potentials in the management of Cardiovascular diseases, diabetes and their complications which might be caused by free radical generation and hyperlipidemia.

Keywords: Antioxidant; hypolipidemic; albino rat; Amarathus viridis; acute toxicity.

1. INTRODUCTION

Hyperlipidemia refers to elevated levels of lipids and cholesterol in the blood, and is also identified as dyslipidemia, to describe the manifestations of different disorders of lipoprotein metabolism. Its existence has posed as an independent and modifiable risk factor for cardiovascular diseases (Atherosclerosis) and mortality alongside with diabetes mellitus [1,2]. This results due to defects or disturbance in carbohydrates, proteins and fats metabolism [3]. The prevalence of hyperlipidemia is growing not only in developed countries but also in developing countries. Treatment of this lipid abnormality reduces cardiovascular events. The modern pharmacological therapy for hyperlipidemia is effective but is costly and associated with side effects leading to patient incompliance [4].

Antioxidants comprises of a range of substances that play a role in protecting biological systems against the deleterious effects of oxidative processes on macromolecules as proteins, lipids and carbohydrates. Many of those substances which contribute to the prevention and treatment of diseases in which reactive species of oxygen are involved are natural molecules of plants. Generation of free radicals or reactive oxygen species during metabolism and other activities beyond the antioxidant capacity of a biological system gives rise to oxidative stress [5]. Thus, the antioxidant status in human reflects the dynamic balance between the antioxidant defense and prooxidant conditions and this has been suggested as a useful tool in estimating the risk of oxidative damage [6].

Nature has been a resource of therapeutic agents for hundreds of years and a remarkable number of recent or novel drugs have been isolated from natural resources [7]. Medicinal plant is a triumph of popular therapeutic diversity and above all other agents, have been used from time immemorial because they have fitted the immediate personal need and are easily accessible and inexpensive. Herbal drugs constitute a major part in all traditional system of medicine especially in the western and eastern Nigeria, where there are many popular native medicine practitioners or traditional doctors [8]. According to the W.H.O, over 80% of the world's population relies on traditional form of medicine, largely plant-based to meet the primary health care needs [9]. Thus, there has been a marked shift towards herbal cures because of the pronounced cumulative and irreversible reactions of modern drugs. One of the many plants which has exhibited some pharmacological potentials is *Amaranthus viridis* Linn.

Amaranthus viridis Linn; belongs to the family 'Amaranthaceae'. *A. viridis* Linn grows annually as an erect, monoecious herb and about 10-75 (-100 cm). *A. viridis* Linn is slender, branched, angular and glabrous. Its leaves are also glabrous, long petiolate, 10 cm lamma deltoid-ovate to rhomboid-oblong. Flowers are green. *A viridis* Linn is known locally in English as 'Slender or green Amaranth'. The plant is traditionally eaten as a vegetable in Bangladesh and South Indian. In Greece, the plant is known as 'vlita' and it is traditionally eaten after boiling. In tropical Africa, *A. viridis Linn* is a widespread and common weed which is occasionally cultivated in Nigeria, Gabon, Dr. Congo and Cote d' voire [10]. In Nigeria, an infusion of the whole plant is used to purify the blood and the pounded root is applied against dysentery. In Cote d' voire, the leaf sap is used as an eye wash to treat infections, convulsions and epilepsy in children. The plant has been used in Indian traditionally to reduce labour pain, treat respiratory and eye problems, asthma and also used for improvement of appetite [11]. The anti-diabetic, hypolipidemic and antioxidant activity of the methanol extract of the *A. viridis* leaves has been reported in alloxan-induced diabetic rat [12,13]. The anti-hyperglycemic and Hypolipidemic activity of the methanol extract of leaves of *Amaranthus viridis* Linn has been shown [14]. *Amaranthus viridis* Linn has been reported to contain tannins, flavonoids, cardiac glycosides and proteins [15].

Despite appreciable progress made in the conventional antilipidemic and oxidative stress management strategies, the search continues for plant-based products for the control of hyperlipidemia and oxidative stress which are associated with a number of pathogens including dyslipidemia, atherosclerosis, diabetes mellitus, heart diseases, neurodegenerative diseases, cancer among others which are risk factors for cardiovascular diseases [16].

The objective and aim of this research is to evaluate if ethanol extract of *Amaranthus viridis* leaves possesses lipid lowering properties and also have in vitro antioxidant activities in hyperlipidemic model of wistar albino rats. If this is positive, the plant could become a suitable candidate for further investigation as source of antioxidant and hypolipidemic drugs in human.

2. MATERIALS AND METHODS

2.1 Collection of Plant Materials

Fresh leaves of *Amaranthus viridis* were collected in May, 2015 from Umuariagha village, umudike in Ikwano LGA of Abia state, Nigeria. The plant materials were authenticated by Mr. Ibeh in the department of forestry, College of Natural Resources and Environmental Management, Michael Okpara University of Agriculture Umudike, Abia State, Nigeria. A voucher specimen (Herbarium No. 1232) was deposited in the Herbarium of the department of plant science and biotechnology, College of Natural sciences.

The leaves were rinsed severally with clean tap water to remove dirt and debris and thereafter shed dried at room temperature. The dried leaves of the plant were pulverized to powder using an electric blender.

2.2 Ethanol Extract of *Amaranthus viridis* Leaves

One hundred grams (100 g) of the pulverized powder of the plant leaves were soaked in 700 ml of absolute ethanol in a covered amber bottle for 72 hrs for complete extraction. The mixture was then filtered using a cheese material (calico white) and thereafter with Whatman No. 1 filter paper, to obtain a homogenous filtrate. The extract (filtrate) was then poured into a beaker of known weight and thus evaporated to dryness using a water bath at 40℃ to obtain the ethanol extract. The extract was weighed and % yield of the plant extract was calculated. The extract was refrigerated at 2-8℃ until use.

2.3 Experimental Animals

Fourteen (14) Wistar albino rats weighing 60 g to 90 g and sixteen (16) swiss mice weighing 18 g to 22 g of either sex obtained from the animal house of the department of zoology, university of Nigeria Nsukka (UNN), were used for the experiment. The animals were housed in clean and only dry plastic cages at room temperature under standard conditions (temperature 25±2℃, relative humidity 45-55%) and were maintained a 12 hrs light-dark cycle. The animals were fed with standard pellet feed (Vital feed, Jos Nigeria) and clean tap water ad libitum during an acclimatization period of 2 weeks before experimentation.

2.4 Induction of Hyperlipidemia

For the induction with high fat diet, the wistar albino rats were fed 15g each of the high fat diet composition; Maize 39%, Egg yolk powder 5.8%, Groundnut cake 13.3%, Crayfish 2.2%, Vitamin mix 2%, Bone meal 2%, CMC 0.4%, Palm kernel oil 6.9%, Corn starch 21.6% and Palm oil 6.9%; for a period of 14 days. For comparison, a group of the wistar albino rat (Negative control) were maintained on normal diet (pelletized feed; vital feed). All the animals had free access to clean tap water and their feed. Body weight of the animals were determined after the period of induction (14 days).

2.5 Experimental Design

2.5.1 Acute toxicity study (LD_{50})

The acute toxicity and lethality (LD_{50}) test of the ethanol extract of *Amaranthus viridis* leaves was determined in swiss mice using Lorke method (1973) with slight modification. Animals in group of four were administered by intraperitoneal route by doubling dilution 2000 mg/kg, 1000 mg/kg, 500 mg/kg and 250 mg/kg of the ethanol extract of *A. viridis* leaves suspended in normal saline after dissolving in DMSO (dimethyl sulphoxide). They were observed for 24 hrs for any overt signs of toxicity or death and further 72 hrs for delayed toxicity. The LD_{50} was calculated as the geometric mean of the highest non-lethal dose (250 mg/kg) and the lowest lethal dose (500 mg/kg) [17].

2.5.2 Sub -acute toxicity study

A total of fourteen (14) wistar albino rat (2 normal; 12 high fat diet-induced rats) were used for the experiment. The albino rats were divided into seven (7) groups of two (2) rats each.

Group A: Normal control rats maintained on normal diet and water ad libitum.
Group B: High fat fed control rats still maintained on high fat diet
Group C: High fat fed rats treated with simvastatin (a standard lipid lowering drug) at a dose of 20 mg/kg B.W and still maintained on high fat diet.
Group D: High fat fed rats treated with EEAVL at a dose of 250 mg/kg B.W and still maintained on high fat diet
Group E: High fat fed rats treated with EEAVL at a dose of 125 mg/kg B.W and still maintained on high fat diet
Group F: High fat fed rats treated with EEAVL at a dose of 62.25 mg/kg B.W and still maintained on high fat diet
Group G: High fat fed rats treated with EEAVL at a dose of 31.125 mg/kg B.W and still maintained on high fat

15 g of both the normal feed and the high fat diet were given to each rat every day for 14 days. The Ethanol Extract of *Amaranthus viridis* Leaves (EEAVL) and the drug were administered to the rats orally by gavage daily for 14 days. After 14 days of treatment, animals were sacrificed by cervical decapitation after a 12hrs fast.

2.6 Blood Plasma Sample Collection and Preparation

Blood samples were collected by cardiac puncture from 12hrs fasted animals. The collected blood samples were centrifuged at 3000 rpm for 20 minutes. The plasma were separated into EDTA bottles and then refrigerated at near 0℃ until biochemical assessment was carried out.

2.7 Biochemical Assessment of Plasma Lipid Profile

The biochemical parameters for the lipid profile notably total cholesterol (TC), triglycerides (TAG) and High-density lipoprotein cholesterol (HDL-C) level in the blood serum were measured by enzymatic method using Randox Diagnostic Kits Spectrophotometrically. Low density lipoprotein was calculated as per Friedwald's equation [18].

$$VLDL = TG/5, \quad LDL = TC - (HDL + VLDL).$$

2.8 Antioxidant Activity

2.8.1 DPPH radical scavenging assay

Radical scavenging activities by antioxidants in the plant extracts were evaluated using DPPH (1, 1- diphenyl-2-picrylhydrazyl) method of assay by Blois (1958). Varying volumes of 0.2 mg/ml of the plant extract were added to 200 μl of (0.36 mg/ml) DPPH solution in methanol. A series of concentration 500 mg/ml, 250 mg/ml, 125 mg/ml and 62.25 mg/ml of the dried plant extract were tested. The mixtures were shaken vigorously and incubated in the dark for 30 minutes after which the reduction of DPPH absorption was measured at 517 nm. Percent inhibition by sample treatment was determined by comparison with the methanol-treated control group. The IC_{50} values denote the concentration of each sample required to give 50% of the optical density shown by the control, using a non-linear regression analysis. All test analysis were run in triplicate and the average values were reported. Vitamin C was used as positive control.

% DPPH Scavenging Activity =

$$\frac{A\ standard - A\ sample}{A\ standard} \times 100\%$$

2.8.2 Nitric oxide scavenging activity

The Nitric oxide scavenging activity was conducted based on the Greiss method by Greiss (1858). 2.0 ml of 10 Mm sodium nitroprusside and 5.0 ml of phosphate buffer were mixed with 0.5 ml of 500 mg/ml, 250 mg/ml, 125 mg/ml and 62.25 mg/ml of the concentrations of the plant extracts and were incubated at 25℃ for 150 minutes. The samples were run as above but the blank was replaced with the same amount of water. After the incubation period, 2 ml of the above incubated solution was added to 2.0 ml of Greiss reagent and incubated at room temperature for a period of 30 minutes. The absorbance of the chromophore formed was read at 540 nm. Vitamin C was used as the positive control and results were expressed as percentage inhibition of nitric oxide. All determinations were performed in triplicates.

2.8.3 Anti-lipid peroxidation activity

The extent of Lipid peroxidation using rat brain homogenate measured in-vitro in terms of formation of thiobarbituric acid reactive substances (TBARS) method of Tamura and Shibamoto [19]. 500 mg/ml, 250 mg/ml, 125 mg/ml and 62.25 mg/ml concentration of the plant extract (EEAVL) were made up with ethanol expressed in terms of dry weight. These samples were individually added to the brain homogenate (0.5 ml). This mixture was incubated with 0.15 M KCL (100 μl). Lipid peroxidation was initiated by adding 100 μl of 15 Mm FeSO4 solutions. The reaction mixture was incubated at 37℃ for 30 minutes. An equal volume of TBA: TCA (1:1, 1 ml) was added to the above solution followed by the addition of 1 ml Vitamin C. This final volume was heated on a water bath for 20 minutes at 80℃ and cooled, centrifuged and absorbance read at 532 nm using a spectrophotometer. The percentage inhibition of lipid peroxidation was calculated by using the formula;

% inhibition of lipid peroxidation =

$$\frac{A\ standard - A\ sample}{A\ standard} \times 100\%$$

The 50% of inhibitory concentration (IC_{50}) was also measured.

2.9 IC_{50} Calculation

IC_{50} values which represented the concentration of *Amaranthus viridis* leaves that caused 50% inhibition were calculated from a scattered plot of % inhibition against the concentration (mg/ml), using the equation $y = mx+c$

Where $y = 50$ (50% inhibition), $x = IC_{50}$ value, m = slope and c = intercept; all from the plot using Ms Excel or graph sheet.

2.10 Statistical Analysis

Values for lipid profile, weight gain/loss and antioxidant activities were expressed as Mean ± Standard Deviation (S.D). The data obtained were statistically analyzed using one way analysis of variance (ANOVA) with Duncan's multiple comparison post Hoc tests (LSD) to compare the level of significance between control and experimental groups. All statistical analysis were evaluated using SPSS version 17.0 software. The values $p< 0.05$ were considered significant.

3. RESULTS

3.1 Plant Extract Yield

The maceration of the powdered plant material (*Amaranthus viridis* leaves) in absolute ethanol gave a total extract yield of 4.17% (4.17 g/100 g).

3.2 Acute Toxicity and Lethality Test (LD_{50})

The acute toxicity study (Testing) of the ethanol extracts of *Amaranthus viridis* leaves (EEAVL) in Swiss mice gave an intraperitoneal LD_{50} (Lethal dose) value of 353.56 mg/kg (Table 1)

Table 1. Acute toxicity study and lethality test

Dose (mg/kg)	Number of animals per group	Number of mortality within 24 hours
2000 mg/kg	4	4
1000 mg/kg	4	4
500 mg/kg	4	4
250 mg/kg	4	0

Geometric mean between the lowest lethal dose and the highest non lethal dose

$$L.D_{50} = (500 \times 250)^{1/2}$$
$$= 353\ mg/kg$$

3.3 Effect of High fat Diet and Normal diet on the Body Weight and Lipid Profile of Experimental Animals (Wistar Albino Rats) for 14 Days

3.3.1 Effect on body weight

The High fat diet induction (Hyperlipidemia) for 14 days on Wistar albino rats increased their body weight (BW) gradually from 75±8 g to 83±8 g while animals fed with normal diet also increased in BW from 72±3 to 81±1 g (Table 2).

Table 2. Effect of high fat diet and normal diet on the BW of wistar albino rat for 14 days

Body weight (g)	Treatment day 0	Treatment day 14
Normal diet (NC)	72±3	81±1
High fat diet (PC)	75±8	83±8

Values represent Mean±SD of; 12 rats (P.C) and 2 rats (N.C)

3.3.2 Effect on lipid profile

The high fat diet induction (hyperlipidemia) increased lipid profile significantly ($p < 0.05$) in experimental animals when compared to control groups. Total Cholesterol increased from 157±4 mg/dl to 224±6 mg/dl, Triglyceride increased from 65±1 mg/dl to 78±5 mg/dl, HDL-C increased from 78±6 mg/dl to 90±3 mg/dl and LDL-C increased from 66±1 mg/dl to 118±7 mg/dl. (Table 4)

3.4 Effect of Daily oral Administration of EEAVL and Simvastatin on the Body Weight and Lipid Profile of High Fat diet (Hyperlipidemic) Induced Albino Rats

3.4.1 Effect on body weight

The oral administration of the plant extract, EEAVL (250 mg, 125 mg/kg, 62.25 mg/kg and 31.13 mg/kg) daily for 14 days to high fat diet-induced (hyperlipidemic) rats, decreased the rate of weight gain slightly, while there was a little decrease in the body weight of simvastatin treated group by 1.62%. (Table 3).

3.4.2 Effect on lipid profile

The effect of daily oral administration of EEAVL at the doses of 250 mg/kg, 125 mg/kg, 62.25 mg/kg and 31.13 mg/kg for 14 days significantly ($p < 0.05$) reduced Total Cholesterol (TC) levels in high fat diet induced experimental animals by 18.3%, 16.5%, 9.4% and 9.4%; reduced Triglycerides by 12.9%, 12.3%, 5.8% and 3.9%; increased HDL-C levels by 8.9%, 5.5%, 14.3% and 4.4%, while LDL-C levels decreased non significantly ($p< 0.05$) by 39.4%, 33.47%, 32.63% and 26.3% respectively, when all were compared to Simvastatin (20mg/kg) that decreased TC (21.9%), Triglyceride (32.9%), HDL-C (6.7%) and LDL-C (31.8%) in the experimental animals. (Table 4).

Table 3. Effect of oral daily administration of EEAVL and simvastatin on the body weight of High fat diet-induced (hyperlipidemic) albino rats for 14 days

Groups & treatment	Body weight (g) day 0	Body weight (g) day 14
N. Control	$81±1^{b}$	$89±4^{a}$
P. Control	$75±6^{c}$	$83±7^{a}$
Simv. (20 mg/kg)	$82±2^{b}$	$80±7^{a}$
250 mg/kg EEAVL	$94±2^{a}$	$95±6^{a}$
125 mg/kg EEAVL	$85±5^{a}$	$86±5^{a}$
62.25 mg/kg EEAVL	$72±4^{c}$	$75±8^{b}$
31.13 mg/kg EEAVL	$87±4^{a}$	$90±5^{a}$

Values are represented as Mean±SD (n = 2); Values with the same superscript have no significant difference ($p < 0.05$) between them

3.5 Antioxidant Activities of *Amaranthus viridis* Leaves Extract

Table 5, depicts the % scavenging activity of *Amaranthus viridis* leaves (500 mg/ml, 250 mg/ml, 125 mg/ml and 62.25 mg/ml) observed with DPPH, Nitric oxide and Anti-lipid peroxidation with Vitamin C (20 mg/ml) used as the positive control. The result showed a considerable linear increase in the % scavenging ±activities with increasing concentration (mg/ml) of the extract. The highest % inhibition of the extract was observed at 500mg/ml for DPPH (96.4±0.5, Fig. 1), Nitric oxide (96.3±0.07, Fig. 2) and Anti-lipid peroxidation (97.6±0.04, Fig. 3) when compared to vitamin C at 20 mg/ml (99.3±0.3) thus varying insignificantly. On a comparative basis, the extract showed better activity in quenching Nitric oxide radical with an IC_{50} value of 72.2 mg/ml compared to lipid peroxidation radicals (78.1 mg/ml) and stable radical DPPH (107.7 mg/ml).

Table 4. Effect of oral administration of EEAVL and simvastatin on the Lipid profile of high fat diet induced (hyperlipidemic) experimental animals for 14 days

Groups	T-CHOL (mg/dl)	TRIG (mg/dl)	HDL-C (mg/dl)	LDL-C (mg/dl)
N. Control	157±4[d]	65±1[c]	78±6[c]	66±1[b]
P. Control	224±6[a]	76±5[a]	90±3[b]	118±7[a]
Simv. (20 mg/kg)	175±4[c]	52±4[d]	84±6[b]	81±2[b]
250 mg/kg EEAVL	183±4[b]	68±1[b]	98±6[a]	72±1[b]
125 mg/kg EEAVL	187±13[b]	68±4[b]	95±1[a]	79±15[b]
62.25 mg/kg EEAVL	196±6[b]	71±4[a]	102±8[a]	80±2[b]
31.13 mg/kg EEAVL	196±9[b]	75±2[a]	94±6[a]	87±14[b]

Values are represented as Mean±SD (n = 2); Values with the same superscript have no significant difference ($p < 0.05$) between them

Table 5. *In vitro* antioxidant activity (% scavenging activity) of *Amaranthus viridis* leaves extract for DPPH, nitric oxide and anti-lipid peroxidation assay

Conc. (mg/ml) *A. viridis* leaves	DPPH (%)	Nitric oxide (%)	Anti-lipid peroxidation (%)
(Vit.C300)	99.3±0.2[a]	99.3±0.1[a]	99.4±0.1[a]
500 mg/ml	96.4±0.5[a]	96.3±0.7[a]	97.6±0.4[a]
250 mg/ml	81.3±4.6[b]	89.5±5.4[a]	94.5±0.7[a]
125 mg/ml	60.1±2.4[c]	68.7±10.1[b]	69.4±5.9[b]
62.25 mg/ml	26.4±9.1[d]	41.2±9.7[b]	36.6±25.0[c]
IC_{50} (mg/ml)	107.8	72.2	78.1

Values are represented as Mean±S.D for triplicate data. Values with the same superscript have no significant difference between them

DPPH (%) Scavenging activity

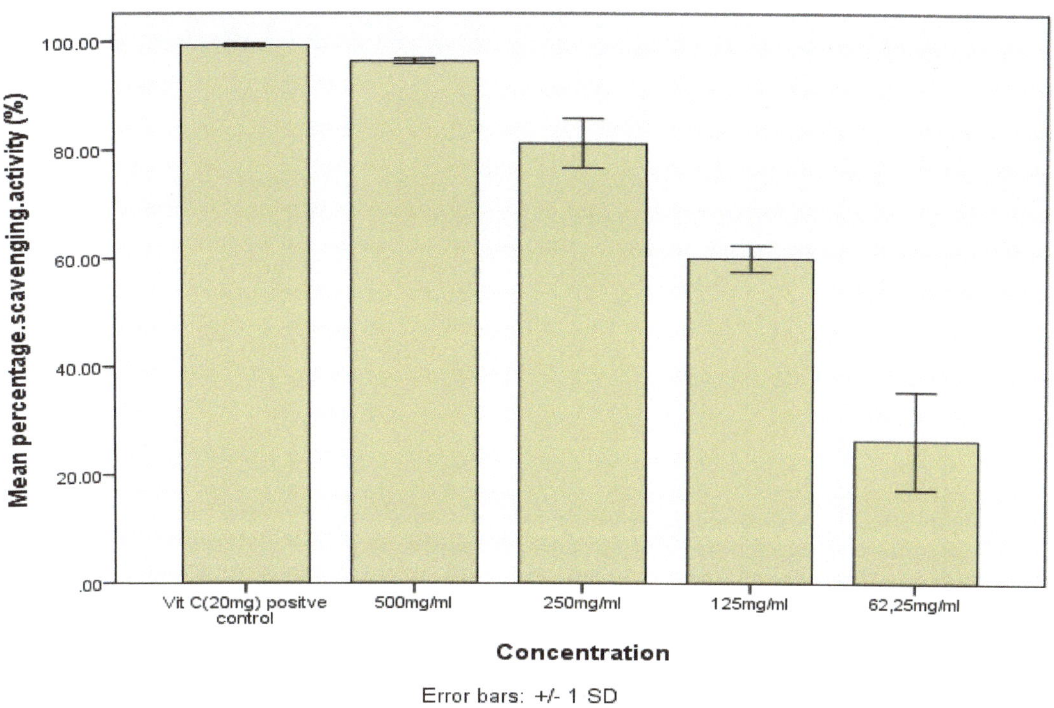

Fig. 1. A bar chart showing DPPH radical % scavenging activity of *Amaranthus viridis* leaves

Nitric oxide (%) inhibition activity

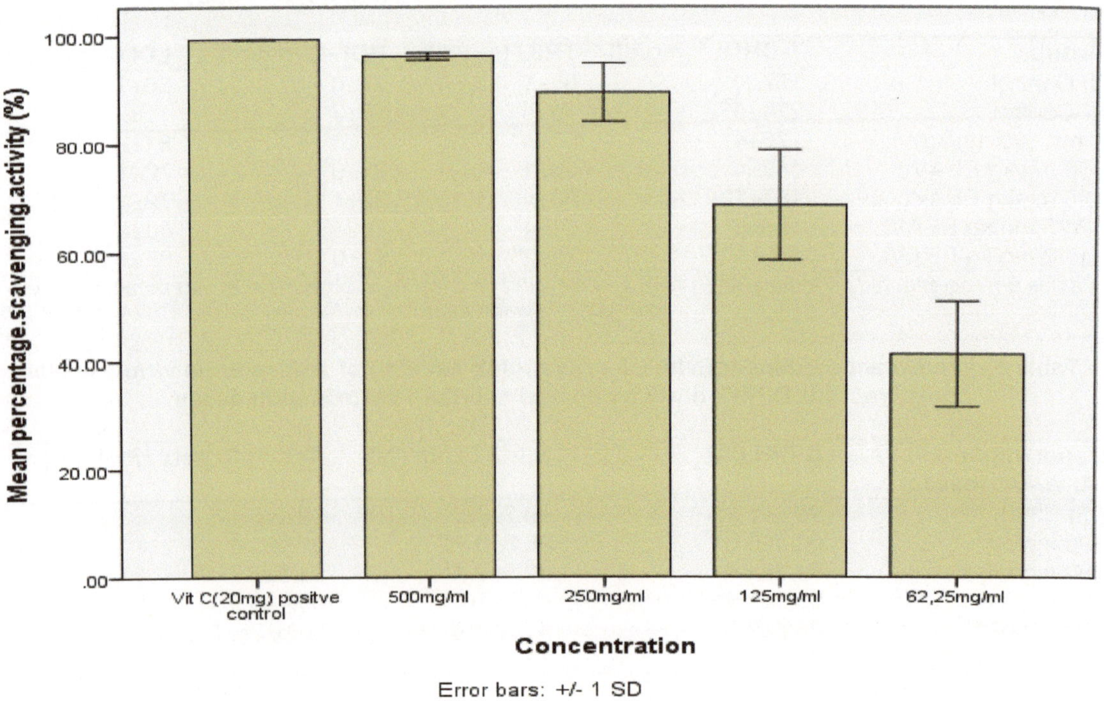

Fig. 2. A bar chart showing Nitric oxide % scavenging activity of *Amaranthus viridis* leaves

Anti-lipid peroxidation activity

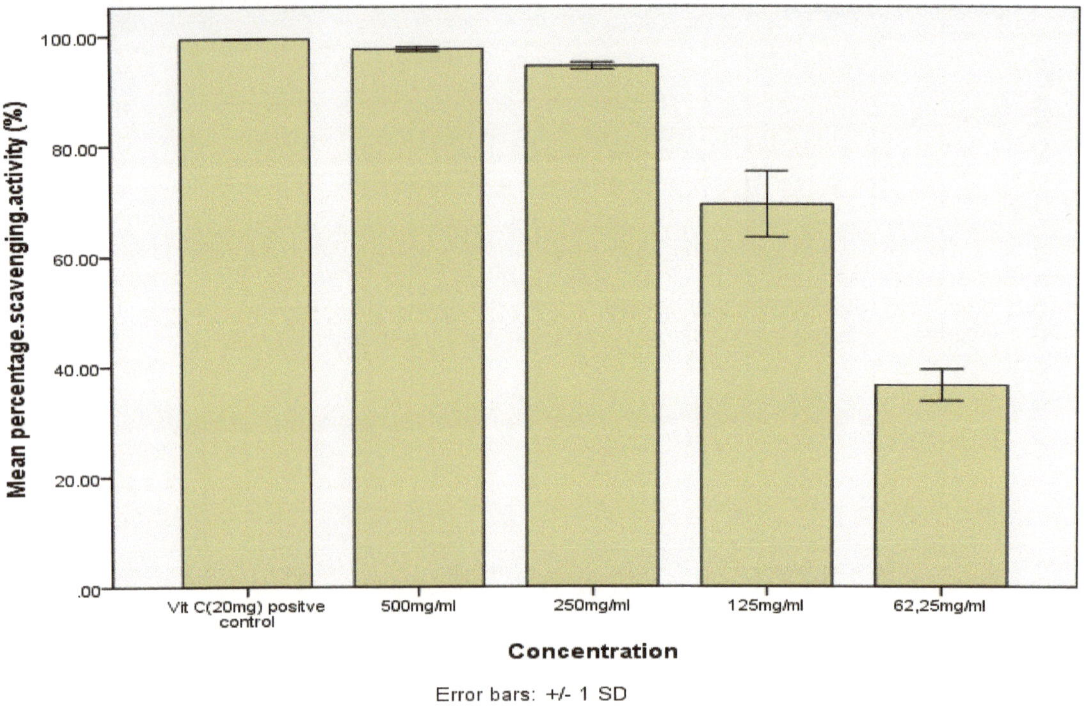

Fig. 3. A bar chart showing Anti-lipid peroxidation activity of *Amaranthus viridis* leaves

4. DISCUSSION

Feeding a high fat diet to experimental animals (wistar albino rats) for up to 28 days caused significant metabolic changes resulting in the development of Hyperlipidemia; 24% increase in body weight, hypercholesterolemia (levels increased by 43%), hypertriglyceridemia (levels increased by 20%), 78% increase in LDL-C and 15% increase in HDL-C. Dietary cholesterol has been shown to reduce fatty acid oxidation, which in turn, increases the levels of hepatic and plasma triglycerides [20]. In humans, hyperlipidemia caused by high fat diet predisposes one to cardiovascular diseases.

A scale proposed by Lorke [17], roughly classified substances according to their LD_{50} as follows; very toxic ($LD_{50} < 1.0$ mg/kg), toxic (LD_{50} up to 10.0 mg/kg), less toxic (LD_{50} up to 100.0 mg/kg) and only slightly toxic (LD_{50} up to 1000.0 mg/kg). Based on this proposal with an Intraperitoneal LD_{50} of 353.56 mg/kg, the extract used is relatively safe, but caution must be taken in administration of the extract.

Results of this study demonstrated that an ethanol extract of the leaves of *Amaranthus viridis* on daily oral administration at different doses showed a significant reduction ($p< 0.05$) in the levels of Total cholesterol, Triglyceride, LDL-C ($p> 0.05$), decreased the rate of weight gain in experimental animals and thus increased HDL-C in experimental animals. These effects were similar to those effects showed by Simvastatin (standard lipid lowering drug) but differs in that, it decreased HDL-C when compared to EEAVL at the doses studied.

It is obvious and hypothesized that the hypocholesterolemic activity of the extract after daily oral dose of administration may be due to a number of mechanisms, some common with simvastatin including a) inhibition of HMG-COA reductase enzyme responsible for synthesis of cholesterol by the liver, b) stimulation of cholesterol-7-alpha-hydroxylase (CYP7A1), which converts cholesterol into bile acids and/or inhibition, c) inhibition of cholesterol absorption from the intestine due to the formation of complexes with compounds such as saponins, glycosides and flavonoids [21,22]. A reduction in Triglyceride levels may be due to decreased lipogenesis, increased lipolytic activity by inhibition of hormone-sensitive lipase or lipogenic enzymes and /or activation of lipoprotein lipase [23] as has been proposed for simvastatin [24] and some plant exhibiting hypolipidemic activity [25]. In other words, the results suggest that the oral administration of EEAVL at different doses studied significantly ($p<0.05$) reduced the plasma triglyceride biosynthesis and favours the redistribution of cholesterol among the lipoprotein molecules. The crucial risk factor for cardiovascular diseases includes a low level of HDL-Cholesterol. The association between a low level of HDL-Cholesterol and an increased risk of cardiovascular diseases has been well established through epidemiological and clinical studies [26]. Since low level of HDL-Cholesterol plays a direct role in the atherogenic process, therapeutic intervention to raise HDL-Cholesterol together with other risk factors is widely encouraged. In this study, treatment with EEAVL led to a significant elevation of plasma HDL-Cholesterol, indicating its promising protective role in cardiovascular diseases. HDL exerts part of its anti-atherogenic effects by counteracting LDL oxidation and recent studies also showed that HDL promotes the reverse cholesterol transport pathway, by inducing an efflux of excess accumulated cellular cholesterol and prevent the generation of an oxidatively modified LDL [27]. On the basis of the result, EEAVL may probably play an anti-atherogenic role through the inhibition of lipids oxidation as well as the elevation of HDL Cholesterol.

LDL-Cholesterol is another primary target of cardiovascular diseases risk-reduction therapy. In this study, EEAVL administered orally at different doses lowered LDL-Chloesterol levels of the hyperlipidemic rat model insignificantly ($p<0.05$). Excess LDL can be deposited in the blood vessel walls and become a major component of atherosclerotic plaque lesions. In view of the result, EEAVL elicited beneficial effects by lowering the plasma levels of cholesterol including low-density lipoprotein of the treated rats. Therefore, with the results investigated, EEAVL may thus, elicit some health benefits through the modulation of physiologic functions including the atherogenic lipid profile.

Oxidative stress has been implicated in the pathology of many diseases conditions including diabetes, cardiovascular diseases, inflammatory conditions, cancer and aging [28]. Antioxidants may offer resistance against the oxidative stress by scavenging the free radicals, inhibiting the lipid peroxidation and by many other mechanisms and thus prevent diseases. The in-vitro antioxidant activity of *Amaranthus viridis* leaves was also evaluated. The percentage (%)

inhibition/scavenging activities by DPPH, Nitric oxide and Anti-lipid peroxidation which showed a linear increase with increasing concentration of the extract depicts a common pattern of inhibition in plant extracts. On a comparative basis, the extract showed better activity in quenching Nitric oxide radical with an IC_{50} value of 72.2 mg/ml compared to lipid peroxidation radicals (78.1 mg/ml) and stable radical DPPH (107.7 mg/ml). IC_{50} value is inversely related to scavenging ability.

Nitric oxide is a free radical produced in mammalian cells, involved in the regulation of various physiological processes. However, excess production of NO is associated with several diseases [29]. In the present study, the nitrite produced by the Incubation of solutions of sodium nitroprusside in standard phosphate buffer at 25℃ was reduced by the ethanol extract of AVL. This may be due to the antioxidant principles in the extract which compete with oxygen to react with nitric oxide thereby inhibiting the generation of nitrite.

The peroxidation of membrane lipids initiated by oxygen radicals may lead to cell injury. Initiation of lipid peroxidation by ferrous sulphate takes place through OH radical by Fenton reaction [30] thereby initiating a cascade of oxidative reactions. The results obtained in the present study may be attributed to several reasons through; scavenging of OH or superoxide radicals or by changing the ratio of Fe^{3+}/Fe^{2+} ; reducing the rate of conversions of ferrous to ferric or by chelation of iron itself [31]. The antioxidant activity of the extract may probably be due to the rapid and extensive degradation of the antioxidant principles.

DPPH is a relatively stable radical. The assay is based on the measurement of the scavenging ability of antioxidants towards the stable radical DPPH. From the present result, it may be postulated that AVL reduces the radical to the corresponding hydrazine when it reacts with the hydrogen donors in the antioxidant principles [32]. DPPH radicals reacts with suitable reducing agents, the electron pairs off and the solution loses colour stoichiometrically depending on the number of electron taken up [33].

Amaranthus viridis leaf extract has been reported to contain alkaloids, tannins, saponins, flavonoids and glycosides [15]. The active constituent responsible for the antioxidant and hypolipidemic actions of AV are not certain but may be mediated by one of its phytochemical component identified as Flavonoids or Saponins [34]. Flavonoids are natural products, which have been shown to possess various biological properties related to antioxidant mechanism [35].

5. CONCLUSION

Oxidative stress and hyperlipidemia has been affecting mankind since ages. Though many drugs are available to treat these, but the problem of increased cholesterol and triglycerides in blood and generation of radicals is still prevailing and has been a cause for many coronary disorders. The observed Hypocholesterolemic and Hypotriglyceridemic effects together with invitro antioxidant potentials of Ethanol leaves extracts of *Amaranthus viridis* (EEAVL) in hyperlipidemic rats (High fat diet-induced), makes it quite important in the management of oxidative stress and hyperlipidemia which is associated with cardiovascular and neurodegenerative diseases and prevent its complications [36]. Further investigations are needed to elucidate the mechanism (s) of action, especially bioactivity guided fractionation, isolation and identification of the constituents of the plant extract responsible for the observed pharmacological activities.

CONSENT

It is not applicable.

ETHICAL ISSUES

All animal experiments were in compliance with the National Institute of Health Guide for care and use of laboratory animals (Pub. No. : 85-23, revised 1985). An approval for the use of animals' experimental protocols was secured from the university committee of ethical and appropriate use of animals.

COMPETING INTERESTS

Authors have declared that no competing interests exist.

REFERENCES

1. Chu NF, Pan WH. Prevalence of obesity and its comorbidities among school children in Taiwan. Asia Pacific Journal of Clinical Nutrition. 2007;16(Suppl. 2):601-607.

2. Jacobson MS. Heart healthy diets for all children: No longer controversial. J Pediatr. 1998;133(1):1-2.
3. Ahmed F, Urooj A. The Anti-hyperglycemic activity of *Ficus glomerata* stem bark in streptoz otocin-induced diabetic rats. Global J Pharmacol. 2008;2(3):41-45.
4. Grundy SM, Balady GJ, Criqui MH. Primary prevention of coronary heart disease: Guidance from Framingham: A statement for healthcare professionals from the Circulation. 2000;97(18):1876–87.
5. Zima TS, Fialova L, Mikulıkova L, Popov P. Oxidative stress, metabolism for ethanol and alcohol-related diseases. Journal of Biomedical Science. 2001;8:59-5.
6. Tiwari AK. Antioxidant: New generation therapeutic base for treatment of polygenic disorders. Curr. Sci. 2004;86:1092-1102.
7. Cragg GM, Newman DJ. Medicinals for the millennia. Ann. NY Acad Sci. 2001;953:3-6.
8. Maduka HCC, Okoye ZSC. Elemental composition of Sacoglottis gabonensis, a Nigeria alcohol beverage additive. Pakistan. J Biol. Sci. 2002;5(1):66-68.
9. Mazid M, Taqi AK, Firoz M. Medicinal plants of Rural India: A review of use by Indian folks. Indo Global Journal of Pharmaceutical Sciences. 2012;2(3):286–304.
10. Costea M, Sanders A, Waines G. Notes on some little known Amaranthus taxa (Amaranthaceae) in United States. Sida, contributions to botany. Sci. 2001;19(4): 975-992.
11. Townsend CC. Amaranthaceae; Flora of Ethopia and Eritrea, Vol.2, Magnoliaceae to flacocurtiaceae, the national herbarium, Addis Ababa University, Addis Ababa, Ethopia; 2000.
12. Krishnamurthy G, Lakshman K, Pruthvi N, Chandrika PU. Antihyperglycemic and hypolipidemic activity of methanolic extract of *Amaranthus viridis* leaves in experimental diabetes. Indian Journal of Pharmacology. 2011;43:450-454.
13. Ashok KBS, Lakshman K, Veerapur VP. Antidiabetic, hypolipidemic and antioxidant activities of methanolic extract of *Amaranthus viridis* Linn in alloxan induced diabetic rats. Exp. Toxicol. Pathol; 2012.
14. Girija K, Lakshman K, Pruthvi N, Chandrika PU. Antihyperglycemic and hypolipidemic activity of methanolic extract of *Amaranthus viridis* leaves in experimental diabetes. Indian J. Pharmacol. 2011;43:450-4.
15. Ahmed SA, Sumarra H, Tehreema I. Phytochemical profiling with antioxidant and the antimicrobial screening of *Amaranthus viridis* leaf and seed extract. Open Journal of Medical Microbiology. 2013;3:164.
16. Krauss RM, Eckel RH, Howard B, Appel LJ, Daniels SR, Deckelbaum RJ. AHA dietary guidelines: Revision, A statement for healthcare professionals from the Nutrition Committee of the American Heart Association. Circulation. 2000;102(18): 2284-2299.
17. Lorke D. A new approach to practical acute toxicity testing. Archieve of Toxicology; 1973.
18. Friedewald WT, Levy RI, Fredrickson DS. Estimation of the concentration of Low density lipoprotein cholesterol in plasma, without the use of preparative centrifuge. Clin Chem. 1972;18:499.
19. Tamura H, Shibamoto. Antioxidant measurement and 4-hydroxylnonenal. J. Am. Oil Chem. Soc. 1991;68:941-943.
20. Fungwe TV, Cagen LM, Cook GA. Dietary cholesterol stimulated hepatic biosynthesis of triglycerides and reduces oxidation of fatty acids in the rat. J Lipid Res. 1993; 34:93-41.
21. Yokogoshi H, Oda H. Dietarytaurine enhances cholesterol degradation and reduces serum and liver cholesterol concentrations in rats fed a high cholesterol diet. Amino Acids. 2002;22: 433-439.
22. Chen W, Matuda K, Nishimura N and Yokogoshi H. The effect of taurine on cholesterol degradation in mice fed a high-cholesterol diet. Life Sciences. 2004;74: 1889-1898.
23. Ahmed M, Shikha HA, Sadhu SK, Rahman MT, Datta BK. Diuretic, and anti-inflammatory principle from *Scoparia dulcis*. Pharmazie. 2001;56:657-660.
24. Kumar H, Singh D, Kushwaha SK, Gupta AK. Centrally acting analgesic activity of grandiflora in triton wr- 1339 induced hyperlipidemic rats. International Journal of Phytomedicine. 2013;2:52.
25. Sharma P, Darte Y, Tej K. (1997). Bhat, Food Chemistry, DPPH antioxidant assay revisited. 2009;113(4):1202–1205.

26. Assman G, Gotto AM. HDL cholesterol and protective factors in atherosclerosis. Circulation. 2004;109.
27. Yokozawa T, Cho EJ, Sasaki S. The protective role of Chinese prescription kangen-karyu extract on diet-induced hypercholesterolemia in rats. Biol Pharm Bull. 2006;29:760-5.
28. Cross CE. Oxygen radicals and human diseases. Annual Int. Med. 1987;107:526.
29. Lalenti A, Moncada S, Di Rosa M. Modulation of adjuvant arthritis by endogenous nitric oxide. Br J Pharmacol. 1993;110:701.
30. Halliwell B. Superoxide-Dependent formation of hydroxyl free radicals in the presence of iron chelates. FEBS Lett. 1978;92:321.
31. Braugghler JM, Duncan CA, Chase LR. The involvement of iron in lipid peroxidation. Importance of ferrous to ferric ratio in initiation. J Biol Chem. 1986;261: 10282.
32. Sanchez-Moreno C. Methods used to evaluate the free radical scavenging in foods and biological systems. Food Sci Tech Int. 2002;8:122.
33. Blois MS. Antioxidant determinations by the use of stablefree radicals. Nature. 1958;26:1199.
34. Duarte-Almeida JM, Negri G, Salatino A, de Carvalho JF, Lajolo FM. Antiproliferative and antioxidant activities of a tricin acylated glycoside from sugarcane *(Saccharumofficinarum)* juice. Phytochemistry. 2007;68:1165-1171.
35. Middleton E. The flavonoids. Trends Pharmacol Sci. 1984;5:335.
36. Onat A, Sari I, Yaziici M, Can G, Hergenic G, Avci GS. Plasma triglycerides, an independent predictor of cardiovascular diseases in men: A prospective study based on a population with prevalent metabolic syndrome. International Journal of Cardiology. 2006;108:89-95.

30

Phytochemical and Pharmacological Basis for the Ethnomedicinal Use of Root Extracts from *Anogeissus leiocarpus* as an Antidiabetic in Eastern Nigeria

Edwin O. Omeje[1*], Patience O. Osadebe[1], Wilfred O. Obonga[1] and Christopher E. Ugwuoke[2]

[1]Department of Pharmaceutical and Medicinal Chemistry, University of Nigeria, 410001, Nsukka, Enugu State, Nigeria.
[2]Department of Pharmacognosy and Environmental Medicine, Faculty of Pharmaceutical Sciences, University of Nigeria, 410001, Nsukka, Enugu State, Nigeria.

Authors' contributions

This work was carried out in collaboration between all authors. Author EOO was largely responsible for the design, collection of plant materials and execution of the experiment as well as writing of the initial draft of manuscript. Author POO was responsible for the overall supervision of the work and editing of manuscript. Author WOO participated in the research design and statistical analysis while author CEU assisted with the plant identification alongside A. O. Ozioko and also formed part of the editorial team. All authors read and approved the final manuscript.

Article Information

Editor(s):
(1) Esam Z. Dajani, Loyola University Chicago, USA.
Reviewers:
(1) Cesar Luiz da Silva Guimaraes, Federal University of Rondônia, Brazil.
(2) Abdullahi M. Nuhu, Kaduna Polytechnic, Kaduna, Nigeria.
(3) Anthony Cemaluk C. Egbuonu, Michael Okpara University of Agriculture, Nigeria.

ABSTRACT

Purpose: To obtain and validate evidence for or against the continued traditional use of *A. leiocarpus* root extract as an antidiabetic.
Methods: Aqueous methanol, ethanol, trona-treated ethanol extracts of the plant whole root, were screened for antidiabetic activity using alloxan-induced diabetic rats at three different oral dose

**Corresponding author: Email: edwin.omeje@unn.edu.ng*

levels (100-500 mg kg^{-1}day^{-1}) against standards. Phytochemical and acute toxicity tests were also carried out on the extracts.

Results: Tannins, saponins, carbohydrates occurred in very high amounts while steroids, terpenoids alkaloids, flavonoids and resins were moderate. The extracts exhibited a dose-dependent potent and statistically significant ($p<0.05$, ANOVA) antidiabetic activities up to the dose of 200 mg kg^{-1} compared to the untreated group with a glucose reduction values of 52.69±5.99% and 66.61±5.79%, respectively, at 12 and 24 h compared to 24.39±1.54% and 38.79±4.06% recorded for the positive control. Above 200 mg/kg dose, the extract did not produce additional activity. The calculated LD_{50} values of all the extracts were above 10,000 mg kg^{-1} in mice.

Conclusion: This study validates the traditional use of root extracts of *A. leiocarpus* as a potent, cheap and alternative antidiabetic remedy.

Keywords: A. leiocarpus; combretaceae; alloxan-induced; aqueous methanol; ethanol; trona-treated.

1. INTRODUCTION

Plants are complex systems capable of making diverse compounds that have complex chemical structures and a variety of physical and biochemical properties. Repeatedly, natural products have been proven as unmatchable sources of molecules for effective treatment and mitigation of disease burdens of man and animal [1]. In fact, Africans foresee future with a fast growing dependence on herbal medicines for the health needs of world's populations, especially with the avalanche of advancing research in science and technology- biotechnology, molecular biology, plant genomics, and recently, metabolomics. Most times, the thrust for drug development from nature is driven by several ethnomedicinal claims of the potencies of plant or animal-derived bioactive substances. The ethno botanical uses of plants are diverse in both traditional and veterinary medical practices [2], and the use of plants for medicinal purposes dates back to antiquity [3]. Therefore, the ethno-based evidences for the use of these medicinal plants must be validated through *in vitro*/*in vivo* proof of concept [4,5]. The high proportion (average of 80%) of diverse populations in several African nations depend largely on crude herbal drugs for their health needs mostly owed to economic factors, hunger, crises, violence and poor distribution of adequate health facilities [6]. These stress factors usually precipitates serious health problems amongst Africans, notable of which are hypertension and other cardiac diseases, malaria, HIV/AIDS and diabetes. Of all these, diabetes account for over 0.06% morbidity and mortality worldwide (population of approximately 7 billion people) and usually occurs with severe complications. This projection is expected to double by the year 2030 [7]. This Figure, which is far higher than that of HIV-related deaths is obviously higher in Sub-Saharan Africa where poverty encourages heavy poor dieting (high sugar-high calorie foods) resulting in a high incidence of this disease at almost an epidemic scale. According to the WHO estimates of 2000 for the African region, diabetes alone accounted for over 10% of both mortality and morbidity [8]. In Africa therefore, several plants are used by herbalists for the treatment of *diabetes mellitus* [9] and some have been scientifically validated [10-12]. Recently, in a continued effort and in collaboration with notable herbalists based in eastern Nigeria for the purpose of finding putative antidiabetic plants in Nigeria, several of the herbalists claimed that a plant which was identified and confirmed by taxonomist (Mr. Alfred Ozioko) as *A. leiocarpus* (DC.) Guill and Perr, (Combretaceae), has highly potent antidiabetic activities in humans (oral conversations; 2010). During the collection, one of the herbalists accompanied us to the site. The taxonomist also affirmed that the plant root was used as anti-diabetic agent in his locality.

A. leiocarpus, also known as 'African birch' or 'Axle-wood tree', is a tall evergreen tree native to African savannas of tropical Africa [13]. It is the sole West African species of the genus *Anogeissus*, a genus otherwise distributed from tropical central and East Africa through tropical Southeast Asia [13]. The leaves serve as a fodder to livestock and small branches with leaves are crushed to make one of the yellow dyes [14]. The gum is used to make ink more viscous or to glue leather and is used occasionally as Arabic gum replacement. The gum was used as food additives mixed with gum Arabic or as a substitute for it [15]. It is used in traditional medicine as a remedy for many ailments of livestock and man, which include: helminthosis, schistosomiasis, leprosy, diarrhea and psoriasis [13,16]. Recently, castalagin, a hydrolysable tannin, was isolated from the plant stem bark and this compound mediated the killing of *Leishmania in vitro* [17]. *A. leiocarpus* is used medically for the treatment of ascariasis, gonorrhea, general body pain, blood clots, asthma, coughing and tuberculosis [18]. It is also used as vermifuges and the leaves decoction is used for washing and fumigation [16]. Uniquely, this plant grows only in swampy areas in Nigeria. Our thorough and intensive literature searches did not show any report of its use as an antidiabetic in folkloric medicine till date. The obvious need to validate this strong folkloric claim became the drive for the present study.

1.1 Aims and Objectives of the Study

The main aim of the present study was to investigate an ethnopharmacological claim that extracts of *A. leiocarpus* possess potent antidiabetic property. In addition, the study had an objective to verify the claim that extraction done in the presence of sodium sesquicarbonate (trona) was better in terms of its antidiabetic activity.

2. MATERIALS AND METHODS

2.1 Collection of Plant Materials

A. leiocarpus roots and leaves were collected by the researchers in the month of October, 2010 from swampy area in Adani, Uzo-Uwani Local Government Area of Enugu State in south eastern Nigeria in collaboration with one of the practicing herbalist. The roots were identified and certified by Mr. Alfred O. Ozioko, a taxonomist with the Bioresources Development and Conservation Programme (BDCP) centre in Nsukka. Voucher specimens of the plant parts have been deposited at the centre and the herbarium unit of the Pharmacognosy and Environmental Medicine Department of our Institution with the numbers BDC-10-032 and PHE-07-2010, respectively. The plant parts were cleaned, shade-dried and pulverized. This was stored in a polyethylene bag at room temperature (27±3℃) prior to use.

2.2 Chemicals/Reagents Used

Glibenclamide (glanil®) and pure sample (Nigerian German Chemicals), Alloxan, Tween 80, Diphenylpicryl hydrazine (DPPH), ascorbic acid, absolute ethanol, absolute methanol, DMSO were obtained from Sigma Aldrich. Normal saline and dextrose saline were obtained from DANA, Nigeria Limited), and trona ("Akanwu") was obtained from a large market near our institution.

2.3 Animals Used

Batches of albino mice (20-33 g) or rats (120-165 g) of both sexes were procured from the animal house, Department of Pharmacology and Toxicology, Faculty of Pharmaceutical Sciences, and from the animal house, Department of Veterinary Parasitology and Entomology, Faculty of Veterinary Medicine, University of Nigeria, Nsukka. The animals were kept in standard laboratory conditions and fed with pelletized rodent commercial diet (vital feed Nig., Ltd) and water *ad libitum* throughout the study. They were exposed to 12 h light-dark cycle. This investigation was conducted following an approval by the relevant ethical Committee on laboratory animal use and international rules were observed. Specifically, the experimental protocols were executed in accordance with the guidelines of the Ethics Committee of the University of Nigeria as registered by the National Health Research Ethics Committee of Nigeria (as per the approved ref: NHREC/05/01/2008B). The animal care and handling was in line with the internationally accepted principles for laboratory animal use and care as found in the European Community guidelines (EEC Directive of 1986; 86/609/EEC) [19].

2.4 Preparation of Crude Aqueous-Methanol Extract

The whole roots *A. leiocarpus* were cleansed and dried under shade for 8 days. They were pulverized in mechanized laboratory grinder (MANESTY-F520, England) to fine powder. A total of 200 g of the powder was extracted in batches with absolute ethanol; first wetted with 200 ml of absolute ethanol and the actual extraction carried out with another 300 ml of aqueous-methanol using Soxhlet extractor for 24 h. The resulting ethanol extract was evaporated to dryness under vacuum at 40±5℃ to afford dry extract which was weighed and its percentage yield was calculated. The trona-treated ethanol extract was obtained similarly except that 2.5% w/w (2.5 g/100 g powdered plant material) was added to the extracting mixture in the Soxhlet. The dry extract was placed in a clean plastic container and stored in a refrigerator until use. This process was repeated for all other host trees.

2.5 Acute Toxicity Tests (LD_{50}) of Extracts

Acute toxicity tests were performed using the Lorke's method (1983) with the aqueous-methanol extracts [20]. Essentially, this method involves an initial dose range determination stage in which nine mice were used (three animals per treatment group). The aqueous-methanol extract was dissolved in 3% tween 20 solution and doses of 10, 100, and 1000 mg/kg were administered intraperitoneally to the respective groups of mice. The animals were then observed for 24 h. No deaths occurred in any of the animal after 24 h and the second stage was carried out. Doses of 5000 and 10000 mg/kg were administered to two groups of one animal per group. The animals were again observed for 24 h. LD_{50} was then calculated as geometric mean of the highest dose that did not kill any animal and the largest dose that killed all the animals. This was done with all the extracts.

2.6 Phytochemical Test

This was carried out as described by Harborne [21]. All reagents for the phytochemical test were freshly prepared following standard procedures.

2.7 Anti-diabetic Evaluation

The effects of the ethanol extract of *A. leiocarpus* containing trona ("akanwu") on alloxan-induced diabetic rats was carried out following a modification of the method by [22]. Briefly, 20 rats were used for the experiment. The animals were acclimatized and fed with water and commercial animal feed (Top Feed Limited, Nigeria) pellets. They were then fasted for 12 h. The basal glucose concentration was checked before the induction of diabetes. Diabetes was induced by intra-peritoneal administration of 140 mg/kg body weight of alloxan monohydrate (90.0 % pure) freshly prepared in normal saline. The rats were then fed normally and dextrose water added to their drinking water until after 48 h of the induction of diabetes. Blood samples were collected from the tail vein of the rats and blood glucose concentration at 0 h was determined using Accu-Chek® Active glucometer. The diabetic rats with blood glucose level greater than 150 mg/dl were grouped into five groups (n=4). The five groups were then treated as follows: The first group (positive control) received 15 mg/kg body weight glibenclamide dissolved in 3% Tween 80 solution, the ethanol extract of *A. leiocarpus* containing trona dissolved in 5%. DMSO was given to the second, third and fourth groups at a dose of 100, 200, and 400 mg/kg body weight, respectively. The last group (negative control) received only 0.5 ml of 5% DMSO solution. Blood samples were collected from the tail vein of the rats and blood glucose concentrations were determined at 0, 1, 3, 5, 6, 12 and 24 h using Accu-Chek® Active glucometer. Similar procedures were repeated for the aqueous methanol and ethanol extracts. The results were recorded accordingly.

2.8 Statistical Analysis

The results obtained were recorded as were the mean values with the standard error in mean (SEM) and statistical significance between treated and control groups were evaluated by the Students' *t*-test and one way analysis of variance (ANOVA; Fischer LSD *post hoc* test). Differences between means of treated and control group and also between solvents at P=.05 was considered significant.

3. RESULTS

The extraction process by Soxhlet method afforded yields of 14.64, 15.76, and 16.80% for the ethanol, trona-treated ethanol and methanol extracts respectively. It is obvious that trona showed negligible effect on the overall yield of extract. The use of trona does not therefore, enhance yield during extraction. The result of the preliminary phytochemical test shows that all the obtained extracts of *A. leiocarpus* contain tannins, glycosides, saponins, carbohydrates, flavonoids, resins, alkaloids, terpenoids, steroids and reducing sugars. Proteins, oils and acidic compounds were generally absent in all tested extracts. These phytoconstituents were present in varying amounts. Remarkably, while tannins, glycosides, saponins, carbohydrates and reducing sugar occurred in very high amounts, steroids, terpenoids alkaloids, flavonoids and resins occurred in moderate amounts in all extracts. The acute toxicity tests of the methanol extract following oral administration and using Lorke's modified method, showed the average LD_{50} value to be above 10,000 mg/kg. Obviously, this value signifies high margin of safety in mice when administered orally. The results of the activities of the different doses (100, 200 and 400 mg/kg) of the crude ethanol, the trona-treated ethanol and the methanol extracts on the alloxan-induced diabetic rat are shown as percentage reductions in glycaemia over 12 h in Tables 1, 2 and 3 respectively.

Table 1. Antidiabetic activities of the ethanolic extract of *A. leiocarpus*

Treatment (mg/kg)	Percentage reduction in blood glucose of rats post treatment (%)					
	1 h	3 h	5 h	6 h	12 h	24 h
100	-19.36±6.02	17.95±0.20*	20.98±2.79*	27.82±1.49	52.69±5.99**	41.41±4.11
200	-13.81±7.62	25.23±4.44*	25.54±1.06*	38.00±1.02*	66.61±5.79**	69.77±6.31**
400	-25.18±3.64	-21.44±3.02	-29.35±1.01	21.51±0.30	9.06±2.38	6.62±4.99
GB (15 mg/kg)	-4.60±3.17	-2.21±2.77	6.53±1.32	23.71±1.54	24.39±1.66**	38.79±4.06**
VH (0.5 ml DMSO)	-28.18±3.21	3.59±1.25	11.24±1.03	11.01±1.01	16.06±0.83	33.41±3.72

**, ** Significant reduction in hyperglycemia at p=.05 and 0.01 respectively the extract compared to the positive control; GB (Glibenclamide); VH (Vehicle)*

Table 2. Antidiabetic activities of the trona-treated ethanolic extract of *A. leiocarpus*

Treatment (mg/kg)	Percentage reduction in blood glucose of rats post treatment (%)					
	1 h	3 h	5 h	6 h	12 h	24 h
100	-21.24±4.09	18.40±1.30*	21.74±2.32*	29.91±2.18*	54.72±4.85**	40.32 ±3.23
200	-23.32±5.13	22.21±2.11*	23.34±1.09*	36.21±2.77*	65.67±3.65**	67.86±6.31**
400	-25.18±3.62	-27.54±4.15	-27.37±2.04	20.65±1.29	10.05±1.08	8.76±3.48
GB (15 mg/kg)	-15.34±3.30	-6.27±1.45	7.22±0.39*	24.83±2.35*	23.42±2.04*	43.65±4.21**
VH (0.5 ml DMSO)	-27.34±4.65	4.61±0.98	10.78±1.07	11.01±1.17	10.13± 0.72	32.35±2.64

**, ** Significant reduction in hyperglycemia at p=.05 and 0.01 respectively the extract compared to the positive control; GB (Glibenclamide); VH (Vehicle)*

Table 3. Antidiabetic activities of the methanolic extract of *A. leiocarpus*

Treatment (mg/kg)	Percentage reduction in blood glucose of rats post treatment (%)					
	1 h	3 h	5 h	6 h	12 h	24 h
100	-55.09±3.75	65.55±5.17	-55.09±3.75	-41.80±1.55	12.32±7.48**	18.02±6.76
200	-53.50±7.08	-19.07±1.22	-14.57±0.46	-10.31±0.43	10.21±3.66**	17.02±4.80
400	-15.05±0.95	13.80±1.15	19.18±0.26	17.17±0.59**	31.76±1.84	27.35±1.11
GB (15 mg/kg)	-8.18±3.22	-3.44±1.29	11.24±0.01	10.86±0.30**	16.20±0.84	33.40±3.71
VH (0.5 ml DMSO)	-24.60±3.14	-12.21±2.57	-16.53±0.03	-23.71±1.56	31.80±2.92	30.34±2.68

*** Significant reduction in hyperglycemia at p< 0.01 by the extract compared to the positive control, GB (Glibenclamide); VH (Vehicle)*

At the third hour post treatment with the ethanol extract, there was observed, a progressive and significant (p=.05) reduction in glycaemia of the rats the at 100 and 200 mg/kg doses of the aqueous ethanol extract of *A. leiocarpus* with the maximum response produced at 24 h by the 200 mg/kg dose (69.77±6.31% reduction) compared to the unstimulated control (33.41±3.72% reduction) and positive control; Glibenclamide (38.79±4.06% reduction). Similar trends were observed for the responses at the 12th h. Surprisingly, repeated experiments showed that a higher dose of 400 mg/kg did not produce reduction in glycaemia as expected. Trona-treated ethanol extract produced similar trend of activities (reduction in glycaemia) but without any obvious advantage as was claimed by the practicing herbalist (Table 2).

The use of methanol as solvent for extraction was found to produce extracts of moderate activity than the ethanol extracts even at comparatively lower doses. However, higher doses of the methanol extract produced a steady incremental reduction in glucose level up till the 5th h (Table 3). This suggests that the herbalist's choice of ethanol as solvent for extraction is reasonable.

4. DISCUSSION

The avalanche of claims of the antidiabetic potency of *A. leiocarpus* in human subjects by several herbalists in South Eastern Nigeria and notably from a renowned middle-aged herbalist from Delta State, Nigeria but resident in Nsukka, south eastern Nigeria in 2010 spurred interest to work on this plant (*A. leiocarpus*). According to him, the extracts usually performed better in the reduction of glycaemia compared to established orthodox antidiabetic drugs. Remarkable from his several years of practice, is that, recalcitrant hyperglycemia to orthodox antidiabetic agents usually responded fastly to the very first two dosing with the extract. These were indeed claims that needed reproducible scientific validation. Spurred by these strong claims, we conducted a field study in early part of 2010 and discovered that several of such herbalists used the plant as either part or main constituent of their antidiabetic concoction. As part of evidence, we also discovered that at the site of collection of the plant parts, most of the tree stands visited had at least a root part collected from them and preliminary inquiries from locals led credence that the collections were for antidiabetic use. Furthermore, the root had very fast regenerative power as usually less than 12 weeks is needed for harvested root part to recover fully. Further evidence from blood glucose measurement showed that indeed, the ethanol extracts had potent antidiabetic activity. Placebo effects of solvent were ruled out accordingly. In response to all these interesting findings established from the field study, we set out into this investigative research work. Although this information was discovered with much excitement, the paramount and primary interest to us became that of toxicity. In response to this concern, the acute toxicity of the extracts was evaluated using the Lorke's approach and found that all the methanol and ethanol extracts were very safe with LD_{50} values generally greater than 10,000 mg/kg. The current data obtained did not suggest that the use of sodium sesquicarbonate (trona) in the extraction produced adverse effect on the safety of the extracts. This is in agreement with the practice in most parts of Nigeria; the use of trona to soften hard cereals and reduce its cooking time considerably has not produced any reported toxicity concern for many centuries. Besides, the trona is usually used in comparatively small quantity compared to the volume of extracts. These findings suggest in strong terms, that the extracts of *A. leiocarpus* have very good (wide) margin of safety. Although these data are suggestive of widely safe extracts, the sub-acute and chronic toxicity profiles as well as the cytotoxicity studies should be established in the near future. The obtained yields of 14.64%, 15.76% and 16.80% for the ethanol, trona-treated ethanol and methanol extracts are fairly high compared to other reported yields from roots of plants [23]. This fairly high yield of extracts is in tandem with the observed rich composition of phytoconstituents of *A. leiocarpus*. The result of the preliminary phytochemical test shows that all the obtained extracts of *A. leiocarpus* contain tannins, glycosides, saponins, carbohydrates, flavonoids, resins, alkaloids, terpenoids, steroids and reducing sugars. Proteins, oils and acidic compounds were generally absent in all tested extracts. These phytoconstituents were present in varying amounts. It is remarkable to note that, while tannins, glycosides, saponins, carbohydrates and reducing sugar occurred in very high amounts, steroids, terpenoids alkaloids, flavonoids and resins occurred in moderate amounts in all extracts. As part of evidence for affirmation of these, several of these constituents (saponins, flavonoids, terpenoids, steroids and alkaloids) which occurred in either high or moderate amounts have been reported to exhibit potent antidiabetic activity [24]. In terms of antidiabetic potencies, the crude ethanol extract of *A. leiocarpus* showed marked activity which was fairly dose-dependent up to the 200 mg/kg body weight dose. Above this dose, there was an aberrant reduction in activity with increasing dose level. At the third hour post treatment with the ethanol extract, there was observed, a progressive and significant ($p<0.05$) reduction in glycaemia of the rats at the 100 and 200 mg/kg doses of the aqueous ethanol extract of *A. leiocarpus* with the maximum response produced at 24 h by the 200 mg/kg dose (69.77±6.31% reduction) compared to the unstimulated control (33.41±3.72% reduction) and positive control; Glibenclamide (38.79±4.06% reduction). This shows that the herbalist claims are supported by the present data as the extracts at these doses performed even better than the positive drug, Glibenclamide. At the dose of 400 mg/kg, the ethanol extract exhibited significant activity at 3 h post treatment but became less active after 12 h. This aberrant behaviour could not be completely explained by the present data but it is well know that certain plant metabolites usually exhibit biphasic pharmacological activities pattern. Although, the methanol extract was higher in yield, it produced a haphazard pattern in the reduction of glycaemia with the 100 mg/kg body weight dose producing the highest reduction at 3 h post treatment. At present, we are unable to explain the basis of this aberrant behavior. Nevertheless, it further supports the use of ethanol as the better extracting solvent as claimed by the herbalist. The activity spectrum of the ethanol extracts is similar to the positive drug, Glibenclamide that has established long duration of action [25]. The present data did not provide concrete evidence to support the use of trona during the extraction stage as there was no marginal advantage recorded from its use. Chemically, the basic nature of trona could enhance the extraction process by sequestering acidic constituents such as flavonoids or enhancing the solubility of basic constituents (like alkaloids) in the plant root and free them for extracting solvent. This however, is a speculation that needs further verification. In summary, the present data represents an exciting finding supporting the use of ethanol extracts of *A. leiocarpus* as a potent antidiabetic in ethnomedicinal practice of eastern Nigeria. This is in addition to other numerous activities associated with this plant root extract.

5. CONCLUSION

In conclusion, the crude ethanol extract of *A. leiocarpus* possesses potent anti-diabetic activities, and therefore can be potentially used as safe alternative in the treatment and management of *Diabetes mellitus*. The use of trona in the extraction process did not yield any statistically significant antidiabetic activity compared to the ethanol extract alone. Its use in the preparation of the extracts is therefore discouraged.

CONSENT

It is not applicable.

ACKNOWLEDGEMENTS

The authors wish to acknowledge the herbalist, Mr. Sam Ejechie who shared with us the secrets of his practice with respect to this plant and physically led our team for the initial collection of the plant material. Mr. Alfred Ozioko, a taxonomist with BDCP, Nsukka is appreciated for identifying the plant material.

COMPETING INTERESTS

The authors declare that there is no conflict and or competition of interest(s) in this research work. Furthermore, the authors have the full support of the herbalist for the present research work and any other work that may emanate from it.

REFERENCES

1. Perry LM. Medicinal plants: Attributed properties and uses. Cambridge: MIT Press. 1980;10-15.
2. Agunu A, Ibrahim NDG, Onyiloyi GA, Abdurrahman EM. Toxicity of stem bark extract of *Steganoteaenia araliacea* in rats. Nigerian J Nat Prod Med. 2003;7:65-67.
3. Ogunyemi AO. The origin of herbal cure and its spread. In: Sofowara A, editor. Proceedings of a Conference on African medicinal plants. Ile-Ife: University of Ife Press. 1979;20-22.
4. Paul C, Arnold J, Vlietinck Dirk VR, Loouis M. Anti-infective potential of natural products: How to develop a strong *in vitro* 'proof-of-concept'. J Ethnopharmacol. 2006;106:290-302.
5. Osadebe PO, Omeje EO. Comparative acute toxicities and immunomodulatory potentials of five Eastern Nigeria mistletoes. J. Ethnopharmacol. 2009;126: 287-293.
6. Bagozz D. WHO report on the use of traditional medicines in Africa; 2011. Available:http://www.allcountries.org/health/traditional_medicine.html. [cited 2011 October 11].
7. Kirigia JM. The economic burden of Diabetes mellitus in the WHO African region. African Health Monitor; 2008.
8. Obatomi DK, Oye AAA, Temple VJ. Reduction in serum glucose and cholesterol level in experimental diabetic rats treated with extracts of African Mistletoe (*Loranthus begwensis*). Med Sci Res. 1997;25:651–654.
9. Augustine KT. Therapeutic values of onions (*Allium sativum).* Indian J Expt Biol. 1996;34:634-640.
10. Kelkar SM, Keckly GS, Bapat VA. Determination of the antidiabetic activities of Allium *cepa* (onions) on tissue cultures. Indian J Biochem Biophysiol. 2001;38: 277-279.
11. Aderibigbe AO, Emudianughe TS, Lawal BAS. Evaluation of anti-diabetic actions of

Magnifera indica in mice. J Phyto Res. 2001;15:456-458.
12. Iwu MM. Anti-diabetic and aldose reductase activities of biflavonoids of *Garcinia kola*. J Pharm Pharmacol. 1990; 42:290-292.
13. Burkill HM. The useful plants of West Africa vol.1, families A.D Royal Botanical Gardens, Kew. 1985;417.
14. Mann A, Gbate M, Umar NA. Medical and economic plants from Nupe land. Bida: Jube Evans Publishers. 2003;1-67.
15. Ahmed SE, Mohamed BE, Karamalla KA. Analytical studies of the gum exudates from *Anogeissus leiocarpus*. Pakistan J Nutr. 2010;8:782-786.
16. Onyeyili PA. Antihelmintic efficacy of some plants used in ethno veterinary practices in the arid zone of north eastern Nigeria. RGA NO 28 project Report; 2000.
17. Shuaibu MN, Pandey K, Wuyep PA, Yanagi T, Hirayama K, Ichinose A, Tanaka T. Castalagin from *Anogeissus leiocarpus* mediates the killing of *Leishmania in vitro*. Parasitol Res. 2008;6:1333-1338.
18. Ibrahim MB, Owonubi MO, Onaolapo JA. Antibacterial effect of the leaf, stem and root bark of *Anogeissus leiocarpus* on *S. aureus, S. pyrogens, E. coli, P. vulgaris*. J Pharmac Res Dev. 1997;2:20-26.
19. EEC. Council Directive 86/609/EEC of 24 November 1986 on the approximation of laws, regulations and administrative provisions of the Member States regarding the protection of animals used for experimental and other scientific purposes. Official J Eur Communities. 1986;L358:1-29.
20. Lorke D. A new approach to practical acute toxicity testing. Arch Toxicol. 1983;54:275-287.
21. Harborne HB. Phytochemical Methods: A Guide to Modern Technique of plant Analysis. 2nd edn; London: Chapman and Hall. 1984;282.
22. Osadebe PO, Okide GB, Akabogu IC. Study on anti-diabetic activities of crude methanol extracts of *Loranthus micranthus* (Linn) sourced from five different host trees. J Ethnopharmacol. 2004;95:133-138.
23. Ali S. Chemical constituents, antimicrobial and antioxidant activity of the hexane extract from root and seed of *Levisticum persicum* Freyn and Bornm. J Med Plant Res. 2011;5:5127-5131.
24. Cristinia H, Pedro MGB, Franklin B, Marienela V, Luis P, Sandra B. Hypoglycemic and anti-hyperglycaemic effects of *Witheringia solanaceae* in normal and alloxan-induced hyperglycaemic rats. J Ethnopharmacol. 2011;133:907-910.
25. Katzung BG, Masters SB, Trevor AJ, Katzung BG (ed). Basic and Clinical Pharmacology, 12th Edition, New York: McGraw-Hill Companies.

Permissions

All chapters in this book were first published in BJPR, by SCIENCE DOMAIN international; hereby published with permission under the Creative Commons Attribution License or equivalent. Every chapter published in this book has been scrutinized by our experts. Their significance has been extensively debated. The topics covered herein carry significant findings which will fuel the growth of the discipline. They may even be implemented as practical applications or may be referred to as a beginning point for another development.

The contributors of this book come from diverse backgrounds, making this book a truly international effort. This book will bring forth new frontiers with its revolutionizing research information and detailed analysis of the nascent developments around the world.

We would like to thank all the contributing authors for lending their expertise to make the book truly unique. They have played a crucial role in the development of this book. Without their invaluable contributions this book wouldn't have been possible. They have made vital efforts to compile up to date information on the varied aspects of this subject to make this book a valuable addition to the collection of many professionals and students.

This book was conceptualized with the vision of imparting up-to-date information and advanced data in this field. To ensure the same, a matchless editorial board was set up. Every individual on the board went through rigorous rounds of assessment to prove their worth. After which they invested a large part of their time researching and compiling the most relevant data for our readers.

The editorial board has been involved in producing this book since its inception. They have spent rigorous hours researching and exploring the diverse topics which have resulted in the successful publishing of this book. They have passed on their knowledge of decades through this book. To expedite this challenging task, the publisher supported the team at every step. A small team of assistant editors was also appointed to further simplify the editing procedure and attain best results for the readers.

Apart from the editorial board, the designing team has also invested a significant amount of their time in understanding the subject and creating the most relevant covers. They scrutinized every image to scout for the most suitable representation of the subject and create an appropriate cover for the book.

The publishing team has been an ardent support to the editorial, designing and production team. Their endless efforts to recruit the best for this project, has resulted in the accomplishment of this book. They are a veteran in the field of academics and their pool of knowledge is as vast as their experience in printing. Their expertise and guidance has proved useful at every step. Their uncompromising quality standards have made this book an exceptional effort. Their encouragement from time to time has been an inspiration for everyone.

The publisher and the editorial board hope that this book will prove to be a valuable piece of knowledge for researchers, students, practitioners and scholars across the globe.

List of Contributors

Patrick Emeka Aba and Chidiebere Peace Okenwa-Ani
Department of Veterinary Physiology and Pharmacology, University of Nigeria, Nsukka, Enugu State, Nigeria

Yemisi Adefunke Jeff-Agboola
Department of Biological Sciences, Ondo State University of Science and Technology, P.M.B 353 Okitipupa, Nigeria

Anthony Kayode Onifade
Department of Microbiology, Federal University of Technology, P.M.B 704, Akure, Nigeria

Nguyen Hai Dang, Pham Thanh Binh, Nguyen Thi Tham, Bui Thi Mai Anh, and Nguyen Tien Dat
Insitute of Marine Biochemistry, Vietnam Academy of Science and Technology, 18-Hoang Quoc Viet, Cau Giay, Hanoi, Vietnam

Nguyen Phuong Dai Nguyen
Department of Biology, Faculty of Natural Science and Technology, Tay Nguyen University, 567 Le Duan, Dac Lac City 630000, Vietnam

Fathy Ibrahim Abd-Allah
Department of Pharmaceutics and Industrial Pharmacy, Faculty of Pharmacy, Al-Azhar University, Nasr City, Cairo, Egypt

K. Kalimuthu, V. Chinnadurai, Y. Sarmila Juliet
Department of Botany, Plant Tissue Culture Division, Government Arts College (Autonomous), Coimbatore-641018, Tamil Nadu, India

R. Prabakaran
Department of Botany, PSG College of Arts and Science (Autonomous), Coimbatore- 641014, Tamil Nadu, India

P. Subramaniam
Government Boys Higher Secondary School, Chinna Thadagam, Coimbatore, India

Lincy Joseph and Mathew George
Pushpagiri College of Pharmacy, Kerala, India

Olajide Sunday Faleye and Ebenezer Oluyemi Dada
Department of Microbiology, Federal University of Technology, Akure, Ondo State, Nigeria

Boushra Mohamed El-Houssieny, and Hussien Mohamed El-Messiry
Department of Pharmaceutics, National Organization of Drug Control and Research, Giza, Egypt

Esmat Zein El-Dein
Department of Pharmaceutical Technology, Faculty of Pharmacy, Tanta University, Tanta, Egypt

Khalid Da'u Khalid, Mustapha Balarabe Idris, Naziru Alhassan Muhammad and Ahmad Bala
Department of Chemistry, Jodhpur National University, Narnadi, Jhanwar Road, Boranada, Rajasthan, India

Anaka Ogochukwu Ngozi and Nwagwu Chinonye Sophia
Department of Pharmacology and Toxicology, Faculty of Pharmacy, Igbinedion University, Okada, Nigeria

Omoti Caroline Edijana
Department of Haematology, University of Benin Teaching Hospital, Benin, Nigeria

Owolabi Omonkhelin Josephine
Department of Pharmacology and Toxicology, Faculty of Pharmacy, University of Benin, Benin, Nigeria

O. Innih Silvanus
Department of Anatomy, School of Basic Medical Sciences, College of Medical Sciences, University of Benin, Nigeria

Md. Razibul Habib
Directorate General of Drug Administration, Bangladesh

Mohammad Mustakim Billah, Kashfia Nawrin, Md. Ibrahim Khalil
Department of Pharmacy, East West University, Dhaka, Bangladesh

Md. Rakibul Hasan
Department of Pharmacy, North South University, Dhaka, Bangladesh

Md. Mominur Rahman
Department of Pharmacy, International Islamic University Chittagong, Bangladesh

I. C. J. Omalu, K. Abdulraman, S. Ibrahim, C. Hassan, S. S. Eke, E. D. Ubanwa, and A. A. Boyi
Department of Biological Sciences, Federal University of Technology Minna, Nigeria

E. C. Egwim
Global Institute for Biotechnology and Exploration, Federal University of Technology Minna, Nigeria

A. Aliyu
Ministry of Livestock and Fisheries, Niger State, Nigeria

Osadebe Patience Ogoamaka and Onugwu Lawrence Ekene
Department of Pharmaceutical and Medicinal Chemistry, Faculty of Pharmaceutical Sciences, University of Nigeria, 41001, Nsukka, Nigeria

Omeje Edwin Ogechukwu
Department of Pharmaceutical and Medicinal Chemistry, Faculty of Pharmaceutical Sciences, University of Nigeria, 41001, Nsukka, Nigeria
Division of Medicinal and Process Chemistry, CSIR-Central Drug Research Institute, Chattar Manzil, P.O.Box 173, 226001, Lucknow, India
Division of Endocrinology, CSIR-Central Drug Research Institute, Chattar Manzil, P.O.Box 173, 226001, Lucknow, India

Deepshika Tewari, Rakesh Maurya, Naibedya Chattopadhyay and Mohd Parvez Khan
Division of Endocrinology, CSIR-Central Drug Research Institute, Chattar Manzil, P.O.Box 173, 226001, Lucknow, India

Okoye Theophine Chinwuba
Department of Pharmacology and Toxicology, Faculty of Pharmaceutical Sciences, University of Nigeria, 41001, Nsukka, Nigeria

Ugwoke Christopher Emeka
Department of Pharmacognosy and Enviromental Medicine, Faculty of Pharmaceutical Sciences, University of Nigeria, 41001, Nsukka, Nigeria

S. O. Ogbonnia, O. E. Akinsande and T. A. Ayeni
Department of Pharmacognosy, Faculty of Pharmacy, University of Lagos, Idi-Araba, Lagos, Nigeria

G. O. Mbaka
Department of Anatomy, Lagos State University College of Medicine, Ikeja, Lagos, Nigeria

D. A. Otah
Department of Physiology, College of Medicine of the University of Lagos, Idi-Araba, Lagos, Nigeria

Akintayo L. Ogundajo and Olamidisun A. Owoyele
Department of Chemistry, Faculty of Science, Natural Products Research Unit, Lagos State University, Badagry Expressway, PMB 0001 LASU Post Office, Ojo, Lagos, Nigeria

Isiaka A. Ogunwande
Department of Chemistry, Faculty of Science, Natural Products Research Unit, Lagos State University, Badagry Expressway, PMB 0001 LASU Post Office, Ojo, Lagos, Nigeria
Department of Chemical Sciences, Faculty of Science, Olabisi Onabanjo University, Ago-Iwoye, Ogun State, Nigeria

Mutiu I. Kazeem
Department of Biochemistry, Faculty of Science, Antidiabetic Drug Discovery Group, Lagos State University, PMB 0001, Ojo, Lagos, Nigeria

Abdul Razak O. Ogunmoye
Department of Chemical Sciences, Faculty of Science, Olabisi Onabanjo University, Ago-Iwoye, Ogun State, Nigeria

Ogbonna Okorie and Ebinyansi Onyinyechi
Department of Pharmaceutics and Pharmaceutical Technology, Faculty of Pharmaceutical Sciences, University of Port Harcourt, Rivers State, Nigeria

E. Omotoso Abayomi
Department of Pharmaceutical and Medicinal Chemistry, Faculty of Pharmaceutical Sciences, University of Port Harcourt, Rivers State, Nigeria

Ritu Aggarwal, Priyanka Yadav and Uma Chaudhary
Department of Microbiology, Pt. B.D. Sharma Institute of Medical Sciences, Rohtak, India

Vipul Kumar
Department of Chest and TB, Pt. B.D. Sharma Institute of Medical Sciences, Rohtak, India

Enemakwu Thomas Andrew, M. M. Adeyemi and L. Salihu
Department of Chemistry, Nigerian Defence Academy Kaduna, Nigeria

Yue Liu, Hewei Shao and Xiaoyan Han
Tianjin Key Laboratory of Chemistry and Analysis of Chinese Materia Medica, College of Chinese Materia Medica, Tianjin University of Traditional Chinese Medicine, Tianjin 300193, China

Yi Zhang
Tianjin Key Laboratory of Chemistry and Analysis of Chinese Materia Medica, College of Chinese Materia Medica, Tianjin University of Traditional Chinese Medicine, Tianjin 300193, China
Department of Experimental Teaching, Tianjin University of Traditional Chinese Medicine, Tianjin 300193, China

Hassan Afify and Mahmoud Nour El-Din
Department of Pharmacology and Toxicology, Faculty of Pharmacy, Egyptian-Russian University, Cairo, Egypt

El-Sayed Akool
Department of Pharmacology and Toxicology, Faculty of Pharmacy, Egyptian-Russian University, Cairo, Egypt
Department of Pharmacology and Toxicology, Faculty of Pharmacy, Al-Azhar University, Cairo, Egypt

Amany Balah and Abdel-Aziz H. Abdel-Aziz
Department of Pharmacology and Toxicology, Faculty of Pharmacy, Al-Azhar University, Cairo, Egypt

Archana Mootha, Sankari Malaiappan, Sheeja S. Varghese and N. D. Jayakumar
Department of Periodontics, Saveetha Dental College and Hospitals, Velappanchavadi, Chennai - 600077, India

N. K. Kortei and V. Appiah
Department of Nuclear Agriculture and Radiation Processing, Graduate School of Nuclear and Allied Sciences, P.O.Box LG 80, Legon, Ghana

G. T. Odamtten
Department of Nuclear Agriculture and Radiation Processing, Graduate School of Nuclear and Allied Sciences, P.O.Box LG 80, Legon, Ghana
Department of Botany, University of Ghana, P.O.Box LG 55, Legon, Ghana

M. Wiafe- Kwagyan
Department of Botany, University of Ghana, P.O.Box LG 55, Legon, Ghana

M. Obodai, D. L. Narh Mensah and P. T. Akonor
Food Research Institute- Council for Scientific and Industrial Research, P.O.Box M20, Accra, Ghana

M. Ayim- Akonor
Animal Research Institute- Council for Scientific and Industrial Research, P.O.Box AH20, Achimota, Ghana

R. M. Adaboro
Ghana Atomic Energy Commission, Applied Radiation Biology Centre, P.O.Box AE 1, Atomic, Ghana

Davoud Balarak and Ferdos Kord Mostafapour
Department of Environmental Health, Health Promotion Research Center, School of Public Health,
Zahedan University of Medical Sciences, Zahedan, Iran

Ali Joghataei
Student Research Committee, Qom University of Medical Sciences, Qom, Iran

Salisu Muhammad Highab and Danjuma Nuhu Muhammad
Department of Pharmacology and Therapeutics, Faculty of Pharmaceutical Sciences, Ahmadu Bello University, Zaria, Nigeria

Musa Aliyu
Department of Pharmacology, Faculty of Clinical Sciences, Bayero University Kano, Nigeria

Bala Yauri Muhammad
Department of Pharmacology and Toxicology, Unaizah College of Pharmacy, Qassim University, Unaizah 51911, Al-Qassim Province, Saudi Arabia

Jessie Idongesit Ndem and Efosa Godwin Ewere
Department of Biochemistry, Faculty of Basic Medical Sciences, University of Uyo, P.M.B. 1017, Uyo, Akwa Ibom State, Nigeria

Akwasi Sougi, Kwabena Ofori-Kwakye, Noble Kuntworbe, Samuel Lugrie Kipo and Mariam El Boakye-Gyasi
Department of Pharmaceutics, Faculty of Pharmacy and Pharmaceutical Sciences, College of Health
Sciences, Kwame Nkrumah University of Science and Technology (KNUST), Kumasi, Ghana

O. E. Famobuwa and U. E. Amuho
Department of Chemistry, Adeyemi Federal University of Education, Ondo, Nigeria

L. Lajide and B. J. Owolabi
Department of Chemistry, Federal University of Technology, Akure, Nigeria

I. B. Osho
Department of Animal Production and Health, Federal University of Technology, Akure, Nigeria

C. T. Onyema, C. E. Ofor, V. C. Okudo and A. S. Ogbuagu
Department of Pure and Industrial Chemistry, Faculty of Physical Sciences, Nnamdi Azikiwe University, Awka, Anambra State, Nigeria

O. D. Omodamiro and P. U. Ezurike
Department of Biochemistry, College of Natural Sciences, Michael Okpara University of Agriculture, Umudike, Abia State, Nigeria

M. A. Jimoh
Department of Plant Science and Biotechnology, College of Natural Sciences, Micheal Okpara University of Agriculture, Umudike, Abia State, Nigeria

Edwin O. Omeje, Patience O. Osadebe, Wilfred O. Obonga
Department of Pharmaceutical and Medicinal Chemistry, University of Nigeria, 410001, Nsukka, Enugu State, Nigeria

Christopher E. Ugwuoke
Department of Pharmacognosy and Environmental Medicine, Faculty of Pharmaceutical Sciences, University of Nigeria, 410001, Nsukka, Enugu State, Nigeria